FEMINIST PERSPECTIVES IN ❖ ❖ ❖ MEDICAL ETHICS

FEMINIST
PERSPECTIVES
IN ❖ ❖ ❖
MEDICAL ETHICS

EDITED BY

HELEN BEQUAERT HOLMES
AND
LAURA M. PURDY

INDIANA UNIVERSITY PRESS
Bloomington and Indianapolis

The paper used in this publication meets the minimum requirements of
American National Standard for Information Sciences—Permanence
of Paper for Printed Library Materials, ANSI Z39.48-1984.

∞™

Manufactured in the United States of America

Library of Congress Cataloging-in-Publication Data

Feminist Perspectives in medical ethics / edited by Helen Bequaert
Holmes and Laura M. Purdy.
    p. cm.
    Includes index.
    ISBN 0-253-32848-9 (cloth). — ISBN 0-253-20695-2 (paper)
    1. Medical ethics. 2. Feminism—Moral and ethical aspects.
3. Women—Health and hygiene. I. Holmes, Helen B. II. Purdy,
Laura Martha.
    R724.F4 1992
    174'.2—dc20   91-17749

1 2 3 4 5 96 95 94 93 92

Dedicated to the memory of
Corinne Guntzel

CONTENTS ❖ ❖ ❖

WOMEN AND CLINICAL EXPERIMENTS

WOMEN AND NEW REPRODUCTIVE "CHOICES"

CONTRACT PREGNANCY

Preface

This anthology, compiled from two special issues of *Hypatia: A Journal of Feminist Philosophy*, has its origins in a request from *Hypatia's* editorial board. When in 1987 the board sought proposals for a special issue on feminist medical ethics, each of us responded. Helen Bequaert Holmes envisioned a medley of papers on feminist ethics in general, on medicine and women's bodies, and on feminist rethinking of any issue in medical ethics. Laura M. Purdy's proposal concentrated on reproductive ethics. In response, the board and Editor Margaret Simons asked us to work together on an issue devoted to the broader approach, with the possibility of a second issue on reproductive ethics if the initial call for papers generated sufficient interest.

Reproduction, after all, has been the major point of intersection between the burgeoning fields of medical ethics and feminist philosophy. There are at least two reasons for this. One is that reproduction is the most obvious place where sex makes a difference. Another reason is that the second wave of feminism was born (perhaps not coincidentally) at a time of accelerating social change and rapid development in reproductive biology.

Thus, we fully expected a deluge of papers on reproduction and that our joint volume would be the end of the story. Imagine, then, our delight as the mailbox filled up with the varied and original papers that now constitute the first of the two special issues, "Feminist Ethics & Medicine," volume 4, number 2 (Summer 1989) of *Hypatia*. But there was no lack of work on reproduction, either, and the survivors of a lengthy process of reading, agonizing, consulting, winnowing, writing, and rewriting now comprise the second special issue, "Ethics & Reproduction," volume 4, number 3 (Fall 1989).

Once the two issues of *Hypatia* had seen the light of day, the possibility of a book to be published by Indiana University Press required further difficult choices. On the one hand, a single volume could not hold all the pieces that had appeared in the earlier publications; on the other, because the essays reflected primarily the interests of individual authors rather than an editorial vision, there were some gaps in subject matter. In the end, we reluctantly decided to drop the book reviews and the papers focusing on theoretical feminist ethics, and commissioned three new papers. One is a response to Fry's piece on nursing, and the others are on fetal abuse laws (Callahan and Knight) and prenatal sex selection (Wertz and Fletcher).

The new collection, like its parent volumes, is an invitation to further reflection and work in feminist ethics. The current outpouring of work is marvelous, even if it is getting harder and harder to keep up. Such, however, is the price of hearing many voices; only thus can we hope to avoid confusing prematurely hardened "feminist lines" on specific issues with fundamental feminist principles such as concern for the welfare of all women. Developing well-argued positions that are sensitive to both difference and similarity among women is a tall order—it will require continuing open-mindedness and thoughtful debate. Let us hope that other journals and publishers will continue to provide the forums we need for developing these exciting ideas.

This book would never have come to fruition without the energy, support, and commitment of many individuals. We are grateful that many of our expenses were covered by the Kirkland Endowment of Hamilton College and by a grant-in-aid from Francis Holmes. Second, we thank those who submitted papers for the original volumes and the authors of the new papers. Next, we send our heartfelt thanks to the some forty-one reader/reviewers who gave so generously of their time and expertise in honing the submissions to the *Hypatia* issues. To *Hypatia*'s past editor, Margaret Simons, go our special thanks for her help and enthusiasm, and especially for her patient tolerance of the intricacies and details generated by such a complicated project; we also appreciate the facilitating work by *Hypatia*'s current editor, Linda Lopez McAlister. We owe considerable thanks, as well, to our editor at Indiana University Press, Joan Catapano, for her patience with this somewhat unwieldy project. Finally, thanks go to our husbands, Francis Holmes and John Coleman, for their strong and constant encouragement and for their kindly tolerance of distracted wives who dance to the *Chicago Manual of Style*, instead of to the hum of clotheswasher and dishwasher.

Helen Bequaert Holmes
Laura M. Purdy

FEMINIST
PERSPECTIVES
IN ❖ ❖ ❖
MEDICAL ETHICS

A Call to Heal Medicine

HELEN BEQUAERT HOLMES ❖ ❖ ❖

Authors in this anthology seem called to heal ethics, medicine, and the new field—medical ethics. After explaining why feminists should feel this calling, I categorize authors' contributions as responses to questions: 1. Why hasn't medical ethics already healed medicine? 2. Are we setting up health as a virtue? 3. What role should caring play? 4. Must we first heal science? 5. How do new developments in reproductive medicine complicate women's reproductive freedom?

Consider the following scenes:

A middle-class, suburban mother paces the floor cuddling her sick toddler, who screams from the pain of earache. Should she call the pediatrician? Since her insurance premium is paid, the resources of modern medicine can be hers: an arsenal of antibiotics, an assemblage of devices and equipment, an inventory of tests—all in the local hospital. Why, then, does she hesitate? Will the pediatrician, busy with "the really serious" cases, simply prescribe an antibiotic over the phone? Will she be told to bring the child to the office in the stormy weather? After that—as happened last time—will her child catch what's "going round"? Will she be asked to "wait and see," as if she isn't already doing that? Then, she meditates about the effects that childhood antibiotics and tonsillectomies have had on some of her friends—wouldn't "wait and see" indeed be better for her child?

A poor, inner-city mother paces the floor cuddling her sick toddler, who screams from the pain of earache. Should she make her way to the clinic at the city teaching hospital? She has friends who were indeed healed when they visited that clinic. But will some unskilled intern use her child to practice a tonsillectomy or eardrum puncture? She knows she'd have to wait on a snowy corner for the bus, to endure the clinic's waiting room while trying to comfort her child, and, finally, to bear a patronizing five minutes with a professional. Wouldn't borrowing a heater or some blankets from a neighbor be better for her child?

Consider other women: the lesbian buddy of an AIDS victim deciding whether to call the ambulance for her friend, whose care has become too complicated for his circle of loving, supportive friends. Or the sixty-year-old caring for her mother with Alzheimer disease, exhausted from the physical care, who learns that at last a bed is available in a nursing home. Or the drug addict who wants to break her habit at the local methadone clinic, but hears that then she'll be required to reveal her sexual contacts. Or the pregnant teenager who fears the scolding she'll get at Planned Parenthood when she appears to request another abortion.[1]

"I go because I must" is often the choice made. Using a utilitarian calculus, most women decide that the benefits of going for medical care may outweigh the risks. A woman may fear *not* going, may hope that pain can be controlled. When a loved one is involved, an unconscious syllogism may inform her decision, something like: medicine is based on science, which in turn is based on truth; therefore medicine can solve problems with the human body; I would be wrong if I didn't give my loved one this chance.

Why is there apprehension and uncertainty about the medical system in the richest nation of the world, in the nation with the most sophisticated medical technology? Is the malaise of modern medicine in large part caused by social conditions, especially the faulty organization of the health care system? In these everyday examples—not the crisis cases found in medical ethics casebooks or blazoned across the front pages of the *Washington Post*—we find ordinary women, ordinary women by the tens of thousands, who confront as "personal" their own bits of the larger "political" questions of medical ethics.

How should medical resources be distributed equitably? How can "care" be given in any "care-giving" profession that has such a tremendous power imbalance between care-giver and -receiver? When are medical technologies truly lifesaving, and when are they given simply because they exist, or because the hospital needs to recoup equipment costs via third-party payment, or because an intern needs to practice? Can promoting public health ever take precedence over personal autonomy and privacy? What is a "good" death and where should it take place?

Note the common theme in the inner questioning of the women above. Surely if a friend would say to any of them, "Go to Dr. X's office—they really care about you there," much indecision would vanish. When someone is deeply distressed about the health of a loved one, the help most wanted is true caring (empathy, a listening ear, concern about comfort and pain, scrupulous assessment of risks/ benefits, etc.)—caring combined, of course, with knowledge about diagnosis and treatment. But can curing be severed from caring?

WHY BRING IN FEMINISTS?

Here, for medicine, I pilfer from Virginia Woolf's statement about science: Medicine, "it would seem, is not sexless; she is a man, a father, and infected too" (Woolf 1938, 139). I sense that the feminist philosophers who have contributed to this issue are concerned about this infection and that they feel called to be healers. They are kindhearted and compassionate critics. Some may believe they owe their health (perhaps even their lives) to the thaumaturgy of modern medicine, such as the "right" antibiotic, a well-run intensive care nursery, or an appropriately used diagnostic test or device. And some feel compromised or inconsistent when they earn their bread teaching ethics simply as it has been taught over the decades.

I see three reasons why feminists should feel called to heal medicine. In the

1980s most feminists have become champions for other oppressed groups, having turned away from an earlier, rather self-centered vision. Sick and disabled people are oppressed in our society; those who are also poor, female, gay, and/or elderly are further oppressed. As members of the globally oppressed majority, we must use what I call "epistemic empathy"[2] toward oppression and offer other oppressed groups our help and insights—in both theory and practice.

A second reason for feminists to be concerned is that women do more than 90 percent of the hands-on sick care: feeding, bathing, cleaning up (vomit, feces, urine, mucus, blood), providing comfort, raising morale. Any infection of the health care system also poisons the care-givers.

A third reason why we ought to try to "dis-infect" medicine is that we may have an epistemic privilege in "caring." If our health care system regularly incorporated true caring about other human beings and genuine feelings of interdependence, many problems might vanish. Caring may be stereotypically assigned to women; it may ghettoize women in the down side of power relationships, but it cannot be thrown out if it is vital to the healing of people and medicine.

A FEMINIST PHARMACOPOEIA

The questions raised by the would-be healers of medicine in this book seem to fall into five categories. Let us consider each.

1. Why hasn't the new field of medical ethics, concerned as it is about the rights and wrongs of medical practice, already healed medicine? Or, put another way, have aspects of the malestream medical ethics pharmacopoeia actually obstructed the healing of the discipline?

Susan Sherwin's analysis begins by praising the field of medical ethics for its sensitivity to the power imbalance between doctor and patient and for developing away from strict utilitarian or deontological reasoning. She commends several male authors who favor considering context when struggling with an ethical dilemma. But then Sherwin points out a very serious defect, the desperate need in medical ethics for political analysis. For medical ethics simply accepts the institution of medicine. The fact that medical ethics, in turn, has itself been accepted almost everywhere in medicine as an appropriate enterprise is evidence that it seldom rocks boats. Indeed, it helps that institution by legitimating norms.

Virginia L. Warren points out two metaproblems with medical ethics: the questions selected and the process used. In her opinion these are sexist. Inappropriate questions (which may be an important factor in the failure of medical ethics to find solutions to the health care crisis) include ones that revolve around competition for power or status or have no validity for those not in the dominant culture. Warren urges us to substitute other categories of questions.

One such category is questions about "housekeeping" issues instead of crisis issues. Glamorous cases make the headlines, but housekeeping issues are the ones that concern everyone, day in and day out, in health care work. One housekeeping question is "How should we foster the conditions which make informed consent possible?" in contrast with a crisis question, "Was informed consent obtained from the patient before this treatment?"

As for the process of discussing ethical dilemmas, Warren is sharply critical of the "Ethics Game" in which opponents argue to win, to prove the superiority of their theory over another's. What I dub her "new games" suggestions include having discussants construct theory from life experience and work on the actual relationships between each other.

Another problem is the use of universal principles in medical (and other applied areas of) ethics. Many of the authors in this book see this use as a source of oppression. Warren, for example, would urge, as Margaret Walker did in our first issue of *Hypatia*, that we strictly avoid the "universalist/impersonalist tradition." According to Walker, we need to "challenge 'principled' moral stances . . . where these are surrogates for, or defenses against, responsiveness in actual relationships" (1989, 21). She also observes that "The rhetoric of universality has been entirely compatible . . . with the most complete (and often intentional) exclusion of women as moral agents from . . . loftily universal constructs" (1989, 24).

Some authors take a more tempered view. Laura Purdy argues that we need principles—not necessarily traditional ones—to guide our thinking and provide consistency. She hopes that feminists will set up as universalizable those principles important to us, to permeate *all* ethics: "What we do not want is another 'special interest' ethics that can be ignored."

Sherwin urges us to maintain a certain level of generalization in a feminist analysis. As a specific example she takes the new techniques for circumventing infertility. Here the conventional focus is already strongly context-specific: each individual should choose what fits her situation. Sherwin argues that a feminist, however, should worry more about the dangers inherent in the ever-increasing medical control over women's lives. Since most interference in women's reproduction in the past has not been physically and emotionally to women's benefit, the expanding dependence of women on male skills and authority should be a crucial concern.

I believe that all our authors would agree that no single theory or no single strategy is adequate for settling every kind of ethical question. Sherwin states, "The important constant is that we must always decide these questions within the wider political context of . . . our general feminist objectives of eliminating oppression in all its forms."

A new threat to women's well-being is the devastating sexually transmitted disease—AIDS. Yet, as Nora Kizer Bell points out, almost totally neglected in the now voluminous literature on this disease is serious consideration of how AIDS-related ethical issues affect women. Among the complicating factors are the mores of female behavior in the drug culture, and society's racial, ethnic, and homophobic biases. Should a pregnant woman who is sero-positive for HIV, from an ethnic group where childbearing will ensure her status as a real woman, "choose" to carry that pregnancy to term? Bell comes to a well-argued conclusion—with which many of our readers may disagree.

In 1989, when Bell's paper was first published, she was among the few Cassandras pointing to the crucial necessity of including women in all considerations of AIDS policy, politics, and ethics. Fortunately, now in 1991, books, articles, and legislative debates show that policy-makers are beginning to listen—but maybe still too little and too late?

Is medical ethics (and its reflection, medicine) ageist? According to Bell in her second contribution, it is indeed, and ageism is a threat to women. Using specific examples from two books by the internationally influential bioethicist Daniel Callahan (1987; 1990), she spells out the danger of setting age limits on health care. Books in the bright new field of medical ethics have been appearing by the dozen— texts, casebooks, single-issue books, proceedings of conferences. Why are they apparently not helping to heal medicine? For one reason, most of these books are implicitly sexist, perhaps unwittingly so. Such books will confirm and further embed sexism in medicine and in ethics. We need more investigative sensitivity like Bell's to expose this subtle sexism.

2. *If we heal medicine so that it can better fulfill its mission of healing, can we do so without setting up health and the perfectly functioning body as virtues?* Or put another way, how can we avoid unintentionally oppressing sick and disabled people still further?

Susan Wendell's contribution reveals the dubious assumptions underlying much of our current theorizing about health care. Many of our authors are critical of medicine as an institution and of the institutionalization of medical ethics. Implicit in such criticism is the assumption that medicine and ethics are not restoring health to enough people in a fair way, that their activities may actually impede attaining health. But there is no criticism of *health itself* as a value or virtue and no questioning of the veneration of the physically perfect body. Wendell shows us that mainstream medicine and society marginalize people whose illnesses cannot be cured, whose bodies cannot be restored to perfect shape. We design society so that only those with perfect bodies can function easily and then discriminate against and blame those who function with difficulty. Can we value and work for health without these consequences?

3. *What precise role should "caring" play in a feminist prescription for the healing of medicine?*

Betty Sichel and Sara Fry are strong activist advocates of "caring" in applied ethics. From her experience on an ethics committee, Sichel first describes how institutional ethics committees can use caring in resolving ethical dilemmas, then argues for their doing so. From her experience as a nurse, Fry argues for caring as *the* fundamental value for nursing ethics. In building her case she describes the advocacy of caring in the writings of nurses Gadow, Watson, and Griffin; she discusses how Noddings's work can apply to nursing, and she shows that two male medical ethicists (Pellegrino and Frankena) have each deviated somewhat from the mainstream in that they include caring as an integral part of their theories. In a response to Fry, Jeannine Boyer and James Nelson ponder how caring can have a *fundamental* character and then answer their own question.

4. If modern medicine is based on science, but science (à la Virginia Woolf) is infected, must we first cure science? Sue V. Rosser and Don Marquis dispel any complacency on this issue. Drawing on her long experience in the assessment of science, Rosser documents the sexism in clinical experimentation—a strange, paradoxical, worst-of-all-worlds history both of failing to consider gender as a variable and of using women unethically as guinea pigs. She describes some hopeful signs of re-vision and urges strong feminist input into the design and implementation of clinical experiments.

Marquis gives a case study analysis of clinical trials on breast cancer therapy, concluding that a study that violated the rights of (many) women will nevertheless benefit all those who get breast cancer in the future. We are left to ponder (and we *must* ponder) whether we want to sanction such experiments. Is there any other way that good data on curing human diseases can be obtained? My commentary attempts to answer this question. First I explore some aspects of the scientific method that may cause the very act of striving for truth to lead to falsehood. Then I describe a few ways in which human subjects of clinical experiments have been or could be directly involved in designing and monitoring experiments to enhance—not reduce—scientific rigor.

5. How have recent developments in reproductive medicine transformed and complicated women's reproductive freedom? The authors in the final two sections of the book call our attention to ways in which recent medical "advances" have challenged women's autonomy in reproduction.

Choice. Rights. Do these terms have any meaning in the era of technological reproduction? Each author in these two sections deals with "choice" and "rights," whether or not he or she explicitly uses the terms. When a technology exists that might (in some cases) help a subfertile couple have a baby, in what sense does that couple "choose" to sign up? Judith Lorber illuminates this issue especially well by discussing what happens in current in vitro fertilization practice when the man in a couple—not the woman—is subfertile.

Expecting a woman to undergo painful drug and surgical treatments to produce a child "for her man" is a high-tech reinforcement of the traditional role required of women. But if high technology could incubate a fetus entirely outside a woman's body, would this liberate women from that role? Numerous useful insights on the relationship between technology and social expectations of women can be found in Julien S. Murphy's careful and nuanced delineation of liberation and oppression involved in this still impossible technique.

A glass womb might be a good idea if the act of giving birth makes women incompetent. Rosalind Ekman Ladd describes how a woman's choice and rights simply vanish at this point in her life. Outside the labor room, experience increases competence—why, then, is a woman in labor incompetent to decide how she wants that labor "managed?" (I shudder whenever medicine uses the term "manage," especially with the normal bodily function of childbirth.)

Mary Anne Warren and Joan C. Callahan/James W. Knight in their respective papers consider other aspects of vanishing choice and rights for pregnant women.

Warren, in her fresh treatment of the philosophical issues in abortion, analyzes the validity of viewpoints that rely on abilities of the fetus (such as viability and sentience) to determine an ethical stance on abortion. To put it baldly, the woman carrying the fetus is nonexistent in those theories. And, as Callahan and Knight show, worse than nonexistent, she can be called a felon for her behavior during pregnancy.

Is it sexist or is it "choice" to use selective abortion to eliminate a child of the sex you don't want? Dorothy Wertz and John Fletcher evaluate existing feminist arguments on both sides and conclude that sex selection is dangerously sexist, but that laws prohibiting it would be more dangerous still.

Our final section considers so-called surrogate motherhood. How did this non-technological process ever become an issue in the age of women's liberation and medical technology? A simple process that has probably been going on for centuries has suddenly become entrepreneurial at the same time that the women's movement has facilitated the opening to women of many formerly male-only professions and trades. Why then take on one of the quintessential roles of women as paid employment? Are surrogate mothers and the wives of contracting sperm donors pawns of patriarchy? Or, to use the rhetoric of the women's movement (as many do elsewhere), do they have the "right" to exercise this "choice"? The authors here (Hilde Lindemann Nelson and James Lindemann Nelson, Kelly Oliver, Sara Ann Ketchum, H. M. Malm) enrich the debate by providing a variety of feminist arguments about the practice.

In sum, this volume demonstrates the glaring inadequacy of mainstream medical ethics. We need persistent attention to the insights of women and a continuing insistence on the value (and values!) of women. Both are essential if we are ever to hope for an accurate and fair assessment of moral issues in medicine.

NOTES

1. I do not wish to give the mistaken impression that all women are wary of the health care system and ponder their own personal bits of these questions whenever they or their loved ones are confronted with illness. Women (and men) may fall into other categories. One, the iatrophile, has faith in medicine as in a god; such a devotee never hesitates to approach a medical practitioner. A second, the iatroholic, is addicted to one or another medical specialty: examples are the person who never misses a weekly visit to the psychiatrist and follows him or her from city to city, and the in-vitro-fertilization patient who comes back again and again for treatment after every failure.

2. Oppressed people have epistemic "privilege" by their "immediate knowledge of everyday life under oppression" (Narayan 1988, 36). However, when I speak of white, middle-class, healthy women understanding the oppression of the sick and disabled, the word "privilege" seems to retain its conventional meaning. There, I use "epistemic empathy" instead, to signify that there are aspects of oppression of the sick that are part of the knowledge of all healthy women.

REFERENCES

Callahan, Daniel. 1987. *Setting limits*. New York: Simon & Schuster.

Callahan, Daniel. 1990. *What kind of life: The limits of medical progress*. New York: Simon & Schuster.

Narayan, Uma. 1988. Working together across difference: Some considerations on emotions and political practice. *Hypatia* 3(2): 31–47.

Walker, Margaret. 1989. Moral understandings: Alternative "epistemology" for a feminist ethics. *Hypatia* 4(2): 15–28.

Woolf, Virginia. 1938. *Three guineas*. London: Harcourt, Brace, Jovanovich.

A Call to Heal Ethics

LAURA M. PURDY ❖ ❖ ❖

It's an exciting time to be in ethics. The need for moral awareness has never been greater. On one hand, we face the 'sleaze factor' of dishonesty that has infested government lately. On the other, we are being ceaselessly assaulted by new tech-nologies (in vitro fertilization, for instance), problems (like AIDS), and possibilities (such as the separation of biological and social parenting). Attempts to address these developments range from presidential commissions to ethics codes for gov-ernment officials, from lead articles in *Time* and *Ms.* to general education require-ments at elite colleges. Meanwhile, scholarship flourishes, continuing its rebound from the legacy of positivism.

Feminists have been drawn, I suspect, in disproportionate numbers to the field known as "applied ethics." For one thing, it has provided a haven for analyzing particular cases with an eye to women's hitherto ignored interests. For another, it has allowed us to do more concrete work, work that has immediate prospects of improving women's lives. In the last few years, however, we have been venturing into more theoretical territory, and there has been an extraordinary explosion of imaginative new ideas. Among them are new models of human interaction and persuasive criticisms of widely accepted assumptions.

Yet philosophers have not quite recovered from the onslaught of various kinds of relativism. There are, in addition, other reasons to worry about where this new research is leading. A major issue in attempting to teach ethics is leading some of us to have doubts about the usefulness of anything like our currently popular theories. As we are all acutely aware, there are several moral theories. Their conclusions about a given case are often incompatible; even where conclusions coincide, justification tends to diverge. We seem therefore compelled to pick only one theory if we wish to be consistent. But which to choose, and why? Although a few seem to me to be downright untenable, there are serious problems with all: whichever we choose opens us up to reproach on theoretical grounds even before we attempt to apply it. Complicating the picture further is the obscurity, and even inconsistency, of some moral theorists (take Kant or Rousseau, for example), so that radically different interpretations of any given theory may be possible. Inter-pretation once chosen, we may discover no help with a particular problem we wish to address. So although we still march our students through the traditional theories, their link with moral problem-solving seems ever more tenuous.

Initially it is tempting to fault our students: they are just not sophisticated enough to grasp the essentials. The issues we face in our own research belie this conclusion, however. Most of us adopt a stable of principles, arranged neatly in our preferred pecking order. But it is hard to have much confidence in any particular ranking, and, as Virginia Warren[1] says, the thrill is gone. Besides, many of us have noticed that attempting to resolve concrete problems brings us nose to nose with difficulties for which the standard theories have no wisdom. What kind of a situation are we dealing with? How is it most appropriately described, and why? Who is to count in the moral deliberations, and why? What are the most relevant facts, and what are the criteria for choosing them? As we grapple with such matters, the question of which moral principle should prevail may recede almost to the vanishing point.

Much feminist theorizing encourages us to attend more carefully to the nuances of particular situations, an attitude one might be tempted to regard as a prerequisite for moral thinking, but which could better be viewed as integral to it. A great deal of work on this aspect of moral thinking clearly awaits us.

Once beyond this stage, what then? Recent feminist work in ethics suggests that "caring" will help: if we care, it will be obvious what matters, what to do. There is much to be said for this view. Many, perhaps most, situations calling for moral decision-making involve choosing between our own selfish desires and others' welfare. Should doctors lie to cover up negligence? Should they suggest unnecessary surgery to make an extra buck? Should we invest in strategic defense initiatives when AIDS patients languish without care? Everybody knows the answers: the question is whether we care enough about others to do the right thing. But not every problem can be resolved in this appealing way. "Caring" cannot show us when we may legitimately say "no" to preserve our own happiness: it seems, on the contrary, to relegate us to our traditional role of self-sacrifice. This injunction might work if everybody did it, but in the meantime, for feminists to embrace it is just business as usual: we perpetuate our own subordination.

Nor can "caring" automatically show us which of two conflicting interests should have priority when not all needs can be met. For instance, how shall we allocate scarce resources between young and old? Caring *will* compel us to consider the kinds of communication, compromise, and concern about long-term effects evident in Amy's resolution of the Heinz case (see Boyer and Nelson, p. 110). It *may* help us rule out practices that belittle or ignore suffering. But it may also narrow our vision to exclude awareness of the broader kinds of social and political context rightly emphasized by Susan Sherwin.

Caring may lead us to focus on particular cases. Concern for particulars is an admirable antidote to the lifeless, overly broad strokes to which we have been so often subjected by moral philosophers. But I think that we must beware of any corresponding tendency to devalue principles excessively. Is our instinct (and is it only that?) for consistency—for principles by which to measure our choices— merely a graduate school artifact, or the product of two thousand years of "mas- culine" philosophizing? "Situation ethics" never caught on, and for good reason: it provided no criterion for judging the quality of moral decision-making. Are *we* in danger of falling into the same trap?

Even those who are skeptical about principles use them. For instance, there seems to be something of an emerging consensus about characteristics of distinc- tively feminist moral thinking. Among them are attention to particular cases, to relationships, to responsibility, to context. These may or may not be traditional moral principles, but they are principles nonetheless: they guide our thinking and provide consistency. Some, eager for a warrant to deny our values, would refuse to recognize their corresponding principles: are we going to collaborate with them?

Without principles, we cannot consistently press the most basic claims motivating moral theories. Thus values like caring are defensible against possible alternatives only if we conceive of ethics as a social institution whose chief function should be to justly promote the well-being of all. Furthermore, only this kind of basic moral assumption safeguards us from the naturalistic fallacy and equips us to wend our way with some art through the moral labyrinth.

Consistency can also be used as a bludgeon, to lump superficially similar cases together, obscuring morally relevant distinctions. The right response to this tendency is not to dismiss the importance of consistency, but rather to patiently show how crudely it cuts.

I think caprice is the only alternative to that critically important form of consistency, universalizability. You may have an abortion, I may not: what is the difference between our two cases? Surely, we do not want to rule such questions out of order. Moreover, it would be misconceived to suppose that the concept of universalizability determines how narrowly to draw distinctions or what their content should be. The kind of close attention to detail, circumstance, and interest we think appropriate to good ethics is not incompatible with universalizability. On the contrary, if we can show why these characteristics are important, universalizability should compel every moral thinker to heed them.

This point is central. Never will we have a decent society without good people; but good people still need guidelines. One of our chief aims as moral philosophers should be to create justifiable formal and material principles that can be understood and used by all. Without such a structure we are in danger of creating yet another ghetto. When the dust settles, there is no telling what feminist ethics will look like. But what we do not want is a "special interest" ethics that can be ignored, or relegated to the already large collection of theories among which people can arbitrarily pick and choose. What I hope for in the long run is that feminism will permeate all ethics, leaving "feminist ethics" to wither away. Only this outcome secures us from "respectable" theories that ignore women's interests.

What can we now say about feminist ethics? I would argue for embracing the very broadest conception of feminism: "recognition that women are in a subordinate position in society, that oppression is an intolerable form of injustice, that there are further forms of oppression in addition to gender oppression . . . that it is possible to change society in ways that could eliminate oppression, and that it is a goal of feminism to pursue the changes necessary to accomplish this" (Sherwin, p. 29n.6).

Feminist ethics might then be taken to include discussions which do the following:

(1) *Emphasize the importance of women and their interests.* Stressing justice for women seems to me to be a minimum condition for describing any work as "feminist." But I think we want, during this time of experimentation and ferment, to avoid any semblance of rigid orthodoxy about the form that this emphasis should

take. We shouldn't be branding some work as "not really feminist" so long as it is premised upon the aforementioned feminist assumptions. This does not mean, of course, that we should not feel free to criticize other views or argue for our own.

Feminist scholars have been documenting in damning detail the invisibility (or worse) of women and their interests in most traditional work. Insisting on gender as a required category of analysis, as Sue V. Rosser and others urge, is a step in the right direction. Studies like Nora Kizer Bell's, which examine mainstream medical ethics theories that fail in their application to women, are good examples of another.

(2) *Focus on issues especially concerning or affecting women.* Although this might seem an obvious category, as we put together this volume quite a bit of disagreement surfaced about whether to consider such work *truly* feminist. My own opinion is that we need to be broadminded here, in part to avoid the kind of sectarian warfare that could undermine our still fragile enterprise. However, subject matter alone is not enough to render work feminist: it should not be classified as such unless it also meets the test suggested under category (1) above. A broad array of narrowly directed case studies such as Don Marquis's piece on breast cancer research fits here. "Unsexy," "housekeeping" issues, such as Rosalind Ekman Ladd's work on competence in pregnant women, that might be ignored as too trivial to merit philosophical treatment by nonfeminists (see Virginia Warren) also belong under this rubric. Last but not least, much of the recent work in reproductive ethics seems to fall most appropriately in this category. The papers in that area chosen for this volume represent a variety of feminist concerns. Among them are papers on women and AIDS, sexist undercurrents in in vitro fertilization and practices surrounding childbirth, the perennial abortion debate, and issues raised by the idea of gestation outside women's bodies. The rest of the reproductive ethics papers present an array of feminist approaches to a newly widespread practice: bearing children for others. Like abortion, contract pregnancy is compelling us to scrutinize our basic beliefs about the relationship between women and children, as well as about the nature and value of women themselves.

(3) *Rethink fundamental assumptions.* Feminists need to reconsider both substantive principles and philosophical methods. Excellent instances of the former are the criticisms of atomism (Jaggar 1983), proposals for new models of human relationships (Held 1987), and discussion of the moral relevance of gender (Okin 1987), as well as the aforementioned principles about detail and context. Valuable examples of the latter are Virginia Warren's criticism of the Gladiator Theory of Truth and the concern about abstraction raised by Sheila Ruth (1981).

(4) *Incorporate feminist insights and conclusions from other fields and disciplines.* Interdisciplinary work like ethics (and medical ethics, in particular) requires substantial general knowledge. It must include awareness of how feminist work is transforming other disciplines; otherwise we will not be able to fit our own contributions into an organic growing whole. Several essays in this volume further this aim by offering us insights from biology (Sue V. Rosser), sociology (Judith Lorber), and law (Sara Ann Ketchum).

These categories are neither exhaustive nor mutually exclusive: surely the future will reveal a fascinating variety of approaches, strategies, arguments, and values.

Let us hope that the rich stream of work we are witnessing, work that is now beginning to include long overdue sensitivity to related oppressions, will steadily broaden its reach to every corner of the moral landscape. In the meantime, we scramble to tackle new problems overwhelming us even as we agonize over the old. We hope that this volume will encourage further dialogue, by informing, provoking, and inspiring debate.

NOTE

1. All references (unless otherwise noted) are to authors in this volume.

REFERENCES

Held, Virginia. 1987. Non-contractual society. *Science, Morality and Feminist Theory*, ed. Marsha Hanen and Kai Nielsen. *Canadian Journal of Philosophy* (supplementary volume 13).
Jaggar, Alison. 1983. *Feminist politics and human nature*. Totowa, N.J.: Rowman and Allenheld.
Okin, Susan Moller. 1987. Justice and gender. *Philosophy and Public Affairs* 16(1).
Ruth, Sheila. 1981. Methodocracy, misogyny and bad faith: The response of philosophy. In *Men's studies modified: The impact of feminism on the academic disciplines*, ed. Dale Spender. Oxford: Pergamon Press.

THE MEDICAL ETHICS COMMUNITY

Feminist Views

Feminist and Medical Ethics:
Two Different Approaches
to Contextual Ethics

SUSAN SHERWIN ❖ ❖ ❖

Feminist ethics and medical ethics are critical of contemporary moral theory in several similar respects. There is a shared sense of frustration with the level of abstraction and generality that characterizes traditional philosophic work in ethics and a common commitment to including contextual details and allowing room for the personal aspects of relationships in ethical analysis. This paper explores the ways in which context is appealed to in feminist and medical ethics, the sort of details that should be included in the recommended narrative approaches to ethical problems, and the difference it makes to our ethical deliberations if we add an explicitly feminist political analysis to our discussion of context. It is claimed that an analysis of gender is needed for feminist medical ethics and that this requires a certain degree of generality, i.e. a political understanding of context.

INTRODUCTION

Feminist ethics and medical ethics are relatively new areas of philosophic specialization; each is developing at a dizzying rate, and some intriguing trends can be seen as common to both. They are both interested in developing the sort of analysis that can offer meaningful guidance in the morally troubling situations of real life. In the literature of each field, we find a sense of frustration with the level of abstraction and generality that characterizes traditional philosophic work on ethics. Both speak of the limitations of restricting ethical analysis to the level of general principles, and they demonstrate a need to focus quite explicitly on the contextual details of life situations that are problematic for morally concerned persons. The use of context is quite different in the two fields, however, and I shall argue that there are important lessons to be learned from the details of contextual focus found in the literature of feminist and medical ethics.

In this essay, I shall explore the ways in which context is appealed to in both feminist and medical ethics, and I shall argue that particular sorts of details should be included in the recommended narrative approaches to ethical problems. In

Hypatia vol. 4, no. 2 (Summer 1989) © by Susan Sherwin

particular, I claim that incorporating an explicitly feminist political analysis in the discussion of context is critical to ethical deliberations. I hope to show that an analysis of gender is an important element of contextually based moral theory and that such analysis requires a degree of generality which ought to be made explicit in discussions of context. By being specific about the sort of context and the degree of generality which should be kept central to analysis in practical ethics, we can begin to define the characteristics of a feminist medical ethics and provide direction to other areas of feminist ethics.

THE ROLE OF CONTEXT IN FEMINIST ETHICS

Turning first to examine the role of context in feminist ethics, we must acknowledge the important influence of Carol Gilligan (1982). In identifying a female tendency to approach ethical problems in a personalized, contextual manner, Gilligan helped articulate the sense of alienation many women have experienced in trying to work within the structures of contemporary moral theory.[1] She identified distinct masculine and feminine voices in ethical reasoning, allowing us to recognize that mainstream ethical theory has been carried on in a voice that is overwhelmingly masculine—the voices of women have been largely excluded or ignored. Feminists stress that it is important in ethics, as in all fields, to include women's moral experiences and reasoning in the deliberations. Hence, most theorists seeking to develop a feminist approach to ethics have given serious consideration to the gender map which Gilligan has provided and have tried to incorporate many of her observations into their approach to ethics.[2]

In her research, Gilligan found that girls and women tend to approach ethical dilemmas in a contextualized, narrative way that looks for resolution in particular details of a problem situation; in contrast, boys and men seem inclined to try to apply some general abstract principle without attention to the unique circumstances of the case. For instance, in Kohlberg's famous Heinz case, Gilligan found that males tended to answer in terms of the logical implications of a general rule, such as that stealing is wrong or that the duty to save a life outweighs other moral rules. In contrast, she found that female subjects tried to preserve relationships and to find new options through better communication and a presumption of cooperation; they tended to respond by seeking more information or by trying to re-conceive the terms set by the example. Gilligan recognized two different patterns of reasoning here: one which pursues universal rules in an endeavour to ensure fairness, and one which is focused on the actual feelings and interactions of those involved. The first approach, which she found to be associated with male moral thinking, she labelled an ethic of justice; the latter, which she found to be more commonly exercised by female subjects, she identified as an ethic of care.

The gender difference she describes is two-fold, characterized by differences in both scope and values: men seem to be preoccupied with developing comprehensive, generalizable, abstract ethical systems which are based on rights, while women seem to be concerned with understanding the specific human dynamics of a situation and, hence, concentrate on particular narrative details with the aim of avoiding hurt and providing care. As a result, we can identify distinct methodological differences between men and women in their approaches to morally troubling questions. But we should be cautious in interpreting the significance of the gender correlations of these differences; much of the discussion in feminist ethics has been occupied with evaluating the implications of developing what might be called a feminine ethics or a woman-centered ethics.[3] Since, in our sexist society, gender is inseparable from oppression, we should be sensitive to the fact that characteristics associated with gender are also likely to be associated with oppression. Obviously, it is important that women's distinctive moral reasoning be (at last) acknowledged as worthy of respect, but many feminists—including Gilligan herself—have expressed caution in interpreting the gender patterns her research reveals in the context of a society that systematically oppresses women. In particular, many feminists are wary of enthusiasm for virtues like caring which are associated with both gender and oppression.[4] Gilligan recommends that we work towards an androgynous ethics that could combine elements of both approaches, but other feminists have pointed out that notions of androgyny seem, themselves, to perpetuate the old gender system.

In any event, Gilligan has helped to identify alternative approaches to ethics from those found in traditional approaches; whatever we might make of the wider claims of her analysis, the focus on context and the value of caring are widely recognized as attractive features to be incorporated in any ethical theory. I would certainly expect these features to play some part in any woman centered (or even woman including) look at ethics and, therefore, in any approach to feminist ethics. It is clear that in doing feminist ethics, it is important to be critical of the maleness of mainstream ethical theory, given its tendencies to demand a very high degree of abstractness and to deny the relevance of concrete considerations, since this orientation restricts the scope and analysis of ethics. If we are to build feminist approaches to ethics, we need to clarify the sort of contextual details that are relevant to an ethical analysis.

The Role of Context in Medical Ethics

The theme of seeking a practical, context-specific approach to ethics is not restricted to feminist literature, however. The literature of medical ethics also contains frequent discussions about the inadequacy of abstract moral reasoning for resolving real moral dilemmas; there, too, we can find evidence of a widespread recognition that we must go beyond "mere theory." Further, there is frequent mention of the need to engage considerations of caring in medical ethics, usually couched in the language of the beneficence which is owed to patients. When placed in context (even if hypothetically), medical dilemmas are often discussed in terms that appear to rank sensitivity and caring ahead of applications of principle.[5]

In the "early days" of philosophical medical ethics (i.e., the 1970s), there was an attempt to try to fit responses to moral dilemmas into the general framework offered by standard moral theories, especially utilitarianism and Kantian deontology. It became apparent quite early on, however, that the simple appeal to theory and principle did not offer satisfying analyses of the sorts of dilemmas that arise in medical ethics. Case studies became a central element in influential journals, in many textbooks, and in individual articles. The texture and the details of cases have become important in trying to decide about perennial issues such as confidentiality, truth-telling, and euthanasia. Clear answers deduced from precise principles are not at hand for most of the topics addressed; many authors now accept the assumption that universal principles cannot be found which will govern such issues in all cases.

Engelhardt, for example, in his basically deontological text, *The Foundations of Bioethics* (1986), claims that

> The obligation to do to others their good is a fundamental one. . . . However, the obligation as such is abstract. Only in concrete contexts can one determine the extent of the obligation, and how to rank the various goods that can be at stake. (Engelhardt 1986, 92)

Ronald Christie and Barry Hoffmaster have been quite explicit about their rejection of a theory-based medical ethics in their text *Ethical Issues in Family Medicine* (1986). They argue that "general moral theory does not illuminate specific cases and therefore is not helpful" since "[t]he principles of moral philosophy are simply too abstract and too formal to contribute to the resolution of concrete cases" (Christie and Hoffmaster 1986, xv). Arthur Caplan's (1980) clear rejection of the notion that moral theories can simply be wheeled on stage and applied without careful attention to the details of a particular case is widely endorsed in the current literature. We can see, then, that the trend in medical ethics is to examine issues in context and avoid dependence on general abstract rules and rights.

Some philosophers still entrenched in mainstream moral theory have difficulty in seeing the distinction being cited here, since surely all moral theories are context sensitive to some degree. Kantian theory, for example, demands an interpretation of context in order to determine which maxim applies in a given case. But Kantian theory does assume that the maxims, once identified, will be universal and our policy on suicide, truth-telling, or confidentiality will be consistent across the full spectrum of relevant cases. It does not direct us to make our ethical assessments in terms of particular details of the lives of the individuals.

Utilitarianism is often espoused precisely as an antidote to such a rigid ethics. It certainly seems to be extremely sensitive to contextual features, in that it recommends we calculate relevant utilities for all possible options in a given set of circumstances. Nonetheless, it discounts some important features which medical ethics and feminist ethics consider important. Utilitarianism requires that we calculate the relevant utility values for all persons (or beings) affected by an action or practice and proceed according to a calculation of the relevant balances. In contrast, those engaged in doing feminist or medical ethics often reflect a desire to take account of the details of specific relationships and to give added weight to some particular utility related qualities like caring and responsibility. Many of those engaged in feminist ethics diverge even further from standard utilitarianism, for they argue that the preferences of the oppressed ought to be counted differently from those of the dominant group. (Feminist objections to pornography, for instance, do not rely merely on the weighing of harms done against pleasure produced but reflect concern about the dehumanizing effect of the message of pornography whatever the utilities involved turn out to be.) In feminist and medical ethics, it is important to consider factors that do not carry any special weight in utilitarianism. There is a need to look at the nature of the persons and the relationships involved in our analysis and not merely to record such values as preference satisfaction or pleasure or pain; while the latter values are specifically held, their importance comes from some abstract sum and not from their attachment to any particular persons in particular situations. Hence, neither Kantian nor utility theory satisfies the requirement of particularity as it is conceived in feminist and medical ethics.

IMPORTANCE OF RELATIONSHIPS AND CHARACTER

The focus on context in feminist and medical ethics helps make evident that the nature of specific relationships is an important element of ethical analysis, i.e., that an ethics of actions is incomplete when evaluation is done in abstraction from the relationship holding between the participants performing them and those affected by them. Within feminist ethics, there is widespread criticism of the assumption that the role of ethics is to clarify obligations among individuals who are viewed as paradigmatically equal, independent, rational, and autonomous (see, for instance, Baier 1987 and Held 1987). Few women conceive of human relationships as being primarily between equal, autonomous beings, for their experience characteristically involves complex relationships of various sorts of interdependencies among persons of widely different degrees of power. From the perspective of feminism, it is clear that the relationships studied in ethics must attend to the interdependent, emotionally varied, unequal relationships that shape our lives. Further, feminist theorists have noted that our ethics must be concerned not only with actions and relationships, but that it should also focus on questions of character and the development of attitudes of trust within those relationships (see Baier 1986).

Similar claims are found within the literature of medical ethics, where it is widely recognized that the relationship between physician and patient is far from equal (especially if the patient is very ill) and that the model of contracts negotiated by independent, rational agents does not provide the ideal perspective on this sort of relationship; in particular, the disadvantaged position of the dependent patient is a major theme in the many discussions of paternalism found throughout the medical ethics literature.

We can also find parallel claims in the literature of feminist and medical ethics regarding the importance of evaluating behaviour in terms of its effect on the quality of relationships. For instance, discussions in medical ethics of the importance of telling patients the truth about their condition often refer to the effect that a discovered lie would have on the patient-physician relationship; these discussions could be redescribed in Baier's language of the place of trust and anti-trust in ethics (Baier 1986).

There seems, then, to be agreement that matters of character, responsibility, and other features that affect trust are recognized as important in both domains. Moreover, as we have seen, medical ethics shares with feminist ethics a commitment to focus on context and an understanding of the significance of inequality within relationships, and some authors in medical ethics express a desire reminiscent of feminism to include caring values in their analysis. Because of all these shared critiques of contemporary moral theory, it might appear that medical ethics is already well on its way to being feminist, yet there are some significant differences in the two approaches which disqualify most of contemporary medical ethics from any claim to feminist ethics.

SOME REQUIREMENTS FOR A FEMINIST ETHICS

For medical ethics to be thought feminist, it must also reflect a political dimension, but this is mostly lacking in the literature to date. Although there are currently many diverse attempts to characterize feminist ethics, all share some political analysis of the unequal power of women and men, of white people and people of colour, of first world and third world people, of rich and poor, of healthy and disabled, etc.[6] Ours is a world structured by hierarchies and a sense of supremacy on the part of the powerful; there are numerous social patterns which shape the people we are and the sorts of relationships we will have with one another. In attending to the quality of actual interactions among people in ethics, we need to account for the influence of social and political factors on the nature of those relationships. From either the caring or the justice perspective (to use Gilligan's language), we can see that empowerment of people who are currently victims of oppression is an ethical as well as a political issue, and ethical investigations of particular problem areas should reflect these dimensions. Many feminist critics have observed that current medical practice constitutes a powerful social institution which contributes to the oppression of women. They have demonstrated that the practice of medicine serves as an important instrument in the continuing disempowerment of women (and members of other oppressed groups) in society and thrives on hierarchical power structures. By medicating socially induced depression and anxiety, medicine helps to perpetuate unjust social arrangements. With its authority to define what is normal and what is pathological and to coerce compliance to its norms, medicine tends to strengthen patterns of stereotyping and reinforce existing power inequalities. It serves to legitimize practices such as woman battering or male sexual aggression that might otherwise be evaluated in moral and political terms.[7]

Nonetheless, the discussion in medical ethics to date has been largely myopic, failing to comment on this important political role of medicine. That is, the institution of medicine is usually accepted as given in discussions of medical ethics, and debate has focused on certain practices within that structure: for example, truth-telling, obtaining consent, preserving confidentiality, the limits of paternalism, allocation of resources, dealing with incurable illness, and matters of re-production. The effect is to provide an ethical legitimization of the institution overall, with acceptance of its general structures and patterns. With the occasional exception of certain discussions of resource allocation, it would appear from much of the medical ethics literature that all that is needed to make medical interactions ethically acceptable is a bit of fine-tuning in specific problem cases.

A good indication of the legitimizing function of medical ethics can be seen by noting its gradual acceptance among those who are influential within the medical profession. Increasingly, medical practitioners seem to be recognizing the value of incorporating discussions of medical ethics within their own work, for they can thereby demonstrate their serious interest in moral matters. Such serious profes-sional concern in matters of medical ethics serves to encourage the public to place even greater trust in their judgement. Keeping the scope of medical ethics narrowed to specific problems of interaction helps physicians maintain their supportive stance towards it.

Feminists must be critical of the fact that medical ethics has remained largely silent about the patriarchal practice of medicine. Few authors writing on medical ethics have been critical of practices and institutions that contribute to the oppres-sion of women. The deep questions about the structure of medical practice and its role in a patriarchal society are largely inaccessible within the framework; they are not considered part of the standard curriculum in textbooks of medical ethics. Consequently, medical ethics, as it is mostly practiced to date, does not amount to a feminist approach to ethics.

There are other important differences, as well. Feminist theory has gone beyond medical ethics in the criticism of traditional ethics by re-conceiving some of the central concepts of ethical theory. It has, for instance, provided grounds for re-jecting an ontology of persons conceived as isolated, fully developed individuals. Rather, it acknowledges the social roots of a person as a being who develops within a specific social context and who is, to a significant degree, a product of that context (or, in the term of Baier 1985 and Code 1987, a "second person"). Al-though we may continue to consider the individual to be a key unit of ethical analysis to the extent that we value persons as unique individuals whose lives are of concern to us, most feminists reject the assumption of individualism underlying contractarian approaches to ethics through which individuals are encouraged to consider themselves and their interests as independent from others. Persons do not exist in abstraction (i.e., not apart from their social circumstances), and moral directives to disregard the details of personal life under some imaginary "veil of ignorance" are actually pernicious for ethical and political analysis because of their trivialization of these important facts. Moral analysis should examine persons and their behaviour in the context of political relations and experiences, but this di-mension has so far been missing from most of the debates in medical ethics.

It is important to explore how the shared precepts of medical and feminist ethics have, in the case of medical ethics, produced a field which is meant to be critical of all morally unacceptable medical practice, but which implicitly supports patriar-chal policies in the medical establishment. In this way, I hope, we can gain insight for feminist ethics into how to develop the commonly held ideas while still preserving their feminist force. I fear that the early formulations of some of these insights in feminist ethics were oversimplified to a degree which makes them dangerous to a feminist program. By contrasting the formulations of these ideas within feminist ethics with their role in the relatively conservative program of medical ethics to date, we will be able to see more clearly what must be added to them to turn existing approaches to medical ethics into feminist medical ethics. In so doing, we will have a clearer idea of how to characterize feminist ethics and, at the same time, we will be able to identify the direction in which medical ethics must move if it is to be truly compatible with feminist ideals.

Understanding Context

In particular, it is important that we add the political dimension of feminist analysis to each of the shared insights previously cited. We must, for instance, be more precise about the view found throughout much of feminist ethics which rejects the notion of an ethics founded on general principles in favour of a context specific ethics.[8] There is a growing tendency in feminist theory to reject any sort of general analysis, arguing that the experiences of women are so varied and diverse we cannot form general conclusions which are inclusive of all women. But I believe that the experience of medical ethics offers grounds for maintaining a certain level of generality in our moral claims.

Consider, for instance, how the methodological concern for contextual specificity is carried out in discussions of reproductive issues in medical and feminist ethics. We can see important differences in their definition and handling of the ethical issues associated with the new reproductive technologies. Those in the secular tradition of medical ethics tend to hold fast to the case by case approach. They seem to think that, barring religious objections to technological intervention in reproduction, the use of such techniques as artificial insemination, in vitro fertilization, embryo transplant, and sex selection are matters best determined in context. They recognize the need for informed consent (though they seem willing to accept remarkably low standards for consent here) and the need to protect confidentiality, etc., but by and large most authors in medical ethics deny that there are any new or unique problems posed by the new reproductive technologies (e.g., Gorovitz 1982).

Feminist theorists, in contrast, recognize that reproductive technologies are a product of existing social patterns and values, and most find reasons to believe that these technologies will shape attitudes and opportunities regarding reproduction in the future. They are unwilling to allow decisions about such practices as in vitro fertilization, sex preselection, or "surrogate" pregnancies to be addressed in isolation from the general pattern constituted by the combined use of these technologies; they resist attempts to decide on the acceptable use of such practices on the merits of each individual case. Surely, if we were to adopt a context specific approach to case analysis, we could identify very strong grounds for allowing individuals to choose such arrangements in specified circumstances, but, because there is a real danger that the increased spread of such practices will contribute to social attitudes that further undermine the social position of women and children in society, we must examine the use of such technology in general. We can and should recognize and sympathize with the desire of affluent, married women to circumvent infertility through techniques such as in vitro fertilization and contractual pregnancy, but we must also evaluate these practices in terms of their effect on other women—including those who are not approved for such medical "assistance" or who are used as medical means to the reproductive interests of others—before making up our minds on such practices. Further, we should be sensitive to the ideology of racism, sexism, classism, or bias against the disabled which often underlies efforts to pursue the production of "quality" babies, for such attitudes are at the heart of many developments in the new reproductive technologies.[9]

A principal ground for concern from a feminist perspective is that the technology is being developed and marketed in such a way as to further increase the control of medical professionals and decrease the control of women over reproduction. A general perspective allows us to see how the new reproductive technologies function within the larger medical pattern of claiming medical authority over an ever expanding sphere of women's personal lives. Historically, male institutions have always sought to control women's reproduction: male religious, political, and economic leaders have used a variety of means to achieve control over women's reproductive capacities. Until very recently, the law in North America ensured that husbands had full sexual access to their wives' bodies; in many cases, men still presume themselves to have de facto claims on women's bodies as is evidenced by the continuing practices of rape, sexual harassment, woman-battering, and other acts of woman-directed violence. The medical profession has claimed its share of this patriarchal control. All phases of a woman's reproductive life, from menstruation through menopause, have been medicalized and subjected to expert control by the male-dominated medical profession. Feminists have documented ample evidence to suggest these arrangements have not all been in the best interest of women (consider, for example, the shockingly high rate of hysterectomies and cesarean sections and the growing tendency to medically initiated, court-ordered cesareans). Many women have suffered serious and unnecessary complications from unwarranted medical interference. The effect of the medicalization of women's reproductive lives has been to make women dependent on male authority for whatever control they can muster over their own reproduction.

Increased reproductive technology generally means increased medical control. In many cases, one technological measure engenders the need for further technological treatment in the future (e.g., the sterility which now drives many women to seek medical means to circumvent it can often be traced to medically prescribed use of the notorious Dalkon Shield or to the absence of safe reversible sterilization techniques). Given the patriarchal bias and authoritarian nature of medicine and the fact that the new reproductive technologies further extend the potential power of this male dominated institution, feminists have grounds for viewing increased medical control of reproduction with alarm.

Thus, from the perspective of feminist ethics, we must evaluate the new reproductive technologies as general practices and not just examine particular applications of them. But the general analysis will not be a purely abstract exercise as it is commonly practiced in mainstream moral theory; it will not look only at abstract properties like rights, autonomy, personhood, or even utility measures— properties which people hold anonymously without regard to their particular circumstances. In doing feminist ethics, we must appeal to contextual details, and the context cited should involve the broad political context of reproduction in a given society. It is not enough to consider merely the details of a particular woman's reproductive situation.

Abortion is the one area of reproduction where discussion in both medical and feminist ethics seems to accept the need to develop a clear, universal moral policy so as not to leave space for evaluation on a case by case basis. Most authors writing on this topic seek to determine some general policy regarding the moral acceptability of abortion or the proper social policy governing access to abortion. Within medical ethics, analyses tend to consist of arguments focusing on such abstract matters as the definition and value of life, the definition of personhood, the scope of human rights, or the social consequences of tolerating or prohibiting abortion on a wide scale; some authors in medical ethics even acknowledge the importance of autonomy for women in controlling their own reproduction. The arguments found in medical ethics tend to focus the debate on the moral status of the fetus and treat the pregnant woman merely as a fetal environment, or else they focus on the property rights of women to expel unwanted invaders (e.g. Thomson 1971).

But the sort of generality appealed to is quite different for feminists than for nonfeminists writing within medical ethics. Feminists see the implications for women's overall freedom and relative power if we accept a policy whereby others are able to coerce women into seeing an unwanted pregnancy through to term. In other words, feminist analyses address questions about the difference it makes to all women's lives if women are free to decide whether or not to continue each pregnancy, whereas many writers in medical ethics try to formulate a general abstract rule about the relative importance of preserving life or protecting autonomy. In both cases, a general position on abortion is sought, but in the tradition of male-dominated medical ethics, the policy is formulated in terms of abstract values and rules which are to be invoked whatever the effect on particular persons' lives. In the case of feminist thought, the analysis links women's freedom from coercion over pregnancy to other aspects of women's relative power in society. Hence, feminist ethics still addresses questions of context, but it does so in terms of a general policy within a society afflicted with patriarchal dominance relations. In medical ethics, abortion is seen as a moral problem for doctors and/or society; in feminist ethics, it is perceived as a choice embedded within women's lives. The tendency in medical ethics to see abortion decisions as isolated from other aspects of women's lives misses the most important feature of the feminist campaign for reproductive freedom for women.

These differences between the analyses developed by theorists working primarily from the perspective of medical ethics and by those working from the perspective of feminist ethics are significant to our understanding of the injunction to avoid general ethical analysis in favour of a contextualized, narrative approach to ethics. Feminism discusses the pervasive nature of sexism and its effects on all human relations; so, issues must be examined in light of their connection with patterns of gender dominance. Clearly, abortion, too, must be addressed in terms of a broadly defined social context which is sensitive to the historical fact that male-dominated institutions have always sought to manipulate women's sexual and reproductive lives. Although pregnancy and childbirth have profound social and economic effects on women, women have not been allowed control over them. Since women's control over their own reproduction is central to all aspects of division of power between women and men, arguments about abortion must be couched in this political recognition.

The arguments surrounding the new reproductive technologies and abortion indicate that feminists should interpret the ideal of considering ethical questions in a contextually based framework quite broadly. There is a need to define context in social and political terms and to consider actions in terms of the practice they are part of, attending to the effect of these practices on women's pursuit of greater power in a society that currently subordinates them.

This is not to say that all questions in feminist medical ethics must be addressed in terms of the practice(s) they represent. Many decisions will still be best carried out by looking to the details of the specific circumstances and people involved. For example, questions about who has the final authority in determining the best interests of a child when there is disagreement between parents and physicians must, I believe, be resolved by considering the details of the particular cases. Sometimes parents are best at identifying their child's interests, e.g. when the child is suffering from a terminal disease and the doctors want to try a painful and largely unsuccessful therapy to provide the child at least with "a chance." In situations where the child has been subject to violent abuse or serious neglect, however, parents are not to be trusted with their child's well-being. To resolve these sorts of controversies, we must look not just to broad social policy (though this is likely to still be an important factor) but also to the details of the relationships among the child, the parents, and the physician. In other words, we must keep in mind the wisdom of Virginia Held's (1984) analysis of ethics, namely that we ought not to expect a single theory or strategy to be adequate for settling all kinds of ethical questions. Different forms of analysis are appropriate to different sorts of moral dilemmas. The important constant is that we must always decide these questions within the wider political context of considering how this analysis effects (if at all) our general feminist objectives of eliminating oppression in all its forms. Which sort of analysis is appropriate to which sort of problem is a matter for feminist medical ethics to explore.

Towards a Feminist Medical Ethics

There are numerous other directions in which work in feminist ethics can inform and transform work in medical ethics and where medical ethics can provide models (both good and bad) for work in feminist ethics. For instance, the literature in both feminist and medical ethics reflects an interest in questions concerning the nature and quality of particular relationships in light of the recognition that rights and responsibilities cannot be assumed to be universal but depend on existing roles and relationships among persons of differing power and status.

In medical ethics, discussions about the ideal form of the doctor-patient relationship have considered various male models: Robert Veatch (1972), for instance, rejected the "engineering model," the "priestly model," and the "collegial model," and found himself left with the "contractual model." Others have observed that the very different power status of patients and physicians makes the contractual model inappropriate and have suggested other contractually based models as alternatives (e.g., Michael Bayles's [1981] suggestion of a fiduciary model).

Feminists, too, have been suspicious of appeals to contractual models in many human interactions. They have also been searching for better models of relationships that are not based in equal power or need, and it is interesting to speculate how discussions of the ideal patient-physician relationship might be modified by discussions in feminist ethics of the place of mother-child relationships (Held 1987, Ruddick 1980, and Whitbeck 1984), or friendship (Code 1987, Stocker 1987, and Raymond 1986). The inclusion of female experiences widens the conceptual map significantly for this long-standing problem in medical ethics. The medical context again demonstrates, though, the need to be cautious in generalizing from certain female experiences, for the models which feminists have focused on are ones suitable to relationships of love and trust, but medicine, from a feminist perspective, is a domain better suited to "antitrust" (Baier 1986).

While feminists have acknowledged the existence and legitimacy of relationships of dependency, they are, nonetheless, concerned to transform medical interactions in such a way as to reduce the power of medical authority. As a result, feminist discussions of medical practice frequently warn of the abuse of medical power in situations that are disempowering to patients. In contrast with authoritarian norms of medical practice, feminists aspire to a system of personal control over health care. They seek to spread health information widely and foster self-help approaches to health matters. Medical expertise ought to be a resource held under the control of patients and their caregivers. The institution of medicine should be transformed from one of crisis management to one of health empowerment. Perhaps the nurse-patient model is worth examining in this context, for, ideally, nurses define their role as one of informing and empowering patients, rather than controlling them. The difficulty, though, is that nurses, like mothers, are limited in the effectiveness of their efforts at empowerment of others because the constraints of hierarchical structures limit their own authority.

A principal task of feminist medical ethics is to develop conceptual models for restructuring the power associated with healing by distributing medical knowledge in ways that allow persons maximum control over their own health. It is important to clarify ways in which dependence can be reduced, caring can be offered without paternalism, and health services can be obtained within a context worthy of trust. A clear understanding of the dynamics of the power structures now inhibiting these processes is an important aspect of our ethical analysis. We must look at the structures of medicine and medical interaction when attempting to understand the details of any particular medical experience. Such lessons from feminist medical ethics are significant to other areas of feminist ethics, suggesting guidance to feminists pursuing ethical theory and its applications. We look to feminist medical ethics to provide a more comprehensive, and fairer, approach to medical ethics than has been evident to date.

NOTES

I wish to express my gratitude to Richmond Campbell, Lorraine Code, Kathleen Martindale, and Debra Shogan for their generous assistance in the development of this paper.

1. For an apt description of the "moral madness" women commonly experience when confronted with patriarchal ethical demands, see Morgan (1987).

2. See, for instance, the various discussions in the collection *Women and Moral Theory*, Kittay and Meyers, 1987.

3. Nel Noddings (1984) has spelled out the full implications of pursuing the feminine approach to ethics exclusively in *Caring*. Though I would not classify her as a feminist, Noddings has given theoretical voice to the ethic of care described by Gilligan, rejecting all aspects of an ethics based in abstract principles in favour of an ethics concerned only with particular relationships based on caring.

4. See, for instance, the arguments put forward by Houston (1987) and Wilson (1988).

5. This tendency seems to me to be especially common in the contributions of physicians to medical ethics; it is less apparent in the philosophical discussions in the field.

6. I am well aware of the rich diversity of views clustered under the label of "feminist analysis," but I think that there are some core views that transcend the differences which divide feminists in their internal debates. For the purposes of this paper, I will focus only on the common themes which include a recognition that women are in a subordinate position in society, that oppression is a form of injustice and hence is intolerable, that there are further forms of oppression in addition to gender oppression (and that there are women victimized by each of these forms of oppression), that it is possible to change society in ways that could eliminate oppression, and that it is a goal of feminism to pursue the changes necessary to accomplish this. I believe that the argument presented in this paper is unchanged however we explain the cause of women's oppression and whatever we imagine is best for bringing about the desired changes. Therefore, I shall speak of a feminist analysis without being specific here about which particular variation I have in mind.

7. See Stark, Flitcraft, and Frazier (1983). For a more far ranging discussion, see the powerful indictment of medicine's contribution to the oppression of women in the survey by Ehrenreich and English (1979).

8. This proposal is found in many places. I made it myself in my first attempts at defining feminist ethics in Sherwin (1984). Annette Baier makes similar claims throughout *Postures of the Mind* (1985); several authors in *Science, Morality, and Feminist Theory* (Hanen and Nielsen, 1987) and *Women and Moral Theory* (Kittay and Meyers, 1987) also present variations on this claim.

9. I spell out this argument more fully in Sherwin (1987).

REFERENCES

Baier, Annette. 1985. *Postures of the mind: Essays on mind and morals.* Minneapolis: University of Minnesota Press.

Baier, Annette. 1986. Trust and antitrust. *Ethics* 96: 231–260.

Baier, Annette. 1987. The need for more than justice. In *Science, morality and feminist theory.* Marsha Hanen and Kai Nielsen, eds. *Canadian Journal of Philosophy* (supplementary volume 13).

Bayles, Michael. 1981. *Professional ethics.* Belmont, CA: Wadsworth Publishing Co.

Caplan, Arthur. 1980. Ethical engineers need not apply: The state of applied ethics today. *Science, Technology, and Human Values* 6 (33): 24–32.

Christie, Ronald J., and C. Barry Hoffmaster. 1986. *Ethical issues in family medicine.* New York: Oxford University Press.

Code, Lorraine. 1987. Second persons. In *Science, morality and feminist theory.* Marsha Hanen and Kai Nielsen, eds. *Canadian Journal of Philosophy* (supplementary volume 13).

Ehrenreich, Barbara, and Deirdre English. 1979. *For her own good: 150 years of the experts' advice to women.* Garden City, N.Y.: Anchor Press, Doubleday.

Engelhardt, H. Tristram, Jr. 1986. *The foundations of bioethics.* New York: Oxford University Press.

Gilligan, Carol. 1982. *In a different voice: Psychological theory and women's development.* Cambridge, MA: Harvard University Press.

Gorovitz, Samuel. 1982. *Doctors' dilemmas: Moral conflict and medical care.* New York: Oxford University Press.

Hanen, Marsha, and Kai Nielsen, eds. 1987. *Science, morality, and feminist theory. Canadian Journal of Philosophy* (supplementary volume 13).

Held, Virginia. 1987. Non-contractual society. In *Science, morality and feminist theory.* Marsha Hanen and Kai Nielsen, eds. *Canadian Journal of Philosophy* (supplementary volume 13).

Held, Virginia. 1984. *Rights and goods: Justifying social action.* New York: The Free Press.

Houston, Barbara. 1987. Reclaiming moral virtues: Some dangers of moral reclamation. In *Science, morality and feminist theory.* Marsha Hanen and Kai Nielsen, eds. *Canadian Journal of Philosophy* (supplementary volume 13).

Kittay, Eva Feder, and Diana T. Meyers, eds. 1987. *Women and moral theory.* Totowa, N.J.: Rowman and Littlefield.

Morgan, Kathryn. 1987. Women and moral madness. In *Science, morality and feminist theory.* Marsha Hanen and Kai Nielsen, eds. *Canadian Journal of Philosophy* (supplementary volume 13).

Noddings, Nel. 1984. *Caring: A feminine approach to ethics and moral education.* Berkeley: University of California Press.

Raymond, Janice. 1986. *A passion for friends: Towards a philosophy of female affection.* Boston: Beacon Press.

Ruddick, Sara. 1980. Maternal thinking. *Feminist Studies* 6 (2): 342–367.

Scheman, Naomi. 1983. Individualism and the objects of psychology. In *Discovering reality: Feminist perspectives on epistemology, metaphysics, methodology, and philosophy of science.* Sandra Harding and Merrill B. Hintikka, eds. Dordrecht, Holland: D. Reidel Publishing Company.

Sherwin, Susan. 1984. A feminist approach to ethics. *Dalhousie Review* 64 (4): 704–713.

Sherwin, Susan. 1987. Feminist ethics and in vitro fertilization. In *Science, morality and feminist theory.* Marsha Hanen and Kai Nielsen, eds. *Canadian Journal of Philosophy* (supplementary volume 13).

Stark, Evan, Anne Flitcraft, and William Frazier. 1983. Medicine and patriarchal violence: The social construction of a "private" event. In *Women and health: The politics of sex in medicine.* Elizabeth Fee, ed. Farmingdale, N.Y.: Baywood Publishing Company.

Stocker, Michael. 1987. Duty and friendship: Towards a synthesis of Gilligan's contrastive moral concepts. In *Women and moral theory.* Eva Feder Kittay and Diana T. Meyers, eds. Totowa, N.J.: Rowman and Littlefield.

Thomson, Judith Jarvis. 1971. A defense of abortion. *Philosophy and Public Affairs* 1 (1): 47–66.

Veatch, Robert M. 1972. Models for ethical medicine in a revolutionary age. *Hastings Center Report* 2 (3): 5–7.

Whitbeck, Caroline. 1984. A different reality: Feminist ontology. In *Beyond domination: New perspectives on women and philosophy.* Carol C. Gould, ed. Totowa, N.J.: Rowman & Allenheld.

Wilson, Leslie. 1988. Is a "feminine" ethics enough? *Atlantis* 5 (17): 15–23.

Feminist Directions in Medical Ethics

VIRGINIA L. WARREN ❖ ❖ ❖

I explore some new directions—suggested by feminism—for medical ethics and for philosophical ethics generally. Moral philosophers need to confront two issues. The first is deciding which moral issues merit attention. Questions which incorporate the perspectives of women need to be posed—e.g., about the unequal treatment of women in health care, about the roles of physician and nurse, and about relationship issues other than power struggles. "Crisis issues" currently dominate medical ethics, to the neglect of what I call "housekeeping issues." The second issue is how philosophical moral debates are conducted, especially how ulterior motives influence our beliefs and arguments. Both what we select—and neglect—to study as well as the "games" we play may be sending a message as loud as the words we do speak on ethics.

We might as well admit it. Medical ethics has grown a bit stale. Hot new topics continue to arise—such as whether to withhold artificial food and fluids from patients, or to "harvest" organs for transplant from fetuses and anencephalic newborns. But calling on the same list of Basic Moral Principles does not produce the thrill it once did, though the issues are as significant and heartbreaking as ever. My aim here is to see whether feminism can suggest some new directions for medical ethics, and for philosophical ethics generally.

I shall begin with two disclaimers. First, I am *not* claiming that a feminist medical ethics must develop in any particular ways, only that certain paths are suggested by feminism. Second, I am *not* claiming that these possibilities could *only* have come from a feminist perspective. These directions may, for example, reinforce some ideas from Marxism or from the holistic health movement. I have no desire to plant a flag on the moon and claim, "Feminists got here first." I do hope, however, that the speculations emerging from the cross-fertilization of medical ethics and feminism will bear fruit.

"SEXIST ETHICS"

Before pondering what a feminist medical ethics might look like, however, muse about what a *Sexist Ethics* might be like (as Overall 1987, 1–13, does). My aim is neither to condemn philosophic ethics through caricature, nor to search for sexist villains. The sexism—of which I, too, am guilty—is mostly unintended. Rather, I want to spur the imagination. What would academic moral philosophy be like if it were sexist? Let us begin with *substance*—with what questions and solutions are discussed. Later we will consider *process*: how moral debates are conducted. And, should the resulting picture fit real life, let us recognize it.

First, a Sexist Ethics would use a male perspective to frame moral questions and to shape solutions. Magicians know to keep the audience's attention away from the action. But moral philosophers may be magicians who have tricked even themselves by concentrating on the topic at hand, without asking which topic most deserves study or what will result from approaching this topic this way. In a Sexist Ethics, moral questions would often involve competitions for power, status or authority. For example, the autonomy-paternalism debate in medical ethics concerns who has the moral authority to make the final decision: patient or physician. And solutions to moral problems would often downplay or ignore the interests of women (and children). For example, when medical costs are contained by sending hospital patients home "quicker and sicker," family members—usually females—must nurse them at home. This unpaid labor—by mothers, wives, daughters, and daughters-in-law—needs to be given more weight. Even now, women's work is often "invisible."

Second, a Sexist Ethics would never appear sexist. It would be clothed in a cloak of neutrality because favoring some group or position would be unthinkable. The dominant trend in philosophical ethics has been to regard people as best able to decide what is moral when least tied to place and time, when least connected through ties of partiality to family and community. Ideal moral decision-makers are viewed as common denominators—e.g., rational egos (Kant) or calculators of utility—who are more likely to adopt the proper universal perspective when the veneer of particularity is stripped away.

Two distortions may result from this approach to ethics. First, although some moral agents may adopt a common denominator moral perspective without feeling that anything of value is lost, others may feel the loss intensely. The reason for this loss is that persons whose unique experiences have been largely omitted from the dominant culture—e.g., women, Blacks, gay males and lesbians—may find the stripping away of particularity from the moral observer to be anathema to self. By subtracting those features that shed light on their experience and life, such individuals may become, at least in part, invisible to themselves.

A second distortion may arise because adopting a universal perspective toward moral situations tends to (although it does not need to) reveal generic persons and relationships whose psychological subtleties have been washed away. Specifically, the fact that human beings are gendered is likely to be deemed irrelevant to moral deliberation. It is too bad if the stereotypic woman—with all her reproductive organs, emotions, and kinship ties to particular others—does not fit the category of Plain Wrap Human Being. Of course, men are also gendered. Sexist Ethics would not take sufficient account of males *qua* males, any more than it does of females *qua* females. Ironically, distortion may be the likely result of our trying so hard not to distort.

Third, a Sexist Ethics would frame the ethical debate so that women would be kept on the defensive. Women would spend much time for little gain. A Sexist Ethics would seduce women to work within its framework by offering hope for improvement—but only if they did not rock the patriarchal boat too vigorously. "Strive for *equality* with men," it would say, "and all will be well. There is no need for more fundamental change." Such a domesticated ethics would, for example, allow women and men to compete equally for the positions of nurse and physician, without questioning the roles themselves, roles which were founded on an unequal power relationship between females and males.

Women might be kept on the defensive in another way: topics chosen for moral debate might have the unintended effect of fanning the flames of sexism. In moral philosophy in the past fifteen years, the two most commonly discussed topics concerning women have been abortion and preferential hiring. In both cases, women's interests and rights are pitted against the interests and rights of "innocent" others: fetuses, and young (white) male applicants to law or medical school who were not principally responsible for the worst sexist practices.

The central place of preferential hiring in the "contemporary moral issues" literature is particularly instructive. Women (and minorities) studying preferential hiring are made to feel how many expectations of males (and whites) they are crushing, and how much hostile backlash awaits, if they push too hard to be let into the club. With sexism (and racism) so prevalent, it borders on the scandalous that so much philosophical energy is focused on preferential hiring. For, while this issue clearly merits attention, it directly affects a relatively small percentage of job-holders for brief periods, mainly in decisions about hiring and promotion. I say this even though I know that believing that one has been, or might be, passed over for a desired job may profoundly affect one's self-conception and self-worth; hence, the *indirect* effects of a policy of preference may extend far beyond the period of hiring.

My point is threefold. First, enough moral philosophers have focused so narrowly on preferential hiring and on whether white males are wronged by it that the full burden on women (and minorities) of sexist (and racist) practices tends to get insufficient attention. (By contrast, Wasserstrom 1977 is a model for portraying the cumulative impact of racism.) Second, the preferential hiring debate is inflammatory because a zero-sum, us-against-them attitude is presupposed, and often goes unchallenged. Alternative, non–zero-sum approaches to ending discrimination and to securing women's (and minorities') rightful interests usually go unexplored. Third, even if the preferential hiring debate (framed now in terms of justice and utility) were resolved one way or the other, that would not help people of different genders (and races) to *relate* to each other better on the job: to respect each other, and to overcome suspicion and hostility.

A strong message is sent by which moral questions are selected for study. Not only are some important issues neglected, but some debates—especially if not prefaced by a patient, thorough probing of the nature and extent of prejudice— may inflame prejudices. Tavris (1982, 131–35) concludes from the experimental evidence that talking out one's anger tends to make one *more* angry at a person, rather than less (as the catharsis theory claims), and the anger endures. Hence, concentrating in the classroom on preferential hiring and abortion as they are now standardly taught may do more than raise the issue of backlash; it may help unleash the lash.

In addition to substantive questions about the rightness of actions, how philosophical ethics is done—the process—is important. First, the theories and arguments of Sexist Ethics would be used as weapons in a competitive power struggle. Participants in the ethical debate would have an ulterior purpose. Over and above seeking the truth about what is morally right, they would want to win the debate, including to look good at someone else's expense. Second, the "star" system would be part of the Sexist Ethics game. In academia, a huge disparity exists between ability and productivity (as judged on a fair merit system), on the one hand, and reputation, on the other. Would-be "stars" aim at advancing their reputations, and at gaining prestige and the power and perquisites which accompany prestige. Thus, over and above any substantive differences between sexist and feminist ethics, we must attend to how the philosophical "ethics game" is played in discussions, at conferences, and in print.

In my view, contemporary philosophical ethics—including medical ethics— has all of the features described under "Sexist Ethics" to *some* degree, even though the intention to be sexist is usually absent. The degree varies dramatically with the topic, the author or speaker, and the occasion. Imagining how philosophical ethics might become increasingly less sexist is the challenge.

FEMINIST MEDICAL ETHICS: WHAT IS STUDIED

Which questions moral philosophers choose to study—and choose not to study—is itself a moral issue, yet one that is hardly ever raised. In this section I will sketch some changes—suggested by feminism—in the questions addressed in medical ethics.

Feminists could add the perspectives of women of different races, classes, sexual preferences, etc., to questions and solutions already discussed in the literature of medical ethics. For example, more weight would be given in cost-cutting debates to the effects on families—especially on female caretakers—of patients released from hospitals earlier.

In addition, feminists could include women's perspectives—along with the perspectives of males *qua* males, and the interests of children—by *posing new questions.* Carol Gilligan (1982) interviewed women who were considering abortion, and listened to how they framed moral questions and to which moral values they appealed. We, too, need to listen. I will discuss four categories of new questions: (1) inequalities, (2) sexist occupational roles, (3) personal issues, and (4) relationship issues that do not involve deciding the winner of power struggles.

(1) *Inequalities.* The treatment of women patients, women physicians, and people in traditionally female occupations such as nursing or social work should be examined. After exposing any unequal treatment of women in health care, solutions could be sought. An example of unequal treatment of female patients is the policy in many *in vitro* fertilization programs of excluding all women who are not married heterosexuals; that is, only women who want to raise a child with a

husband need apply. When this policy is criticized, one response is to point out the scarcity of places in IVF programs—with no attempt to defend this particular allocation of scarce resources. The issue is deflected, but not taken seriously; and male privilege is protected, but not justified.

(2) *Sexist occupational roles*. Historically, the roles of physician and nurse were designed for males and females, respectively. Tasks were assigned based on what was appropriate masculine and feminine behavior, with nurses expected to defer to physicians (see Stein 1967). So far, the basic question in nursing ethics has been what hospital nurses should do when their moral views clash with those of physicians, who have more institutional and legal power.

Moreover, physicians' training is largely theoretical and technological, and they have final decision-making authority for patient treatment. The role of nurse has always included nurturing patients' psyches (and although much knowledge and skill is required to perform nurturing tasks well, that is often overlooked and labeled "intuition"); and nurses' decision-making authority is subordinated to "doctor's orders." This division of labor in health care—based on which gender the role was designed for—remains, even though an increasing number of physicians are now female. (Male nurses remain a rarity.)

A second type of new question would go further, examining sexism in occupational roles. We need to stop segregating nurturing from theory—whether in health care (the work of nurses and social workers from that of physicians) or in academia (undergraduate teaching from research). Giving females and males equal opportunity to enter occupations in which nurturing and theory are pulled apart does not solve the problem. The answer is not to have fifty percent of nurses be caring, responsive males, while fifty percent of physicians are oriented toward technology and research and are professionally distant—but are female. Nor is the answer to have RNs imitate the higher paid, higher status, traditionally male occupations; for then the caring tasks would be delegated to others (e.g., to licensed vocational nurses). Nurturing needs to be valued more highly, including monetarily, and integrated with technical and theoretical expertise, particularly in medicine. (Nursing is already attempting such integration.) We need to redefine the roles and relationships of all members of the "health care team," making roles more androgynous.

(3) *Personal issues*. A third type of new moral question examines issues which usually are not elevated to the status of the serious in academic contexts, although they matter considerably to health care professionals. For example, medical ethics has been virtually silent about problems influenced (to varying degrees) by job-related stress. One is on one's own. However, the incidence of drug and alcohol abuse by physicians and nurses—people who know the health risks—is much higher than that of the general population. Divorce and suicide rates are also high. Families of health care professionals are also harmed by this stress. We need to probe social and institutional causes (e.g., the nature of medical education—including the 24- and 36-hour shifts residents work), and to seek solutions that address more than one person's private failure.

Moreover, philosophical ethics routinely ignores the little—and not so little— domestic problems of life, which I call "*housekeeping issues*." These "personal" issues contrast with the *"crisis issues"* (e.g., abortion or withdrawal of life-support) that are the bread and butter of contemporary moral philosophy. Perhaps an analogue to the feminist slogan, "The personal is political," is needed: "The personal is professional." That is, what is "merely" personal may profoundly affect how one acts on and off the job, and thus should play a significant role in professional ethics.

An example of an important housekeeping issue is how to help people *use* such valuable legislation (in California and some other states) as the Durable Power of Attorney for Health Care. Should one become incompetent, a Durable Power specifies what medical treatment one does and does not want, and invests a designated person (e.g., spouse, friend) with the legal authority to make one's other medical decisions. While bioethicists have discussed moral reasons for and against passing such legislation (a crisis issue), they rarely address problems of implementation (housekeeping issues). Nor do physicians raise the possibility of signing such a document with patients very often. When physicians do think of it, they may fear that even raising the issue with terminal patients will cause despair and hasten death. Often it is thought of too late: when patients are already comatose, or weakened by illness and confused by drugs. Nor do we help families learn how to discuss such grave matters openly and "before need" (the phrase used in cemetery commercials). If most laypeople are unaware that such legislation exists, they cannot raise the issue of signing a Durable Power with physicians. And few physicians are raising it with them. (Nurses sometimes do, but risk being criticized for encroaching on the physician's prerogative.)

These two categories of moral issues—crisis and housekeeping issues—contrast in several ways.

First, with crisis issues, moral decisions are more or less final. A moral problem arises; one decides; one moves on and feels a sense of progress. With housekeeping issues, however, *the problematic situation is ongoing, rather than resolved once and for all*; and decisions need to be made continually. Job stress, for example, can be contained but not eliminated.

Second, the significance of crisis issues immediately catches our attention. We take pride in facing a difficult challenge. By contrast, housekeeping issues *seem trivial*. Even if we handle these problems well, we feel we have not accomplished much, and others are unlikely to laud our efforts. For example, we discuss crisis issues related to AIDS, such as whether AIDS antibody testing should be mandatory in some cases. But few are discussing housekeeping issues, e.g., how sexually active persons can raise the question of AIDS exposure and protection with prospective sexual partners, while trying to respect privacy and avoid manipulation. Even if housekeeping issues were trivial when considered one at a time, their collective impact on individuals and institutions would be anything but trivial.

Third, crisis issues usually involve a narrow range of alternative actions. By contrast, housekeeping issues commonly *require us to reassess large parts of our lives*: our character traits, how we think about ourselves, and how we relate to others. Their impact is thus felt long after a particular crisis is past.

But do not some crisis issues, such as abortion, also require us to reassess our lives? Yes, a woman's life will probably be dramatically affected by whichever alternative to an unwanted pregnancy she chooses, especially raising the child. My point is that while crisis issues may indeed have far-reaching consequences, house-keeping issues force us to examine an issue in a wide context, calling into question an intertwined web of everyday activities and relationships that is usually taken for granted.

For example, informed consent is standardly interpreted as a crisis issue: "Was an autonomous and informed consent obtained from the patient before this treat-ment, or did the physician withhold relevant information or pressure the patient?" Compare this to informed consent interpreted as a housekeeping issue: "How should we foster the conditions which make informed consent more likely?" The whole physician-patient relationship is thereby called into question: How much time should physicians spend with patients, and on whose terms—when it is convenient for the doctor or when the patient is well-rested and psychologically prepared? How involved should physicians be with patients' value choices and anguish? Should the relationship between physicians and nurses be changed so that they can work together more effectively to encourage patient autonomy?[1]

Fourth, crisis issues are more readily handled using such standard moral prin-ciples as justice, autonomy, beneficence and non-maleficence, and utility. *Applying these principles to housekeeping issues helps only up to a point.* These principles do not deal satisfactorily with psychological subtleties, especially with the intricacies of longer-term relationships. For example, autonomy and beneficence will offer only rudimentary guidance to a health professional deciding whether and how to ap-proach a specific patient about signing a Durable Power of Attorney. Utilitarians, it is true, hold that the Utility Principle always applies. Yet, reducing character traits and relationships to how much happiness and unhappiness they can be ex-pected to produce seems to me to drain them of much of their significance.

Overall, what are we to make of these housekeeping issues, which refer to one's everyday life and to ongoing relationships, and which are routinely overlooked? On a given topic, should housekeeping issues replace crisis issues? Not necessarily. I view it as an open question whether, for a given area, both crisis and housekeeping issues need to be discussed, or whether one of these sets of issues is sufficient. What matters is that we neither ignore important questions, nor distort the moral debate by asking questions in the wrong way—for we sometimes turn housekeeping issues into crisis issues just so they will be resolved.

(4) *Relationship issues that do not involve deciding who wins various power struggles.* The main relationship questions in medical ethics now involve competitions for power, status or authority. Who should have the moral authority to make the final decision: the patient or the physician (in the autonomy-paternalism debate), the physician or the nurse (in nursing ethics)? Relationships are incorrectly assumed to be fine when there is no overt struggle for power.

Moral philosophers should consider ways of resolving power conflicts other than declaring a winner. For example, a strategy of "preventive ethics" could be adopted. Instead of asking who should be "King of the Hill"—physician or patient—ask how the conflict might be prevented in the future. Changes might be needed in medical education or in the social organization of hospitals.

On a larger scale, I believe that the feminist goal of eliminating conflicts over power can be permanently attained only by solving this problem: How can people be helped to develop a sense of self and of self-worth (identity) that is not based on putting down or controlling someone else (power over others)? This question is important because simply trying to eliminate one form of discrimination—against women, gays and lesbians, the disabled—and then another will never have an end. We will be playing musical chairs: there will always be an odd person out. To eliminate discrimination across the board, a radical strategy is needed: educating people to value themselves in a way that does not depend on branding anyone else inferior.

In addition to preventing or eliminating power struggles, other questions about relationships might be asked by a feminist medical ethics. Relationship ethics should discuss openness, responsiveness and caring. For example, how personally involved with patients should health care professionals be in different situations? In order to encourage more sensitivity to their patients and co-workers, how should health care professionals—including physicians—be trained, and what should their working conditions be?

Some issues in medical ethics have been much debated but, in those discussions, crucial questions about relationships have been downplayed or ignored. For example, in the philosophical literature, abortion is often interpreted as a power struggle. Whose rights are more important: the fetus's right to life, if it has one, or the mother's right to autonomously guide her life? What is usually left out of the abortion debate is a network of issues surrounding the parent- (especially mother-) child relationship.[2]

I have been amazed by the casualness with which many opponents of abortion offer adoption as an alternative. Nor have moral philosophers considered the following question in any depth: If a pregnant woman has decided not to abort, when is it morally permissible for her to give up the newborn for adoption? Whenever she wants to? Is adoption permissible only if the baby would be better off being raised by someone else—and, then, only if the mother is unwed? (Can you imagine telling your parents or in-laws that you and your partner have decided to give up their grandchild for adoption? Or telling an older child that its sibling-to-be will be given up for adoption?) Is it permissible for a woman to conceive *in order* that the child be adopted—if everyone, including the child and the adoptive parents, benefit? If it is, then surrogate motherhood (money issues aside) would have a more solid moral foundation. My point is that, regarding abortion and adoption (as well as child custody disputes during divorce), we need to get to the heart of matters of the heart: relationships between parents and children, between life partners, between siblings, between grandparents and grandchildren. At present, we have not identified what the important relationship issues are, nor do we know how to weigh these values against such standard ones as rights, autonomy, and beneficence/utility.

One way to move health care relationships away from the issue of power struggles is to downplay the traditional view of the physician as authority, and to emphasize their role as *educators*. In most fields, teaching non-experts has traditionally been viewed as a female task. Not surprisingly, patient education is often delegated to the predominantly female occupations of nursing and social work.

Observe what happens when informed consent is viewed in terms of an educational model, with the physician as teacher, instead of a medical model, in which treating disease is paramount. Using the medical model, many physicians relate to patients based on whether the interaction will promote patient health. Thus, information is given to patients only if it will not harm the patient's medical condition. For example, a physician might ponder, "Will these facts depress the patient, thereby lowering her immune response?" Moreover, using the medical model, when a patient fails to understand the risks and benefits of alternative treatments, the first explanation is probably psychiatric: the patient is in denial, unable to accept disturbing facts. Maybe, maybe not. Of course people sometimes refuse to hear frightening facts. But, as a teacher, I know how hard it is to communicate even when the subject is emotionally bland, as in logic. Teachers need to repeat, to connect with *this* student's experience, and to get feedback from students so that inaccuracies can be corrected. Teaching skills are hard-won—requiring practice, experimentation, and sensitivity to audience. The medical model downplays the difficulties of teaching well, tends to attribute failures of communication to patients, and lets physicians who are poor teachers off the hook.[3]

In sum, there are many ways to add the perspectives of women to the questions asked in medical ethics. Existing questions can be rethought. And new questions can be posed: about inequality, occupational roles, "housekeeping issues," and relationship issues other than power struggles.

FEMINIST MEDICAL ETHICS: HOW ETHICS IS DEBATED

Over and above which questions are studied, how discussions in moral philosophy are conducted is crucial. I will briefly discuss three feminist themes which suggest directions for how academic medical ethics might be done: (1) diversity, (2) relationships, and (3) basing theory on ordinary experience.

(1) The first theme is _diversity._ Women (and other groups) have had their perspectives and interests minimized or omitted from textbooks and theories. After devising theories that take account of women's experiences, feminist theorists are often ambivalent about establishing these ideas as the paradigm for all humanity. (For example, Gilligan 1987 is still working out to what degree the "justice perspective" and the "care perspective" in ethics are both needed, and to what degree they compete.) And rightfully so: feminists know that "one size fits all" usually does not. We need fully to explore the degree to which philosophical ethics should accommodate multiplicity.

One way of fostering diversity in ethics is finding ways to ask more moral questions from many different perspectives. Currently, medical ethics is overwhelmingly physician ethics. But, from the philosophical armchair, we might ask what questions about health care an Hispanic woman from the barrio would want answered. Or, leaving the armchair, an ethicist might observe on her own—or team up with social scientists to observe—the moral issues which different sorts of people grapple with.[4] I do not underestimate the difficulty of interpreting such data, but facing these difficulties is better than continuing to ignore important moral questions. In medical ethics, we need to do a lot more listening.

We need to explore not only new questions, but also alternative moral principles or values. Those we have now (except in virtue ethics) are best suited to handling conflicts over power and authority. I believe that autonomy, in particular, needs to be reconceived. In medical ethics, the principle of autonomy is most frequently used to fend off others' attempts to make one's decisions. But it may prove wanting as a positive conception of human agency at its noblest. Alternative conceptions might include self-expression (as opposed to self-mastery) or effortlessness (that is, not needing to "make laws for oneself"). More radically, we should question whether the aim is to find one, rather small, set of moral principles or values for everyone (all races, genders, cultures, etc.) at all times in their lives. Some feminists (e.g., Noddings 1984; Sommers 1987; Held 1987) have questioned universalizability or have otherwise tried to find room in moral theory for caring for particular others. Universalizability may indeed be compatible with caring for particular persons. Still, we may seek a tolerable, even desirable, amount of diversity in ethics—both in the normative principles themselves and in the solutions they yield when applied to specific situations—that will not lead to chaos.

(2) A second feminist theme is *relationships*. Accordingly, a feminist approach might examine *how* people in academia relate to each other when discussing ethics.

First, the social interaction occurring during academic debates (written or oral) about ethics should itself be morally evaluated. Did people treat each other with respect? Was good will fostered among the participants? Motives are important. Sometimes, people simply serve as sounding boards for each other as they try to discover what the right response to a morally complex issue is. However, the absence of ulterior motives in ethics discussions is, I suspect, at least as rare in academia as in the rest of life—that is, rare indeed. When participants in moral dialogues have ulterior purposes co-existing with (and sometimes overshadowing) the desire to seek the truth about right and wrong, they are playing a "game": *The Ethics Game*.

In academia, the Ethics Game is sometimes played to one-up the opposition. The goals include proving oneself right (about what is morally right) *and* proving the "opposition" wrong. Moral theories and arguments are used as weapons. Philosophical reputations are at stake: who can poke holes in the opponent's position and defend an alternative position against all objections—for all to see?[5] Winning may take precedence over truth. Most women and some men feel demeaned by playing this game; they feel sullied when they win, foolish when they lose.

When we think of ulterior motives—anything besides simply seeking the truth about right and wrong—we usually think of bad motives, especially of manipulating others in ways that harm their interests. However, playing the Ethics Game need not be bad; both the intentions and the results may be good. For example, during classroom ethics discussions, teachers often desire (an ulterior motive) that students will learn to express their ideas more confidently in public and increase their self-esteem. Here the Ethics Game is played to encourage trust and respect among participants, instead of scoring points at others' expense. Feminists could explore the moral merits of different variations of the Ethics Game.

Destructive forms of competitiveness—which are part of how the academic Ethics Game is often played—might be avoided by experimenting with how papers are authored. Collective authorship (a rarity in philosophy) could be encouraged. Authors could devise ways of minimizing the problems of collaboration. And the process which the authors go through in working together might inform the topic studied (especially if the topic concerns relationships). The collaborative process might even change the authors' lives for the better.[6] Anonymous authorship is another possibility. Each feminist, singly or with others, could—once in a career— write an article under the same pseudonym. Later authors would not need to be consistent with prior writings published under this name. My favorite candidate for identifying this collective feminist identity is "Sue D. Nym." This pseudonym would deliver both a political statement and a Kierkegaardian invitation: the reader should consider the ideas and look within, without considering the author's reputation.

Second, when we are writing or teaching about ethics, we should address not only the intellect but the entire personality of the moral decision-maker. Moral arguments advance reasons for a conclusion, but there is more to do. Learning about the lives of people—real or fictional—can inspire; and others can serve as models for solving moral problems. For example, I once found it immensely helpful to ask myself: "If Gandhi were in my shoes (sandals, of course), how would he deal with the Dean of the Faculty on this matter?"

Moreover, we are often ambivalent about which position is morally correct. It is tempting to reduce internal conflict by aligning with one side, and by projecting the feelings and beliefs we deny onto an opponent—whom we then try to grind into the dust. On different occasions, we may even align with opposite sides— depending on our mood, and on what positions others have already staked out. Helping people—students, readers, and ourselves—to claim all of their ambivalent voices as their own (through role-playing, writing journals, etc.) may be one of the biggest contributions we can make as teacher-scholars to increasing both self-understanding and social harmony.

(3) A third feminist theme is that *theory should be constructed from one's life experience*, that life precedes theory. In the 1960s and '70s, small consciousness-raising groups were pivotal in spreading the feminist spirit. Accepted ideas in politics, morality, science, and everyday living had to be reexamined; and the bedrock of this critique and exploration was to be each woman's experience. It was thought that feminist theory should *not* come down from on high by "experts" and famous authors, even if they were feminists.

The belief that feminist theory should be grounded on the experiences of ordinary women is not a naive philosophical claim. Feminists know that our experience is shaped, even constructed, by our system of (patriarchal and other) beliefs. Rather, it is a political commitment which accomplishes two things. First, one learns to trust one's own judgment, listening to oneself and to other ordinary folk, even if all the books say otherwise. (Not until I taught my first Philosophy of Women course did I realize that *my* conception of God was based on my mother— not on my father, as Freud had said.) Second, the authority of established experts— and one's relationship to them—is challenged. If knowledge is power, "life precedes theory" is social revolution.

This social revolution could be extended to academic ethics. Moral philosophy would not be assumed mainly to trickle down from the experts to students. (See Harding 1987, 8–10, on alternatives to "trickle down" in feminist social science research.) Despite the fact that we philosophers champion "critical thinking," our students are expected, to a great degree, to accept their teachers' framework, methods, and basic assumptions—which form the criteria for doing good philosophy. (How many times did I force students, when they offered moral reasons, to "identify the relevant moral principle" from a short list, before I realized how many of their reasons simply did not fit, unless mutilated?) I have no desire to expel the philosophical baby with the bathwater, but maybe, all along, we have been discarding only part of the water after each bath. It may be time for moral philosophers to question not only the power relationship between physicians and patients, but that between themselves and those they would instruct; and that between themselves and the philosophers (from Plato to Rawls) they turn to for guidance.

Coda

I have described some directions which a medical ethics inspired by the insights of feminism might take. Two overall points will, I believe, prove useful in rethinking philosophical ethics, particularly medical ethics. First, *moral philosophers should decide which moral issues merit attention.* Neglect is not always benign. And raising certain questions—especially in the absence of a wider context—may deeply influence people's beliefs and attitudes. Second, *we need to consider how philosophical moral debates should be conducted,* including how ulterior motives influence us. What we select—and neglect—to study as well as the "games" we play may be sending a message as loud as the words we do speak on ethics.

These two points are instances of the claim that *doing philosophy—including moral philosophy—is a part of life, and so may be evaluated morally.* Working on a particular philosophical issue in a particular way should be part of a search for truth, but it is more. It may influence our relationships with students and colleagues; it may affect how well our readers and students listen to themselves and treat others. We are responsible for all of our choices.

NOTES

I read earlier versions of this paper at the Society of Women in Philosophy, Pacific Division meetings in Los Angeles in April, 1988, and at the conference on "Explorations in Feminist Ethics: Theory and Practice," in Duluth, MN, in October, 1988. I thank the members of both audiences for their comments, and Gregory S. Kavka, who commented on an early version.

1. In our prior non-medical example, the crisis question is: "When hiring, should preference be given to women/minorities?" The housekeeping question is: "How can I behave at work to help end sexism/racism?" The latter invites an examination of discriminatory attitudes and goes far beyond whether preference to women/minorities should be given in

the final hiring decision. Reexamination of the entire job search is needed, and of how the new employee (of whatever gender or race) will be treated on a daily basis in years to come. Moreover, faculty treatment of students should be addressed. For example, should classroom procedures be changed? (Letting the big talkers speak whenever they want to may favor male students and—if the school is predominantly white—whites). And are faculty members more likely to encourage male (white) students to attend graduate school or to try for prestigious jobs?

2. While some authors have discussed these issues, as yet they have had relatively little influence in changing the terms in which the debate is framed. See Addelson 1987, Callahan 1986, Harrison 1984, and Whitbeck 1982; Tooley and Purdy 1974 give a utilitarian perspective.

3. Perhaps preventive medicine would gain more prominence if the physician-patient relationship were viewed more in terms of teaching and guiding, and less as a contest for final decision-making authority (the autonomy-paternalism debate).

4. I would like to ask people which moral questions in health care they want most to *avoid*—and then to study those. In my experience, the most explosive issue does not concern when to withhold life-support, or other crisis issues, but a housekeeping issue: the hospital's own hierarchical social structure. In particular, should the dramatically unequal power distribution between physicians and nurses (social workers, etc.) be maintained?

5. See Lakoff and Johnson (1980, 61–65 and 77–81) on the "rational argument is war" metaphor.

It might be objected that the best way to get to the truth is for others to try their mightiest to slay one's arguments; an idea's survival is purported to be evidence of its truth. In a conciliatory moment, I might reply that different styles of argument may work better for some people, and for some topics, than others. However, my considered opinion is harsher. Though schooled to accept the Gladiator Theory of Truth, I have never found it to be the only way to get to the truth. Moreover, I have often found it to distort truth and to crush creativity. Do not take my word for it; ask your students about it.

6. These and other issues about academic competition are discussed in Miner and Longino 1987; many of the articles are jointly authored.

REFERENCES

Addelson, Kathryn Pyne. 1987. Moral passages. In *Women and moral theory*. Eva Feder Kittay and Diana T. Meyers, eds. Totowa, N.J.: Rowman and Littlefield.

Callahan, Daniel. 1986. How technology is reframing the abortion debate. *Hastings Center Report* 16 (1): 33–42.

Gilligan, Carol. 1982. *In a different voice*. Cambridge, MA: Harvard University Press.

Gilligan, Carol. 1987. Moral orientation and moral development. In *Women and moral theory*. Eva Feder Kittay and Diana T. Meyers, eds. Totowa, N.J.: Rowman and Littlefield.

Harding, Sandra. 1987. Introduction: Is there a feminist method? In *Feminism and methodology: Social science issues*. Sandra Harding, ed. Bloomington: Indiana University Press.

Harrison, Beverly Wildung. 1984. *Our right to choose: Toward a new ethic of abortion*. Boston: Beacon Press.

Held, Virginia. 1987. Feminism and moral theory. In *Women and moral theory*. Eva Feder Kittay and Diana T. Meyers, eds. Totowa, N.J.: Rowman and Littlefield.

Kittay, Eva Feder, and Diana T. Meyers, eds. 1987. *Women and moral theory*. Totowa, N.J.: Rowman and Littlefield.

Lakoff, George, and Mark Johnson. 1980. *Metaphors we live by*. Chicago: University of Chicago Press.

Miner, Valerie, and Helen Longino, eds. 1987. *Competition: A feminist taboo?* New York: The Feminist Press at the City University of New York.

Noddings, Nel. 1984. *Caring: A feminine approach to ethics & moral education*. Berkeley: University of California Press.

Overall, Christine. 1987. *Ethics and human reproduction: A feminist analysis*. Boston: Allen & Unwin.

Sommers, Christina Hoff. 1987. Filial morality. In *Women and moral theory*. Eva Feder Kittay and Diana T. Meyers, eds. Totowa, N.J.: Rowman and Littlefield.

Stein, Leonard I. 1967. The doctor-nurse game. *Archives of General Psychiatry* 16 (6): 699–703.

Tavris, Carol. 1982. *Anger: The misunderstood emotion*. New York: Touchstone, Simon & Schuster.

Tooley, Michael, and Laura Purdy. 1974. Is abortion murder? In *Abortion: Pro and con*. Robert L. Perkins, ed. Cambridge, MA: Schenkman.

Wasserstrom, Richard. 1977. Racism, sexism, and preferential treatment: An approach to the topics. *UCLA Law Review* 24 (3): 581–622.

Whitbeck, Caroline. 1982. The moral implications of regarding women as people: New perspectives on pregnancy and personhood. In *Abortion and the status of the fetus*. William B. Bondeson, H. Tristram Engelhardt, Jr., Stuart F. Spicher, and Daniel H. Winship, eds. Dordrecht: D. Reidel.

Women and AIDS:
Too Little, Too Late?

NORA KIZER BELL ❖ ❖ ❖

Many authors examine the governmental, the scientific, and the sexual politics of AIDS. Many of these same authors tell the AIDS story within the context of decrying homophobia. The implications of that story, however, have a troubling significance for women. This essay proposes to move the discussion of the sexual politics of AIDS beyond the confines of homophobia and to highlight issues not widely discussed outside of AIDS activist circles— issues which are having, and will continue to have, profound effects on women.

> *But should these swallows, indulging their lust, lose heart, or dissolve their plots and singly depart, breaking the bonds that bind them together, then know them as the worst birds that ever wore feathers.* (Lysistrata)

Helen Singer Kaplan argues that *Lysistrata*, Aristophanes' erotic and political satire, is "a fitting parable for our AIDS-crisis time" (Kaplan 1987). She believes that because of their "strategic" position in the course of this primarily sexually transmitted disease, "women have the power and the obligation to guard the general population from the infestation." Women can actually halt the epidemic, she suggests, if "like Lysistrata's women, we do not have sex with infected men. We must form an impenetrable barrier" (Kaplan 1988).

While such a claim is an obvious oversimplification of the problem of AIDS transmission, and while it is both objectionable and inappropriate to make any argument that would lead people to hold women responsible for spreading human immunodeficiency virus (HIV),[1] Kaplan's thesis does call attention to one of the dimensions of AIDS that has been widely ignored: the complexities of the impact of AIDS on women.

In *And the Band Played On*, Randy Shilts describes an incident late in the book in which a female prostitute is revealed by the news media to be HIV seropositive:

> The uproar illuminated that profoundly heterosexual male bias that dominates the news business. After all, thousands of gay men had been infecting each other for years, but attempts to interest news organizations to pressure the city for an aggressive AIDS education campaign had yielded minimal interest. A single fe-

Hypatia vol. 4, no. 3 (Fall 1989). © by Nora Kizer Bell

male heterosexual prostitute, however, was a different matter. She might infect a heterosexual man. That was someone who mattered; that was news (Shilts 1987, 510).

As careful as Shilts is to chronicle the "untold stories" of AIDS and to describe the scientific, the governmental, and the sexual politics of AIDS, he, like so many other authors, tells the story within the context of decrying homophobic hysteria. The implications of that story also have a troubling significance for women.

In what follows, I propose to move the discussion of the sexual politics of AIDS beyond the confines of homophobia and to highlight issues not widely discussed outside of AIDS activist circles—issues which are having, and will continue to have, profound effects on women.

AIDS RISK GROWING

The AIDS risk is growing. On June 14, 1988, Associated Press wire service reports of the Fourth International Conference on AIDS being held in Stockholm, Sweden, quoted Dr. James Curran of the Centers for Disease Control (CDC) in Atlanta as saying that by 1992 AIDS cases in the United States could number between 365,000 and 450,000. Previously, the Public Health Service had predicted that by 1991 the numbers of persons with AIDS would approach 270,000, of whom 140,000 would have died (Morgan and Curran 1986). In the June wire service release Curran was also reported to have advised conferees that as heterosexual transmission continues to grow, more women are acquiring the disease through heterosexual contact (Associated Press 1988).

Since 1981, over 72,000 cases of AIDS have been reported to the CDC, and an estimated 1.5 million persons are believed to be infected with the human immunodeficiency virus (HIV). (Leads from MMWR 1988, 478; AIDS Weekly Surveillance, 8/88) The most recent projections about the spread of the virus, however, have raised the level of public awareness of the presence of HIV and indicate that AIDS/HIV is considerably more widespread than previous estimates suggested.

As a matter of fact, although 90 percent of reported AIDS cases continue to occur among homosexual men or intravenous drug users, a 1987 study notes a disproportionate increase in cases of AIDS over the past three years among women who are heterosexual partners of bisexual men (16%) or of intravenous drug users (67%). From 1981 to 1986 reported cases of AIDS in women increased in parallel with cases in men, and although men with AIDS still clearly outnumber women with AIDS, there is one risk category in which women with AIDS outnumber men with AIDS by a significant margin: persons whose *only* risk factor is heterosexual contact with a person at risk (Guinan and Hardy 1987).

The primary mode of transmission of HIV to women discerned by this study was intravenous drug use (52%). However, the second most common route of transmission to women (21%) was heterosexual contact with someone with AIDS. This compares to a mere 1% of nonhomosexual/bisexual men with AIDS who had this risk factor. Of a total of 456 adults with AIDS whose only risk factor was heterosexual contact with someone at risk, 84 percent were women. It is noteworthy that the proportion of women with AIDS in that risk category increased from 12% in 1982 to 26% in 1986 (Guinan and Hardy 1987, 2040).

As Des Jarlais explains, since approximately 75 percent of IV drug users in the United States are males and since fully 95 percent of those males are predominantly heterosexual,

> there simply are not enough female IV drug users for the majority of the group to have their primary sexual relationships with other IV drug users. The number of females who do not inject drugs themselves but are regular sexual partners of IV drug users has been estimated to be at least half as large as the number of IV drug users. These figures indicate that a large number of persons may become infected with the AIDS virus through the IV user without involvement with IV drugs themselves (1988, 3).

Acknowledging the decrease in HIV transmission among homosexual men, and in light of data such as the above, Guinan and Hardy argue that in the United States, at the present time, "a heterosexual woman is at greater risk for acquiring AIDS through sexual intercourse than is a heterosexual man" (1987, 2041).

As of August 29, 1988, there were 5840 cases of AIDS reported in women in the United States (*AIDS Weekly Surveillance* 8/88), and, given the most recent Public Health Service projections, by 1992 there will be between 29,000 and 36,000 women with AIDS.[2] Furthermore, 70 percent of the women presently ill with AIDS have been diagnosed in the past two years (Murphy 1988, 65).

Such an observed increase suggests that the risk of HIV infection in heterosexual persons is growing, especially among those heterosexuals who have multiple sex partners or who engage in high risk behaviors, leading some researchers to conclude that the spread of HIV infection into new populations in the United States may first be detected among female prostitutes and persons seeking treatment in clinics for sexually transmitted diseases (Quinn, Glasser, et al. 1988, 197).

The increase in the numbers of heterosexually acquired cases of HIV among women is thought to be the result of two factors: 1) because there are more men than women who are infected, women are more likely than men to encounter an infected partner, and 2) it appears that the efficiency of transmission of the virus is greater from man to woman than from woman to man (Guinan and Hardy 1987; Curran and Jaffe 1988).

Other researchers agree that the evidence is mounting that HIV is effectively spread by vaginal intercourse, primarily from men to women. Some acknowledge that the proportion of AIDS cases attributable to heterosexual transmission is "increasing more rapidly than the proportion of cases in any other category of risk" (Friedland and Klein 1987, 1128). In a study conducted in the San Francisco Bay Area, serum samples were collected from women in sexually transmitted disease (STD) clinics and premarital testing sites and those samples were tested for the presence of HIV antibodies using both the ELISA and Western Blot tests. Preliminary results of those tests reported in the *Journal of the American Medical Association* indicated seroprevalence rates in women as high as 6% (Del Tempelis, Shell, et al., 1987). Guinan and Hardy had already reported rates in women as high as 6.9%, and as already noted, the August 1988 *AIDS Weekly Surveillance* report notes a seroprevalence rate in women of 8%.

"The message for individuals engaging in heterosexual intercourse outside of longstanding mutually monogamous relationships is clear. Human immunodeficiency virus infection is present in the heterosexual community. . . . Since the prevalence has reached this level, it would behoove both men and women to protect themselves" (Del Tempelis, Shell, et al. 1987, 475).

Sexism and Homophobia

Randy Shilts, Julien Murphy, Michael Simpson and others argue that the societal response to AIDS has been shaped by a notion of public health "entangled in social biases" (Murphy 1988, 65). As traditionally conceived, "public health" is a concept growing out of philosophical utilitarianism: response to disease is guided by a principle that affirms a policy of protecting the health of the greatest number of persons. Because the first cases of AIDS, then called GRID (Gay Related Immune Disorder), were diagnosed in homosexual men, it is alleged that guardians of the "public health" hardly responded. AIDS failed to meet the public health criterion: a disease that affected the accepted majority (Woods 1987, 193).

> The difference, Curran knew, was media attention. Once Toxic Shock Syndrome hit the front pages, the heat was on to find the answer. . . . Back in 1976, the newspapers couldn't print enough pictures of flag-draped coffins of dead American Legionnaires. However, the stories just weren't coming for the gay syndrome. . . . There was only one reason for the lack of media interest, and everybody in the task force knew it: the victims were homosexuals. Editors were killing pieces, reporters told Curran, because they didn't want stories about gays and all those distasteful sexual habits littering their newspapers. (Shilts 1987, 110)

Spending on research for AIDS was "niggardly" compared to spending on other public health initiatives. In 1982, for example, the CDC budget for AIDS was $2 million (as contrasted with $135 million spent on the Swine Flu fiasco in 1976) (Thompson 1988, 201). Yet the number of cases of AIDS reported between April of 1982 and December of 1982 grew from 300 to 900 (Shilts 1987, 138 and 214).

Unfortunately, because AIDS was first recognized in the United States in the male homosexual population, the disease was stigmatized as a "gay disease," referred to, even among male homosexuals, as the "gay plague." The cause of the disease was believed to be rooted in practices associated exclusively with the gay lifestyle: use of "poppers," frequenting bathhouses, anal intercourse, and so on. In more than one publication it was referred to as "divine retribution" (Woods 1987, 193).

Many believe that homophobia and the systematic expression of anti-gay sentiment also helped contribute to the lack of public awareness and public response to women with AIDS. Since AIDS continued to be characterized essentially as a problem for gay men, not only was it unthinkable that a gay disease should be a public health priority but it was unthinkable that women would become infected with the virus.

Homophobia can be blamed as well for efforts to oppose wide scale AIDS education and safe sex education. Many persons have argued that discussions of the routes of transmission of HIV will expose young people to sexual practices that are deviant and perverse. In arguing that sex education should emphasize (even preach) abstinence rather than safe sex, some legislators even pressed for the prohibition of any reference to condom use in the classroom.

Such an attitude not only adversely affected women, but also meant that implications for their offspring were ignored. Shilts reports that in 1982,

> Dr. Ayre Rubinstein was trying in vain to get his colleagues to believe that the sick babies he was seeing were also victims of GRID. Rubinstein had sent his research paper to the *New England Journal of Medicine*, but he received no reply. He knew this was not unusual given the snail's pace of scientific publishing. But other scientists were saying that Rubinstein's hypothesis was improbable if not altogether impossible. By its very name, GRID was a homosexual disease, not a disease of babies or their mothers. (Shilts 1987, 124)

Until recently, the fact that women were becoming ill with AIDS was rarely mentioned in the mainstream press. In fact, numerical projections and statistics on AIDS have been based, by and large, on data pertaining to transmission between males. As Murphy argues, many people have not been aware both that women can be infected with HIV and that women have been among those struck down by the virus from the very beginning of the epidemic (1988, 65).

> January 7, 1983: The Morbidity and Mortality Weekly Report on AIDS among female sexual partners of male AIDS sufferers established what would be the last major risk group for Acquired Immune Deficiency Syndrome. Mary Guinan had been railing about "semen depositors" for more than a year, but the publication of the two case histories of the New York women with AIDS finally put a "heterosexual contact" category on the CDC's official list of AIDS risk groups. . . . The account also noted that the CDC had received reports of forty-three other previously healthy women who had developed either Pneumocystis or other AIDS-related opportunistic infections, mainly after having had sexual relations with intravenous drug users. (Shilts 1987, 225)

In spite of the fact that cases of AIDS in women have been documented from the early stages of the epidemic in this country and elsewhere, their plight and their place in the epidemic received very little attention. Women weren't educated about their risk factors or about the possible risks to the developing fetus; they themselves wanted to avoid the stigma associated with having a "gay" disease (Ledger 1987, 5). Women were, and still are, "omitted from AIDS brochures and media coverage, and eclipsed in medical research" (Murphy 1988, 65). In campaigns promoting safe sex, men weren't reminded of their responsibilities to their *female* sex partners (Patton 1988). Even today few persons are aware that AIDS is now the leading cause of death among women aged 25 to 29 in New York City (Bacon 1987, 6).

Even though anti-gay sentiment generated a response to AIDS that overshadowed concerns affecting women, attempts to *combat* homophobia have also been disadvantageous to women.[3] Early in the epidemic, it became clear that disclosure of one's seropositivity had devastating psycho-social effects: job and housing discrimination, increased suicide rates, ostracism, termination of women's parental rights, refusal of health care workers to treat, and so on. For that reason, efforts were begun to develop policy that would be responsible to the privacy rights of persons with AIDS. As important as these efforts were, they had the effect of slowing public health efforts to institute partner notification and contact tracing (both public health strategies long acknowledged as effective in combatting the spread of other sexually transmitted diseases).[4] A recognition of the psycho-social effects of a disclosure of one's seropositivity also led (rightfully) to a fear of any form of selective or mandatory testing, thus ruling out premarital or prenatal testing. In truth, it would have made more sense to expend resources on combatting the underlying discrimination that made protection of confidentiality so important. However, even the time required to confront homophobia among policy makers and the public at large has led to an eclipse of the needs of women with AIDS.

Racism, unfortunately, is also implicated in the neglect of issues affecting women. A report from the CDC in October of 1988 indicated that 26 percent of AIDS cases were among blacks and another 15 percent among hispanics (CDC, 1988). In addition, 53 percent of the women with AIDS are black and approximately 51 percent of them are engaged either in intravenous drug use or prostitution (Murphy 1988, 66; Curran and Jaffe et al. 1988, 611). Researchers report further that while 78 percent of the reported cases of AIDS in children younger than six years old are in children of color, children of color constitute only 21 percent of the nation's population in that age group (Osterholm and MacDonald 1987).

The disparities in the risk for AIDS among blacks and hispanics must be examined within the context of the social fabric in which AIDS infection occurs, and at the core of that fabric one finds the problems of poverty, drug abuse, teen pregnancy, lack of education, inadequate health care and social support services, prostitution, and child and spouse abuse. These social problems are not only deplorable, but as Osterholm and MacDonald point out, they are very complex. For example, while needle-sharing activities continue to be a problem among the urban poor, especially persons of color, the United States continues to lead the industrialized world in rates of teen pregnancy and birth rates. "In particular, the rate of black, never married women aged 15 through 19 years who are sexually active is almost 35% higher than that of white women" (Osterholm and MacDonald 1987, 2737). Because the social and economic realities for women of childbearing age in the inner cities are not easily remedied, the great weight of female and pediatric AIDS will continue to fall on the communities of color, particularly in these urban settings.

The charges of racism and the complexity of class politics cannot be ignored in attempting to understand and combat the effect of AIDS on women, for women with AIDS represent the least advantaged groups in American society. Already disenfranchised, these women lack the means to command the public's attention to their lot. These women are *not* the idealized "victim" woman. They represent yet another segment of society that has traditionally been considered "disposable." As Murphy concludes, "[s]mall wonder, then, that their plight has received so little attention" (1988, 66).

There are, therefore, important ethical issues relating specifically to women with AIDS that remain to be addressed. In the concluding portions of this discussion I propose to enumerate and examine three of those: issues related to recommending condom use, issues related to transmission by intravenous drug use, and issues surrounding birth control and reproduction.

CONDOM USE AND WOMEN

Michael Simpson, in his work on feminist thanatology, has written of the "nearly universal and persistent relationship between women, sex, and danger" (1988, 202). Historically, women have been subject to dangerous sex; "the risks of pregnancy, childbirth, abortion, miscarriage, and the puerperium have limited woman's potential across the centuries" (Simpson 1988, 202). Women have had to be the principal advocates for improved methods of contraception, for male contraception, for legalization of abortion, and so on.

Knowledge of women's social and moral history underlies the anger some women feel about the place given to their role in the AIDS epidemic. It is no wonder that Kaplan argues,

> if men and boys find out that women are united in feeling entitled to protection, that *all* women expect men to behave responsibly, and that we *all* insist on making sure that a man is not infected before we will sleep with him; if he knows that he is not going to get the kind of sex he wants unless he proves that he is not infected, then men's behavior will change. When the majority of women insist on safe sex or hold out on sex until they and their partners are ready to commit themselves to an exclusive relationship or marriage, when we stop buying the nonsense that asking him to wear a condom is healthy assertiveness, then men's behavior will change (Kaplan 1988, 82).

Unfortunately, the concepts of "safe sex" and "just say no" (to sex and drugs) portend a blurring of the sex/death boundaries for women. Condom use is touted as a reasonable method for the prevention of HIV transmission during penetrative sex (Freidland and Klein 1987, 1130), and promoting the use of condoms is said to be a "potentially useful" intervention for preventing HIV infection (Quinn, Glasser, et al. 1988, 202). A great deal of the education concerning condom use has been directed at women, and women have been advised to carry their own condoms. Some authors report that women now constitute 70 percent of the con- dom-buying market (Patton 1988). Yet researchers discovered in one study that only 3 percent of men and 4 percent of women reported consistent use of condoms.

Unfortunately, many of the recommendations for AIDS education and condom use fail to take the experience of women into account. Male machismo is reported to lead some men to refuse condom use, preferring, in their words, "the greater thrill of unprotected sex" (Zucker, interview, 1988). While the lure and the excitement of the forbidden and the dangerous are familiar themes in literature and in philosophy, sexual intercourse during the AIDS epidemic can be seen to perpetuate the inequality of women's risk in heterosexual relationships.

In some cultural contexts, a woman's acquiescence to sex on demand is both expected and enforced. Hence, for many women, "just saying no" to sex (or to unprotected sex) has turned into a prescription for battering and other forms of abuse (Bacon 1987, 6). Among the women who are most affected by AIDS, the fact that they are still in situations of unequal power has meant that they now face additional obstacles in ensuring their own bodily safety.

Long aware that condom use was *not* recognized as an effective means of birth control, women are *now* being told that condom use will effectively prevent AIDS transmission. Yet the rate of the condom's failure to protect against pregnancy was measured in a monthly cycle during which most women were fertile only a few days. Women are justifiably concerned that condoms are not a reasonable protection against a disease that can be transmitted every day of the month. Furthermore, many brochures on "safe sex" concentrate on describing ways to make the condom more palatable to the male sexual experience than they do either on ways to ensure the safety of the woman receptor or on sexual practices that are non-penetrative. The many public health messages recommending condom use have conveyed the impression that the male sexual experience is the primary focus. Lisa Bacon notes as well that reliable safe sex information for lesbians is neither widely distributed nor widely known to be available (1987, 6).

The noticeable absence of research efforts to develop better barriers to transmission for women and to publicize alternative methods of expressing one's sexuality is troubling and remains an important issue in the ethics of AIDS.

Women and IV Drug Use

Because intravenous drug use is playing such an important role in the transmission of HIV infection in the United States, and because intravenous drug users represent the largest pool of HIV infected heterosexuals in the United States, dilemmas surrounding illicit drug use have a special significance for women.

Complicating matters further is the fact that 90 percent of IV drug users are heterosexuals, 30 percent of whom are women, and 90 percent of those women are still in their childbearing years. In addition, 30 to 50 percent of female IV drug users are also engaged in prostitution (Freidland and Klein 1987, 1127).

Because women have been forced to assume the responsibility for the control of sex and contraception, and because cultural pressures affecting women likely to acquire AIDS are such that they often have little power "to control the sexual expectations and preferences of their male partners" (Wofsy 1987, 33), many of the issues surrounding IV drug use are unusually difficult to address. Furthermore, as Freidland and Klein indicate, the nature of intravenous drug use is "woven into a pattern of inner-city poverty and minority racial and ethnic status" (1987, 1127) and is characterized by the same lack of community organization and advocacy that has defined the history of women.

A disturbing finding in one study was that one-third of HIV infected men and almost one-half of infected women denied knowledge of having engaged in any high-risk behavior. Among women under 25 years of age, 68 percent denied knowledge of exposure to any risk factor associated with HIV transmission. "Our data suggest that if HIV testing in our clinics were limited only to subjects who acknowledged or perceived high-risk behavior, then half the infected women, and one third of the infected men would not have been tested" (Quinn, Glasser, et al. 1988, 202). Yet counseling programs throughout the course of the epidemic have emphasized the importance of infected persons' informing all persons with whom they share needles or have sexual intercourse of their infectivity.

What is particularly alarming about such a finding is not just what it suggests about the necessity of expanded programs of AIDS education, but what it suggests about perceived cultural responsibilities among high-risk males to their female sexual partners. Voluntary partner notification is apparently not perceived as a strong moral obligation, particularly when it involves informing a woman.

Although there is some evidence that risk reduction measures are being taken seriously by drug users (Des Jarlais 1988, 4), the nature of IV drug use and the profile of the IV drug user are such, unfortunately, that sharing needles continues to be a common practice (Des Jarlais 1988, 3). "Many who use drugs do not perceive of themselves as users. Those who do not understand the health risks and the need to clean needles may continue to share because they erroneously consider their partner to be nonrisk. Sharing is socially expected; the urgency of the fix exceeds the risk" (Wofsy 1987, 33). Sharing also often occurs as part of initiation into drug use and is viewed as an important part of social interaction with other users (Des Jarlais 1988, 3).

Existing efforts at counseling and education have failed to protect women in other ways as well. Prostitution has become intimately interwoven with the drug culture, making prostitutes at risk of acquiring AIDS through both routes. Up to now, the prevalence of HIV infection in female prostitutes has paralleled the cumulative incidence of AIDS in women. Black and hispanic prostitutes, however, have a higher prevalence of HIV infection than do their white counterparts (Leads 1987, 2011). This corresponds to the prevalence of IV drug use among black and hispanic men.

While many in society express little compassion for the prostitute who acquires AIDS from her customer, few economic alternatives exist for women in prostitution, and even fewer exist for the drug-addicted prostitute. A dehumanizing aspect of prostitution is that it is essentially an involuntary form of labor that grows out of the economically disadvantaged position in which women find themselves. Prostitution is a manifestation of a lack of respect for persons, primarily because those who must prostitute themselves have not been accorded the freedom of choice that accompanies being treated fully as a person.[5] In addition, because prostitutes are at the bottom of the heap in all these other ways, they are among those persons who are often least able to organize to protect themselves. It compounds the moral insult to allow women prostitutes to fall prey to HIV infected "johns" and to believe that that is their due.

Surgeon General Koop and others have suggested that one way of reducing the risk of transmission to women via IV drug use is to begin a needle exchange program that would provide addicts legal access to sterile "works." In that way, HIV infected addicts could be helped to stop endangering themselves, their sexual partners, and their offspring.

Such a proposal is problematic, however, because it takes place in a society where drug use of that type is illicit and where drug use often accompanies other illicit behaviors such as prostitution. Offering clean needles to addicts is viewed by some as a tacit endorsement of illegal and self destructive behavior. Because of the cultural web in which addicts and their partners are caught, it is unclear how one should think about the establishment of such a program. At least one thing seems clear: just as it is unproductive and unjustified from a moral point of view to argue that prostitutes who acquire AIDS "get what they ask for," it is unjustified to claim that drug addicts and their sexual partners and offspring "get what they deserve" if they become HIV infected.

Needle exchange programs have been operating successfully in Holland and Australia, and New Jersey is the first state in the United States to begin such a program (Murphy 1988, 66). Successfully combatting AIDS in the contexts of prostitution and illicit drug use will require emotional and intellectual flexibility that most policy makers up to now have failed to exhibit.

BIRTH CONTROL AND REPRODUCTION

Women with AIDS pose further complex ethical issues that involve examining both their reproductive options and their obligations in exercising those options. One such issue grows out of the fact that researchers have found that trends in women with AIDS are good predictors of trends in pediatric AIDS cases, especially among mothers in identifiable risk groups (Guinan and Hardy 1987).

In approximately two-thirds (65%) of the pregnancies of women who are in-fected with the virus, infection is passed on to the infant, and close to 50 percent of those infants will have the disease within two years. The outlook for these children is almost certain death (Koop 1987, 4; Ledger 1987, 5; Piot, Plummer, et al. 1988). Furthermore, about two-thirds of pediatric AIDS cases are the result of transmission from infected mother to child[6] (Koop 1987, 4). More importantly, not only women with AIDS, but also women with ARC and women who are asymptomatic carriers of HIV infection have the potential to transmit the virus perinatally.

HIV infection can be passed from mother to infant in three ways: to the fetus in utero through fetal-maternal circulation, to the infant during labor and delivery, and to the infant through infected breast milk (Freidland and Klein 1987, 1130; Curran, Jaffe, et al. 1988, 614; Piot, Plummer, et al. 1988, 575).

Further complicating this issue is the fact that AIDS not only adversely affects the child born to an infected mother, it also seems to accelerate the progression of disease in the pregnant woman herself (Murphy 1988, 73). Sadly, for many women, especially those who are culturally and economically deprived, childbearing sometimes provides a sense of self-esteem and is sometimes culturally expected. Hence, many women who have borne an infected child continue to reproduce "despite intensive culturally specific counseling" (Wofsy 1987, 33). A second pregnancy in an HIV infected mother, however, is even more likely to move her into full blown AIDS at the same time that it produces an infected infant (Murphy 1988, 73). A tragic irony of these findings is that oral contraception is also a factor thought to increase a woman's susceptibility to sexually acquired HIV infection (Piot, Plummer, et al. 1988, 575).

In addition to the risk of infection by vaginal intercourse, women undergoing artificial insemination (AI) are in some danger of HIV infection. Although not a widely published fact, there are close to 10,000 AI births per year in the United States (Murphy 1988, 73). This form of transmission can easily be eliminated by instituting procedures for testing donor sperm; the ejaculate of first time donors can be frozen and the donor retested for antibody two to three months before the sperm is used (Ledger 1987, 5). Such testing would continue to ensure that AI remains a legitimate reproductive option for women while protecting them and their unborn fetuses from HIV infection.

As one might expect, the more difficult questions in this category of issues affecting women have to do with the rights of prospective mothers and fetal rights. Although Surgeon General Koop believes the number to be underestimated, the Public Health Service has predicted that, by 1991, 3000 children will be afflicted with AIDS (Koop 1987, 3). For that reason, several authors have suggested that prior to becoming pregnant, women who believe that they may have been exposed should be tested for antibody and, if found to be seropositive, should be counseled against becoming pregnant (Del Tempelis, Shell, et al. 1987, 475). Some authors have suggested that in order to forestall pregnancy in infected mothers, premarital or pre-pregnancy testing ought to be mandated. Antibody testing, done within the context of prenatal obstetrical visits, has also been recommended (Quaggin 1987, 192).

Premarital testing, it is argued, allows the potential couple the information they need about their serological status as they contemplate future pregnancies. It also allows the woman in the potential couple information about the man's serological status that could affect a decision to undertake a marital commitment at all (Ledger 1987, 6). Pre-pregnancy testing has been suggested for similar reasons; it would allow a woman information about her own seropositivity that could determine whether she would decide to begin a pregnancy.

These suggestions raise the questions that are the hardest to address.

Given the facts of transmission from infected mother to fetus, given the etiology of the disease, and given the hideousness of a death from AIDS, most persons would agree that there are strong moral reasons for avoiding pregnancy if one is HIV infected. While one might not quarrel with a woman's choosing to risk suffering and death for herself, the argument goes, choosing a 65% possibility of inflicting such harm on another seems morally impermissible.

The conflict generated by such an argument, even under ordinary circumstances, is complicated in the discussion of AIDS/HIV by the fact that most of the women infected at this point are women of color who have far fewer sources of gratification in life than other women. For these women, choices concerning their own reproduction are perhaps the only choices over which they can exercise any control. Attempts to dissuade these women from reproducing might be seen as a strategy for effecting a form of genocide.

One option, abortion, is itself a volatile issue that promises to "increase the difficulty of dealing with HIV infection in the population of pregnant women" (Osterholm and MacDonald 1987, 2737). Contrary to what many right-to-life advocates might argue, there are quite compelling moral grounds for advocating that an infected woman is justified in aborting a fetus she might be carrying: a prospective mother might be said to have an obligation to any potential child to spare it a certain and gruesome death, a prospective mother might be said to have an obligation to ensure and protect her own health for as long as she can (both for her own sake as well as for the sake of others, including the unborn fetus), and a prospective mother might be said to have an obligation to society not to bear children for whom society may have to provide.

The flip side of that argument, however, might suggest that, in the black context, for example, a prospective mother could be said to have a responsibility *to bear* her child, even with only a 35% survival possibility, in order to maintain the integrity of the black community.

However, while I acknowledge the necessity of understanding the political and cultural implications of testing and of counseling HIV infected women against reproducing, I believe it is equally important to the racial integrity of communities of color that transmission to their offspring be avoided where that is possible.

A real worry underlying both of these arguments is mandatory testing. For many women, mandatory testing carries with it the specter of forced celibacy, prohibitions against procreation (accompanied by the potential of sanctions against violators), and even the threat of forced abortion.

Apart from evidence that suggests that mandatory testing would have the effect of driving underground those most in need of testing and counseling, it is unclear both what gains could be expected from forced testing in this context and whether such testing even has the potential of reaching those it purports to reach. Many of the women in populations identified as "at risk" either don't marry those who have fathered their offspring or can't afford prenatal care. There is the additional question of determining how such options might be enforced or punished. By imprisonment? By steep fines? By terminating parental rights? By the time an accurate diagnosis were made and the appropriate causal link established, those found to be violators (and victims) would likely be dead or dying. Further, given the current state of the art with respect to testing, the test results themselves may give women a false sense of security about their serological status. Under such circumstances, if testing were mandated, the end hoped for still might not be realized.

In short, that there are strong moral reasons for preventing further spread of

AIDS to newborns and for preventing pregnancy in infected women does not imply that policy be *mandated* for accomplishing that end. Some authors even express concern over the domino effect such mandated policies would have on the logic for testing other groups (Patton 1988).

There is yet another argument that needs to be examined, one that will be more familiar to those who have a long-standing interest in issues affecting women: a woman must be allowed to weigh for herself the risks inherent in continuing a pregnancy if she is found to be seropositive—only she can evaluate the moral validity of her options.

Preserving women's rights to exercise reproductive choice is said to be important for the reason that the HIV status of the fetus of an infected mother, as well as of asymptomatic mothers who have infected partners, is still highly uncertain and often cannot be determined until some time after birth. Hence, this argument goes, while a woman might elect to terminate a pregnancy if she or her partner is discovered to be HIV infected, she might also justifiably choose to continue the pregnancy. If the prospective mother were carrying the child of a beloved and dying spouse, she might legitimately reason that the risk to the unborn is one that is justified in order to have a part of her spouse live on, or in order to give her own life more meaning, or for sociological and cultural reasons noted above (Murphy 1988, 75).

While I do not believe that mandatory testing is either morally appropriate or enforceable, I do believe that it is morally irresponsible to argue in this case for preserving women's rights to exercise reproductive choice. It seems important to come down hard on someone who would choose a 65% risk of spreading AIDS.[7] Sentimentalism and sexism aside, it seems unconscionable for a person knowingly to risk transmitting a lethal disease to another. Imagine our anger if an HIV infected man or woman were to engage intentionally in unprotected sexual relations with an uninfected partner. It seems uncontroversial to claim that we would feel moral outrage at such an act. It seems equally uncontroversial to claim that we would find it morally objectionable for an infected person knowingly to donate blood. The risk of infecting others with a lethal disease is simply too great. It seems even more objectionable when one doesn't consent to exposing oneself to the risk. For that reason, in the case of a prospective mother who risks transmitting HIV to her fetus, electing to continue the pregnancy seems an even greater abuse of one's moral and sexual responsibility.

Some states have already acknowledged the moral force of claims such as the above by enacting legislation that would make it a criminal act for an individual to engage in intercourse with another without informing that partner of his/her seropositivity[8] (Dickens 1988, 583). Of course, apart from the fact that I'm unsure how to evaluate the enforceability of such laws, it is unrealistic to believe that their payoff will be found in dramatic behavior change. Given the social and cultural context in which most of these women find themselves, it is even less clear what would effect behavior change in seropositive women who continue to conceive. Even so, such laws represent important expressions of a public attitude that such behaviors are wrong and that personal accountability is part of an accepted public morality. Such laws will help shape the moral climate of AIDS.[9]

POLICY IN THE FUTURE

One of the great tragedies of the epidemic is that AIDS is affecting populations that have historically been disadvantaged. Sadly, what seems to emerge from the foregoing discussion is the fact that we really have fewer options for averting these disastrous consequences than we would like to admit.

Many persons sensitive to the politics of AIDS have argued that AIDS must be approached like any other public health issue. Had AIDS first been recognized in American society in the heterosexual community, they argue, our response to this disease would have resembled more closely our response to other communicable diseases. We would have tested, developed counseling and education programs, responded quickly with new monies for research, and so on. Now, they advise, we need all of those things. Most importantly, we need greatly expanded programs of education and counseling, programs that will reach hitherto ignored populations.

Most people argue that education about AIDS must be even more broadly conceived. It must take the shape of preventive education carried into all corners of our communities. Furthermore, if such programs are to be effective, they must take into account the cultural, economic, and social realities of the communities that are at risk. They must talk plainly and openly about sex, about prostitution, and about drug use, and they must involve community-based groups of the very people they are designed to reach (Bacon 1987, 6).

Because it is difficult to identify and target a large proportion of those women who are at serious risk of acquiring HIV through heterosexual intercourse, "it is important to educate all women about their risk of sexually acquired AIDS and to encourage risk-reducing sexual behavior" (Guinan and Hardy 1987, 2042). As some point out, these programs can teach safe *and fulfilling* sex practices.

In addition, because data indicate that a large number of infected persons are unaware of or do not acknowledge their risk for infection, and because "clinic patients who are seronegative for HIV may actually represent a group at increasing risk for acquisition of HIV infection" (Quinn, Glasser, et al. 1988, 202), it is recommended that screening for HIV and counseling and education programs should be in place and *offered to all patients* who attend STD clinics.

As Murphy argues, we are just now beginning to confront the issues generated by women with AIDS. By 1991, the number of documented AIDS cases in women will nearly equal the number of men presently diagnosed with disease (Murphy 1988, 76). Policymakers will have to look more closely at the solutions as they affect women.

Protecting women from AIDS means understanding the following: Women with AIDS lack the natural "community" that lent essential support to many gay men during the early stages of the epidemic. Many women learn their diagnosis second-hand, i.e., at the death of a spouse or at the birth of an infected baby. For women the paucity of available medical care and counseling services is especially burden-some because they carry the double burden often of their own and their offspring's illness. Policies providing for child care, housing, and other special services are issues crucial to helping women with AIDS. Infected women, perhaps even more than men, experience extreme isolation from family and friends, and particularly from other infected women. Often they must watch alone as a child dies, feeling guilt for a child's disease at the same time that they are struggling with their own pain and suffering and disease. They experience a grief that is even more profound when it involves losing their own health and the health of a loved one. Women continue to struggle with the societal assumption that they shoulder the responsibility for sex, conception, and contraception; they carry the burden as well of deciding whether to initiate, continue, or terminate a pregnancy. Both formally and informally, women still constitute the bulk of the country's caregivers and teachers (Wofsy 1987, 34).

For a variety of reasons, women will play a central role in the future of AIDS. Future public health policy needs to take that role seriously. We may have to elect to implement some programs with the knowledge that their gains against AIDS will be admittedly modest: needle exchange programs, mandatory premarital and prenatal testing, abortion counseling, child care and mother-assistance programs, counseling to teach coping skills and "saying no" skills, job counseling and retraining for prostitutes, unemployment assistance for seropositive mothers, among others. For the time, even though some of these programs may be thought to be undesirable, they may be the best we can do under the circumstances.

Meanwhile, there are important public policy reasons for pursuing even more vigorously those programs for social and economic change that impact HIV transmission. It is important to attempt to reshape attitudes about morality and sexual responsibility where they concern AIDS transmission. It is important to advocate that there are certain things that morally and sexually responsible persons just don't do. It is important to demand accountability on the part of persons who refuse personal responsibility in halting AIDS transmission. Finally, it is important to pursue a variety of programs that teach both safe sex and safer sex practices.

NOTES

An earlier, much shorter statistical version of this paper appears in *AIDS Education and Prevention*. In this paper I have chosen to address the more philosophical issues surrounding AIDS/HIV in women.

1. After all, *any person* who engages in behaviors identified as high-risk for HIV transmission has the potential to spread infection.

2. These figures assume that of the 365,000 to 450,000 cases that Dr. Curran estimates for 1992, approximately 8 percent will continue to be women with AIDS. This figure represents the percentage of women with AIDS reported in the August 29, 1988 *AIDS Weekly Surveillance Report*.

3. It is important to understand here that I do not lay the blame for this at the feet of the gay community. On the contrary, the gay community historically has been supportive of efforts to secure a higher moral and political status for women.

4. I have argued elsewhere that AIDS does not fit the traditional communicable disease model. Hence, I am aware that partner notification and contact tracing have little in the

way of treatment (and nothing in the way of a cure) to offer to those traced and notified. What contact tracing does offer is the information that one may have been exposed to the virus, and that, I would argue, is information essential for both men and women to have.

5. I am aware that there are a number of feminist analyses of prostitution that discuss how racism keeps black and Latino women on the streets and lets white women work less conspicuously indoors, and a number of discussions of prostitution as a legitimate form of employment. Although there are important similarities between anti-prostitute sentiment and homophobic sentiment, I don't have the space in this paper, unfortunately, to do more than note that fact.

6. Other pediatric cases result from sexual abuse, drug abuse, adolescent intercourse, and hemophilia.

7. I am extremely grateful to my colleague Ferdinand Schoeman for discussing the difficulties inherent in taking any position other than this. His suggestions throughout this section were most useful and illuminating.

8. Although Dickens notes that Florida and Idaho have introduced such legislation, I am personally aware that South Carolina has enacted such legislation. Dickens also notes that most jurisdictions have chosen to rely on existing criminal statutes to proscribe some behaviors of the HIV infected person.

9. There are seropositive people who knowingly have unprotected sex, however, just as there are cases of persons who know they have serious risk factors for HIV infection and who aren't seeking to learn their HIV status, yet continue to share sexual and drug using behaviors. I consider this to be morally irresponsible behavior.

REFERENCES

Ammann, A. J. 1987. Pediatric acquired immunodeficiency syndrome. *Information on AIDS for the Practicing Physician* 1: 17–23.

Bacon, Lisa. 1987. Lessons of AIDS: Racism, homophobia are the real epidemic. *Listen Real Loud* 8(2): 5–6.

Centers for Disease Control. 1988. August 29. *AIDS weekly surveillance report.*

Curran, J., Jaffe, H., Hardy, A., Morgan, W., Selik, R., & Dondero, T. 1988. Epidemiology of HIV infection and AIDS in the United States. *Science* 239: 610–616.

Coolfont report: A public health service plan for prevention and control of AIDS and the AIDS virus. 1986. *Public Health Report* 101: 465.

Del Tempelis, C., Shell, G., Hoffman, M., Benjamin, R., Chandler, A., & Francis, D. 1987. Human immunodeficiency virus infection in women in the San Francisco Bay area (letter). *Journal of the American Medical Association* 258(4): 474–475.

Des Jarlais, D. and Hunt, D. 1988. AIDS and IV drug use. *AIDS Bulletin* Feb. 1988: 3.

Dickens, B. M. 1988. Legal rights and duties in the AIDS epidemic. *Science* 239: 580–585.

Fleming, D., Cochi, S., Steece, R., & Hull, H. 1987. Acquired immunodeficiency syndrome in low-incidence areas: How safe is unsafe sex? *Journal of the American Medical Association* 258(6): 785–787.

Freidland, G. H., and Klein, R. S. 1987. Transmission of human immunodeficiency virus. *New England Journal of Medicine* 317(18): 1125–1135.

Growing AIDS risk reported. 1988. June 14. *The State* 2.

Guinan, M. E., and Hardy, A. 1987. Epidemiology of AIDS in women in the United States: 1981–1986. *Journal of the American Medical Association* 257(15): 2039–2042.

Kaplan, H. S. 1987. *The real truth about women and AIDS.* New York: Simon & Schuster.

Kaplan, H. S. 1988. No sex this year. *New Woman* January: 81–82.

Koop, C. E. 1987. *Report of the surgeon general's workshop on children with HIV infection and their families.* (Excerpts from keynote address.) Public Health Service: US Dept. of Health and Human Services. HRS-D-MC 87-1.

Leads from the *Morbidity and Mortality Weekly Report*: Antibody to human immunodeficiency virus in female prostitutes. 1987. *Journal of the American Medical Association* 257(15): 2011–2013.

Leads from the *Morbidity and Mortality Weekly Report*: Human immunodeficiency virus infection in the United States. 1988. *Journal of the American Medical Association* 259(6): 785–787.

Ledger, W. A. 1987. AIDS and the obstetrician/gynecologist: Commentary. *Information on AIDS for the Practicing Physician* 2: 5–6.

Minkoff, H. L. 1987. Care of pregnant women infected with human immunodeficiency virus. *Journal of the American Medical Association* 258(19): 2714–2717.

Morgan, W. M., and Curran, J. W. 1986. Acquired immunodeficiency syndrome: Current and future trends. *Public Health Report* 101: 459–465.

Murphy, J. S. 1988. Women with AIDS: Sexual ethics in an epidemic. In *AIDS: Principles, practices, and politics.* I. Corless and M. Pittman-Lindemann, eds. Washington: Hemisphere.

Osterholm, M., and MacDonald, K. L. 1987. Facing the complex issues of pediatric AIDS: A public health perspective. *Journal of the American Medical Association* 258(19): 2736–2737.

Patton, C. 1988. Resistance and the erotic: Reclaiming history, setting strategy as we face AIDS. *Radical Teacher* 68–78.

Piot, P., Plummer, F., Mhalu, F., Lamboray, J., Chin, J., & Mann, J. 1988. AIDS: An international perspective. *Science* 239: 573–579.

Quaggin, A. 1987. Get prepared for more cases of AIDS during pregnancy. *Canadian Medical Association Journal* 136(2): 192–193.

Quinn, T., Glasser, D., Cannon, R., Matuszak, D., Dunning, R., Kline, R., Campbell, C., Israel, E., Fauci, A., & Hook, E. 1988. Human immunodeficiency virus infection among patients attending clinics for sexually transmitted diseases. *New England Journal of Medicine* 318(4): 197–203.

Rossellini, L. 1988. May 30. Rebel with a cause: Koop. *US News & World Report* 104(21): 55–63.

Shilts, R. 1987. *And the band played on.* New York: St. Martin's Press.

Simpson, M. 1988. The malignant metaphor: A political thanatology of AIDS. In *AIDS: Principles, practices, and politics.* I. Corless and M. Pittman-Lindemann, eds. Washington: Hemisphere.

Update: Acquired immunodeficiency syndrome–United States. 1987. *Morbidity and Mortality Weekly Report* 36: 522–526.

Wofsy, C. 1987. Intravenous drug abuse and women's medical issues. *Report of the surgeon general's workshop on children with HIV infection and their families.* Public Health Service: US Dept. of Health and Human Services. HRS-D-MC 87-1.

Woods, D. 1987. Poor media coverage hurting AIDS fight, conference told. *Canadian Medical Association Journal* 136: 193.

Zucker, L. 1988. Interview. University of South Carolina. Columbia, SC.

Toward a
Feminist Theory of Disability

SUSAN WENDELL ❖ ❖ ❖

We need a feminist theory of disability, both because 16 percent of women are disabled, and because the oppression of disabled people is closely linked to the cultural oppression of the body. Disability is not a biological given; like gender, it is socially constructed from biological reality. Our culture idealizes the body and demands that we control it. Thus, although most people will be disabled at some time in their lives, the disabled are made "the other," who symbolize failure of control and the threat of pain, limitation, dependency, and death. If disabled people and their knowledge were fully integrated into society, everyone's relation to her/his real body would be liberated.

In 1985, I fell ill overnight with what turned out to be a disabling chronic disease. In the long struggle to come to terms with it, I had to learn to live with a body that felt entirely different to me—weak, tired, painful, nauseated, dizzy, unpredictable. I learned at first by listening to other people with chronic illnesses or disabilities; suddenly able-bodied people seemed to me profoundly ignorant of everything I most needed to know. Although doctors told me there was a good chance I would eventually recover completely, I realized after a year that waiting to get well, hoping to recover my healthy body, was a dangerous strategy. I began slowly to identify with my new, disabled body and to learn to work with it. As I moved back into the world, I also began to experience the world as structured for people who have no weaknesses.[1] The process of encountering the able-bodied world led me gradually to identify myself as a disabled person, and to reflect on the nature of disability.

Some time ago, I decided to delve into what I assumed would be a substantial philosophical literature in medical ethics on the nature and experience of disability. I consulted *The Philosopher's Index*, looking under "Disability," "Handicap," "Illness," and "Disease." This was a depressing experience. At least 90% of philosophical articles on these topics are concerned with two questions: Under what conditions is it morally permissible/right to kill/let die a disabled person and how potentially disabled does a fetus have to be before it is permissible/right to prevent its being born? Thus, what I have to say here about disability is not a response to

Hypatia vol.4, no. 2 (Summer 1989) © by Susan Wendell

philosophical literature on the subject. Instead, it reflects what I have learned from the writings of other disabled people (especially disabled women), from talking with disabled people who have shared their insights and experiences with me, and from my own experience of disability. It also reflects my commitment to feminist theory, which offers perspectives and categories of analysis that help to illuminate the personal and social realities of disability, and which would, in turn, be enriched by a greater understanding of disability.

We need a theory of disability. It should be a social and political theory, because disability is largely socially-constructed, but it has to be more than that; any deep understanding of disability must include thinking about the ethical, psychological and epistemic issues of living with disability. This theory should be feminist, because more than half of disabled people are women and approximately 16% of women are disabled (Fine and Asch 1988), and because feminist thinkers have raised the most radical issues about cultural attitudes to the body. Some of the same attitudes about the body which contribute to women's oppression generally also contribute to the social and psychological disablement of people who have physical disabilities. In addition, feminists are grappling with issues that disabled people also face in a different context: Whether to stress sameness or difference in relation to the dominant group and in relation to each other; whether to place great value on independence from the help of other people, as the dominant culture does, or to question a value-system which distrusts and de-values dependence on other people and vulnerability in general; whether to take full integration into male dominated/able-bodied society as the goal, seeking equal power with men/able-bodied people in that society, or whether to preserve some degree of separate culture, in which the abilities, knowledge and values of women/the disabled are specifically honoured and developed.[2]

Disabled women struggle with both the oppressions of being women in male-dominated societies and the oppressions of being disabled in societies dominated by the able-bodied. They are bringing the knowledge and concerns of women with disabilities into feminism and feminist perspectives into the disability rights movement. To build a feminist theory of disability that takes adequate account of our differences, we will need to know how experiences of disability and the social oppression of the disabled interact with sexism, racism and class oppression. Michelle Fine and Adrienne Asch and the contributors to their 1988 volume, *Women and Disabilities*, have made a major contribution to our understanding of the complex interactions of gender and disability. Barbara Hillyer Davis has written in depth about the issue of dependency/independence as it relates to disability and feminism (Davis 1984). Other important contributions to theory are scattered throughout the extensive, primarily experiential, writing by disabled women;[3] this work offers vital insights into the nature of embodiment and the experience of oppression.

Unfortunately, feminist perspectives on disability are not yet widely discussed in feminist theory, nor have the insights offered by women writing about disability been integrated into feminist theorizing about the body. My purpose in writing this essay is to persuade feminist theorists, especially feminist philosophers, to turn more attention to constructing a theory of disability and to integrating the experiences and knowledge of disabled people into feminist theory as a whole. Toward this end I will discuss physical disability[4] from a theoretical perspective, including: some problems of defining it (here I will criticize the most widely-used definitions—those of the United Nations); the social construction of disability from biological reality on analogy with the social construction of gender; cultural attitudes toward the body which oppress disabled people while also alienating the able-bodied from their own experiences of embodiment; the "otherness" of disabled people; the knowledge that disabled people could contribute to culture from our diverse experiences and some of the ways this knowledge is silenced and invalidated. Along the way, I will describe briefly three issues discussed in disability theory that have been taken up in different contexts by feminist theory: sameness vs. difference, independence vs. dependency, and integration vs. separatism.

I do not presume to speak for disabled women. Like everyone who is disabled, I have a particular standpoint determined in part by both my physical condition and my social situation. My own disability may be temporary; it could get better or worse. My disability is usually invisible (except when I use a walking stick). I am a white university professor who has adequate medical and long-term disability insurance; that makes me very privileged among the disabled. I write what I can see from my standpoint. Because I do not want simply to describe my own experience but to understand it in a much larger context, I must venture beyond what I know first-hand. I rely on others to correct my mistakes and fill in those parts of the picture I cannot see.

WHO IS PHYSICALLY DISABLED?

The United Nations offers the following definitions of and distinctions among impairment, disability and handicap:

> "*Impairment*: Any loss or abnormality of psychological, physiological, or anatomical structure or function. *Disability*: Any restriction or lack (resulting from an impairment) of ability to perform an activity in the manner or within the range considered normal for a human being. *Handicap*: A disadvantage for a given individual, resulting from an impairment or disability, that limits or prevents the fulfillment of a role that is normal, depending on age, sex, social and cultural factors, for that individual."
>
> Handicap is therefore a function of the relationship between disabled persons and their environment. It occurs when they encounter cultural, physical or social barriers which prevent their access to the various systems of society that are available to other citizens. Thus, handicap is the loss or limitation of opportunities to take part in the life of the community on an equal level with others. (U.N. 1983:I.c. 6–7)

These definitions may be good enough for the political purposes of the U.N. They have two advantages: First, they clearly include many conditions that are not always recognized by the general public as disabling, for example, debilitating chronic illnesses that limit people's activities but do not necessarily cause any visible disability, such as Crohn's disease. Second, the definition of "handicap" explicitly recognizes the possibility that the primary cause of a disabled person's inability to do certain things may be social—denial of opportunities, lack of accessibility, lack of services, poverty, discrimination—which it often is.

However, by trying to define "impairment" and "disability" in physical terms and "handicap" in cultural, physical and social terms, the U.N. document appears to be making a shaky distinction between the physical and the social aspects of disability. Not only the "normal" roles for one's age, sex, society, and culture, but also "normal" structure and function, and "normal" ability to perform an activity, depend on the society in which the standards of normality are generated. Paradigms of health and ideas about appropriate kinds and levels of performance are culturally dependent. In addition, within each society there is much variation from the norm of any ability; at what point does this variation become disability? The answer depends on such factors as what activities a society values and how it distributes labour and resources. The idea that there is some universal, perhaps biologically or medically describable paradigm of human physical ability is an illusion. Therefore, I prefer to use a single term, "disability," and to emphasize that disability is socially constructed from biological reality.

Another objection I have to the U.N. definitions is that they imply that women can be disabled, but not handicapped, by being unable to do things which are not considered part of the normal role for their sex. For example, if a society does not consider it essential to a woman's normal role that she be able to read, then a blind woman who is not provided with education in Braille is not handicapped, according to these definitions.

In addition, these definitions suggest that we can be disabled, but not handicapped, by the normal process of aging, since although we may lose some ability, we are not handicapped unless we cannot fulfill roles that are normal *for our age*. Yet a society which provides few resources to allow disabled people to participate in it will be likely to marginalize *all* the disabled, including the old, and to define the appropriate roles of old people as very limited, thus handicapping them. Aging is disabling. Recognizing this helps us to see that disabled people are not "other," that they are really "us." Unless we die suddenly, we are all disabled eventually. Most of us will live part of our lives with bodies that hurt, that move with difficulty or not at all, that deprive us of activities we once took for granted or that others take for granted, bodies that make daily life a physical struggle. We need an understanding of disability that does not support a paradigm of humanity as young and healthy. Encouraging everyone to acknowledge, accommodate and identify with a wide range of physical conditions is the road to self-acceptance as well as the road to liberating those who are disabled now.

Ultimately, we might eliminate the category of "the disabled" altogether, and simply talk about individuals' physical abilities in their social context. For the present, although "the disabled" is a category of "the other" to the able-bodied, for that very reason it is also a politically useful and socially meaningful category to those who are in it. Disabled people share forms of social oppression, and the most important measures to relieve that oppression have been initiated by disabled people themselves. Social oppression may be the only thing the disabled have in common;[5] our struggles with our bodies are extremely diverse.

Finally, in thinking about disability we have to keep in mind that a society's labels do not always fit the people to whom they are applied. Thus, some people are perceived as disabled who do not experience themselves as disabled. Although they have physical conditions that disable other people, because of their opportunities and the context of their lives, they do not feel significantly limited in their activities (see Sacks 1988); these people may be surprised or resentful that they are considered disabled. On the other hand, many people whose bodies cause them great physical, psychological and economic struggles are not considered disabled because the public and/or the medical profession do not recognize their disabling conditions. These people often long to be perceived as disabled, because society stubbornly continues to expect them to perform as healthy people when they cannot and refuses to acknowledge and support their struggles.[6] Of course, no one wants the social stigma associated with disability, but social recognition of disability determines the practical help a person receives from doctors, government agencies, insurance companies, charity organizations, and often from family and friends. Thus, how a society defines disability and whom it recognizes as disabled are of enormous psychological, economic and social importance, both to people who are experiencing themselves as disabled and to those who are not but are nevertheless given the label.

There is no definitive answer to the question: Who is physically disabled? Disability has social, experiential and biological components, present and recognized in different measures for different people. Whether a particular physical condition is disabling changes with time and place, depending on such factors as social expectations, the state of technology and its availability to people in that condition, the educational system, architecture, attitudes towards physical appearance, and the pace of life. (If, for example, the pace of life increases without changes in other factors, more people become disabled simply because fewer people can keep up the "normal" pace.)

THE SOCIAL CONSTRUCTION OF DISABILITY

If we ask the questions: Why are so many disabled people unemployed or underemployed, impoverished, lonely, isolated; why do so many find it difficult or impossible to get an education (Davis and Marshall 1987; Fine and Asch 1988, 10–11); why are they victims of violence and coercion; why do able-bodied people ridicule, avoid, pity, stereotype and patronize them?, we may be tempted to see the disabled as victims of nature or accident. Feminists should be, and many are, profoundly suspicious of this answer. We are used to countering claims that insofar as women are oppressed they are oppressed by nature, which puts them at a disadvantage in the competition for power and resources. We know that if being biologically female is a disadvantage, it is because a social context makes it a disadvantage. From the standpoint of a disabled person, one can see how society could minimize the disadvantages of most disabilities, and, in some instances, turn them into advantages.

Consider an extreme case: the situation of physicist Stephen Hawking, who has had Amyotrophic Lateral Sclerosis (Lou Gehrig's disease) for more than twenty-seven years. Professor Hawking can no longer speak and is capable of only the smallest muscle movements. Yet, in his context of social and technological support, he is able to function as a professor of physics at Cambridge University; indeed he says his disability has given him the *advantage* of having more time to think, and he is one of the foremost theoretical physicists of our time. He is a courageous and talented man, but he is able to live the creative life he has only because of the help of his family, three nurses, a graduate student who travels with him to maintain his computer-communications systems, and the fact that his talent had been developed and recognized before he fell seriously ill (*Newsweek* 1988).

Many people consider providing resources for disabled people a form of charity, supererogatory in part because the disabled are perceived as unproductive members of society. Yet most disabled people are placed in a double-bind: they have access to inadequate resources because they are unemployed or underemployed, and they are unemployed or underemployed because they lack the resources that would enable them to make their full contribution to society (Matthews 1983; Hannaford 1985). Often governments and charity organizations will spend far more money to keep disabled people in institutions where they have no chance to be productive than they will spend to enable the same people to live independently and productively. In addition, many of the "special" resources the disabled need merely compensate for bad social planning that is based on the illusion that everyone is young, strong, healthy (and, often, male).

Disability is also frequently regarded as a personal or family problem rather than a matter for social responsibility. Disabled people are often expected to overcome obstacles to participation by their own extraordinary efforts, or their families are expected to provide what they need (sometimes at great personal sacrifice). Helping in personal or family matters is seen as superogatory for people who are not members of the family.

Many factors contribute to determining whether providing a particular resource is regarded as a social or a personal (or family) responsibility.[7] One such factor is whether the majority can identify with people who need the resource. Most North Americans feel that society should be organized to provide short-term medical care made necessary by illness or accident, I think because they can imagine themselves needing it. Relatively few people can identify with those who cannot be "repaired" by medical intervention. Sue Halpern makes the following observation:

> Physical health is contingent and often short-lived. But this truth eludes us as long as we are able to walk by simply putting one foot in front of the other. As a consequence, empathy for the disabled is unavailable to most able-bodied persons. Sympathy, yes, empathy, no, for every attempt to project oneself into that condition, to feel what it is like not to be ambulatory, for instance, is mediated by an ability to walk (Halpern 1988, 3).

If the able-bodied saw the disabled as potentially themselves or as their future selves, they would be more inclined to feel that society should be organized to provide the resources that would make disabled people fully integrated and contributing members. They would feel that "charity" is as inappropriate a way of thinking about resources for disabled people as it is about emergency medical care or education.

Careful study of the lives of disabled people will reveal how artificial the line is that we draw between the biological and the social. Feminists have already challenged this line in part by showing how processes such as childbirth, menstruation and menopause, which may be represented, treated, and therefore experienced as illnesses or disabilities, are socially constructed from biological reality (Rich 1976; Ehrenreich and English 1979). Disabled people's relations to our bodies involve elements of struggle which perhaps cannot be eliminated, perhaps not even mitigated, by social arrangements. *But,* much of what is *disabling* about our physical conditions is also a consequence of social arrangements (Finger 1983; Browne, Connors, and Stern 1985; Fine and Asch 1988) which could, but do not, either compensate for our physical conditions, or accommodate them so that we can participate fully, or support our struggles and integrate us into the community *and our struggles into the cultural concept of life as it is ordinarily lived.*

Feminists have shown that the world has been designed for men. In North America at least, life and work have been structured as though no one of any importance in the public world, and certainly no one who works outside the home for wages, has to breast-feed a baby or look after a sick child. Common colds can be acknowledged publicly, and allowances made for them, but menstruation cannot. Much of the world is also structured as though everyone is physically strong, as though all bodies are "ideally shaped," as though everyone can walk, hear and see well, as though everyone can work and play at a pace that is not compatible with any kind of illness or pain, as though no one is ever dizzy or incontinent or simply needs to sit or lie down. (For instance, where could you sit down in a supermarket if you needed to?) Not only the architecture, but the entire physical and social organization of life, assumes that we are either strong and healthy and able to do what the average able-bodied person can do, or that we are completely disabled, unable to participate in life.

In the split between the public and the private worlds, women (and children) have been relegated to the private, and so have the disabled, the sick and the old (and mostly women take care of them). The public world is the world of strength, the positive (valued) body, performance and production, the able-bodied and youth. Weakness, illness, rest and recovery, pain, death and the negative (de-valued) body are private, generally hidden, and often neglected. Coming into the public world with illness, pain or a de-valued body, we encounter resistance to mixing the two worlds; the split is vividly revealed. Much of our experience goes underground, because there is no socially acceptable way of expressing it and having our physical and psychological experience acknowledged and shared. A few close friends may share it, but there is a strong impulse to protect them from it too, because it seems so private, so unacceptable. I found that, after a couple of years of illness, even answering the question, "How are you?" became a difficult, conflict-ridden business. I don't want to alienate my friends from my experience, but I don't want to risk their discomfort and rejection by telling them what they don't want to know.[8]

Disabled people learn that many, perhaps most, able-bodied people do not want to know about suffering caused by the body. Visibly disabled women report that curiosity about medical diagnoses, physical appearance and the sexual and other intimate aspects of disability is more common than willingness to listen and trying to understand the experience of disability (Matthews 1983). It is not unusual for people with invisible disabilities to keep them entirely secret from everyone but their closest friends.

Contrary to what Sue Halpern says, it is not simply because they are in able bodies that the able-bodied fail to identify with the disabled. Able-bodied people can often make the imaginative leap into the skins of people physically unlike themselves; women can identify with a male protagonist in a story, for example, and adults can identify with children or with people much older than themselves. Something more powerful than being in a different body is at work. Suffering caused by the body, and the inability to control the body, are despised, pitied, and above all, feared. This fear, experienced individually, is also deeply embedded in our culture.

THE OPPRESSION OF DISABLED PEOPLE IS THE OPPRESSION OF EVERYONE'S REAL BODY.

Our real human bodies are exceedingly diverse—in size, shape, colour, texture, structure, function, range and habits of movement, and development—and they are constantly changing. Yet we do not absorb or reflect this simple fact in our culture. Instead, we idealize the human body. Our physical ideals change from time to time, but we always have ideals. These ideals are not just about appearance; they are also ideals of strength and energy and proper control of the body. We are perpetually bombarded with images of these ideals, demands for them, and offers of consumer products and services to help us achieve them.[9] Idealizing the body prevents everyone, able-bodied and disabled, from identifying with and loving her/his real body. Some people can have the illusion of acceptance that comes from believing that their bodies are "close enough" to the ideal, but this illusion only draws them deeper into identifying with the ideal and into the endless task of reconciling the reality with it. Sooner or later they must fail.

Before I became disabled, I was one of those people who felt "close enough" to cultural ideals to be reasonably accepting of my body. Like most feminists I know, I was aware of some alienation from it, and I worked at liking my body better. Nevertheless, I knew in my heart that too much of my liking still depended on being "close enough." When I was disabled by illness, I experienced a much more profound alienation from my body. After a year spent mostly in bed, I could barely identify my body as my own. I felt that "it" was torturing "me," trapping me in exhaustion, pain and inability to do many of the simplest things I did when I was healthy. The shock of this experience and the effort to identify with a new, disabled body, made me realize I had been living a luxury of the able-bodied. The able-bodied can postpone the task of identifying with their *real* bodies. The disabled don't have the luxury of demanding that their bodies fit the physical ideals of their culture. As Barbara Hillyer Davis says: "For all of us the difficult work of finding (one's) self includes the body, but people who live with disability in a society that glorifies fitness and physical conformity are forced to understand more fully what bodily integrity means" (Davis 1984, 3).

In a society which idealizes the body, the physically disabled are marginalized. People learn to identify with their own strengths (by cultural standards) and to hate, fear and neglect their own weaknesses. The disabled are not only de-valued for their de-valued bodies (Hannaford 1985), they are constant reminders to the able-bodied of the negative body—of what the able-bodied are trying to avoid, forget and ignore (Lessing 1981). For example, if someone tells me she is in pain, she reminds me of the existence of pain, the imperfection and fragility of the body, the possibility of my own pain, the *inevitability* of it. The less willing I am to accept all these, the less I want to know about her pain; if I cannot avoid it in her presence, I will avoid her. I may even blame her for it. I may tell myself that she *could have* avoided it, in order to go on believing that I *can* avoid it. I want to believe I am not like her; I cling to the differences. Gradually, I make her "other" because I don't want to confront my real body, which I fear and cannot accept.[10]

Disabled people can participate in marginalizing ourselves. We can wish for bodies we do not have, with frustration, shame, self-hatred. We can feel trapped in the negative body; it is our internalized oppression to feel this. Every (visibly or invisibly) disabled person I have talked to or read has felt this; some never stop feeling it. In addition, disabled women suffer more than disabled men from the demand that people have "ideal" bodies, because in patriarchal culture people judge women more by their bodies than they do men. Disabled women often do not feel seen (because they are often not seen) by others as whole people, especially not as sexual people (Campling 1981; Matthews 1983; Hannaford 1985; Fine and Asch 1988). Thus, part of their struggle against oppression is a much harder version of the struggle able-bodied women have for a realistic *and positive* self-image (Bogle and Shaul 1981; Browne, Connors, and Stern 1985). On the other hand, disabled people who cannot hope to meet the physical ideals of a culture can help reveal that those ideals are not "natural" or "normal" but artificial social creations that oppress everyone.

Feminist theorists have probed the causes of our patriarchal culture's desire for control of the body—fear of death, fear of the strong impulses and feelings the body gives us, fear of nature, fear and resentment of the mother's power over the infant (de Beauvoir 1949; Dinnerstein 1976; Griffin 1981). Idealizing the body and wanting to control it go hand-in-hand; it is impossible to say whether one causes the other. A physical ideal gives us the goal of our efforts to control the body, and the myth that total control is possible deceives us into striving for the ideal. The consequences for women have been widely discussed in the literature of feminism. The consequences for disabled people are less often recognized. In a culture which loves the idea that the body can be controlled, those who cannot control their bodies are seen (and may see themselves) as failures.

When you listen to this culture in a disabled body, you hear how often health and physical vigour are talked about as if they were moral virtues. People constantly praise others for their "energy," their stamina, their ability to work long hours. Of course, acting on behalf of one's health can be a virtue, and undermining one's health can be a vice, but "success" at being healthy, like beauty, is always partly a matter of luck and therefore beyond our control. When health is spoken of as a virtue, people who lack it are made to feel inadequate. I am not suggesting that it is always wrong to praise people's physical strength or accomplishments, any more than it is always wrong to praise their physical beauty. But just as treating cultural standards of beauty as essential virtues for women harms most women, treating health and vigour as moral virtues for everyone harms people with disabilities and illnesses.

The myth that the body can be controlled is not easily dispelled, because it is not very vulnerable to evidence against it. When I became ill, several people wanted to discuss with me what I thought I had done to "make myself" ill or "allow myself" to become sick. At first I fell in with this, generating theories about what I had done wrong; even though I had always taken good care of my health, I was able to find some (rather far-fetched) accounts of my responsibility for my illness. When a few close friends offered hypotheses as to how *they* might be responsible for my being ill, I began to suspect that something was wrong. Gradually, I realized that we were all trying to believe that nothing this important is beyond our control.

Of course, there are sometimes controllable social and psychological forces at work in creating ill health and disability (Kleinman 1988). Nevertheless, our cultural insistence on controlling the body blames the victims of disability for failing and burdens them with self-doubt and self-blame. The search for psychological, moral and spiritual causes of illness, accident and disability is often a harmful expression of this insistence on control (see Sontag 1977).

Modern Western medicine plays into and conforms to our cultural myth that the body can be controlled. Collectively, doctors and medical researchers exhibit very little modesty about their knowledge. They focus their (and our) attention on cures and imminent cures, on successful medical interventions. Research, funding and medical care are more directed toward life-threatening conditions than toward chronic illnesses and disabilities. Even pain was relatively neglected as a medical problem until the second half of this century. Surgery and saving lives bolster the illusion of control much better than does the long, patient process of rehabilitation or the management of long-term illness. These latter, less visible functions of medicine tend to be performed by nurses, physiotherapists and other low-prestige members of the profession. Doctors are trained to do something to control the body, to "make it better" (Kleinman 1988); they are the heroes of medicine. They may like being in the role of hero, but we also like them in that role and try to keep them there, because *we* want to believe that someone can always "make it better."[11] As long as we cling to this belief, the patients who cannot be "repaired"—the chronically ill, the disabled and the dying—will symbolize the failure of medicine and more, the failure of the Western scientific project to control nature. They will carry this stigma in medicine and in the culture as a whole.

When philosophers of medical ethics confine themselves to discussing life-and-death issues of medicine, they help perpetuate the idea that the main purpose of medicine is to control the body. Life-and-death interventions are the ultimate exercise of control. If medical ethicists looked more closely at who needs and who receives medical help, they would discover a host of issues concerning how medicine and society understand, mediate, assist with and integrate experiences of illness, injury and disability.

Because of the heroic approach to medicine, and because disabled people's experience is not integrated into the culture, most people know little or nothing about how to live with long-term or life-threatening illness, how to communicate with doctors and nurses and medical bureaucrats about these matters, how to live with limitation, uncertainty, pain, nausea, and other symptoms when doctors cannot make them go away. Recently, patients' support groups have arisen to fill this gap for people with nearly every type of illness and disability. They are vitally important sources of knowledge and encouragement for many of us, but they do not fill the cultural gulf between the able-bodied and the disabled. The problems of living with a disability are not private problems, separable from the rest of life and the rest of society. They are problems which can and should be shared throughout the culture as much as we share the problems of love, work and family life.

Consider the example of pain. It is difficult for most people who have not lived with prolonged or recurring pain to understand the benefits of accepting it. Yet some people who live with chronic pain speak of "making friends" with it as the road to feeling better and enjoying life. How do they picture their pain and think about it; what kind of attention do they give it and when; how do they live around and through it, and what do they learn from it? We all need to know this as part of our education. Some of the fear of experiencing pain is a consequence of ignorance and lack of guidance. The effort to avoid pain contributes to such widespread problems as drug and alcohol addiction, eating disorders, and sedentary lives. People with painful disabilities can teach us about pain, because they *can't* avoid it and have had to learn how to face it and live with it. The pernicious myth that it is possible to avoid almost all pain by controlling the body gives the fear of pain greater power than it should have and blames the victims of unavoidable pain. The fear of pain is also expressed or displaced as a fear of people in pain, which often isolates those with painful disabilities. All this is unnecessary. People *in* pain and knowledge *of* pain could be fully integrated into our culture, to everyone's benefit.

If we knew more about pain, about physical limitation, about loss of abilities, about what it is like to be "too far" from the cultural ideal of the body, perhaps we would have less fear of the negative body, less fear of our own weaknesses and "imperfections," of our inevitable deterioration and death. Perhaps we could give up our idealizations and relax our desire for control of the body; until we do, we maintain them at the expense of disabled people and at the expense of our ability to accept and love our own real bodies.

DISABLED PEOPLE AS "OTHER"

When we make people "other," we group them together as the objects of *our* experience instead of regarding them as fellow *subjects* of experience with whom we might identify. If you are "other" to me, I see you primarily as symbolic of something else—usually, but not always, something I reject and fear and that I project onto you. We can all do this to each other, but very often the process is not symmetrical, because one group of people may have more power to call itself the paradigm of humanity and to make the world suit its own needs and validate its own experiences.[12] Disabled people are "other" to able-bodied people, and (as I have tried to show) the consequences are socially, economically and psychologically oppressive to the disabled and psychologically oppressive to the able-bodied. Able-bodied people may be "other" to disabled people, but the consequences of this for the able-bodied are minor (most able-bodied people can afford not to notice it). There are, however, several political and philosophical issues that being "other" to a more powerful group raises for disabled people.

I have said that for the able-bodied, the disabled often symbolize failure to control the body and the failure of science and medicine to protect us all. However, some disabled people also become symbols of heroic control against all odds; these are the "disabled heroes," who are comforting to the able-bodied because they re-affirm the possibility of overcoming the body. Disabled heroes are people with visible disabilities who receive public attention because they accomplish things that are unusual even for the able-bodied. It is revealing that, with few exceptions (Helen Keller and, very recently, Stephen Hawking are among them), disabled heroes are recognized for performing feats of physical strength and endurance. While disabled heroes can be inspiring and heartening to the disabled, they may give the able-bodied the false impression that anyone can "overcome" a disability. Disabled heroes usually have extraordinary social, economic and physical resources that are not available to most people with those disabilities. In addition, many disabled people are not capable of performing physical heroics, because many (perhaps most) disabilities reduce or consume the energy and stamina of people who have them and do not just limit them in some particular kind of physical activity. Amputee and wheelchair athletes are exceptional, not because of their ambition, discipline and hard work, but because they are in better health than most disabled people can be. Arthritis, Parkinsonism and stroke cause severe disability in far more people than do spinal cord injuries and amputations (Bury 1979). The image of the disabled hero may reduce the "otherness" of a few disabled people, but because it creates an ideal which most disabled people cannot meet, it *increases* the "otherness" of the majority of disabled people.

One recent attempt to reduce the "otherness" of disabled people is the introduction of the term, "differently-abled." I assume the point of using this term is to suggest that there is nothing *wrong* with being the way we are, just different. Yet to call someone "differently-abled" is much like calling her "differently-coloured" or "differently-gendered." It says: "This person is not the norm or paradigm of humanity." If anything, it increases the "otherness" of disabled people, because it reinforces the paradigm of humanity as young, strong and healthy, with all body parts working "perfectly," from which this person is "different." Using the term "differently-abled" also suggests a (polite? patronizing? protective? self-protective?) disregard of the special difficulties, struggles and suffering disabled people face. We are dis-abled. We live with particular social and physical struggles that are partly consequences of the conditions of our bodies and partly consequences of the structures and expectations of our societies, but they are struggles which only people with bodies like ours experience.

The positive side of the term "differently-abled" is that it might remind the able-bodied that to be disabled in some respects is not to be disabled in all respects. It also suggests that a disabled person may have abilities that the able-bodied lack in virtue of being able-bodied. Nevertheless, on the whole, the term "differently-abled" should be abandoned, because it reinforces the able-bodied paradigm of humanity and fails to acknowledge the struggles disabled people face.

The problems of being "the other" to a dominant group are always politically complex. One solution is to emphasize similarities to the dominant group in the hope that they will identify with the oppressed, recognize their rights, gradually give them equal opportunities, and eventually assimilate them. Many disabled people are tired of being symbols to the able-bodied, visible only or primarily for their disabilities, and they want nothing more than to be seen as individuals rather than as members of the group, "the disabled." Emphasizing similarities to the able-bodied, making their disabilities unnoticeable in comparison to their other human qualities may bring about assimilation one-by-one. It does not directly challenge the able-bodied paradigm of humanity, just as women moving into traditionally male arenas of power does not directly challenge the male paradigm of humanity, although both may produce a gradual change in the paradigms. In addition, assimilation may be very difficult for the disabled to achieve. Although the able-bodied like disabled tokens who do not seem very different from themselves, they may *need* someone to carry the burden of the negative body as long as they continue to idealize and try to control the body. They may therefore resist the assimilation of most disabled people.

The reasons in favour of the alternative solution to "otherness"—*emphasizing difference* from the able-bodied—are also reasons for emphasizing similarities among the disabled, especially social and political similarities. Disabled people share positions of social oppression that separate us from the able-bodied, and we share physical, psychological and social experiences of disability. Emphasizing differences from the able-bodied demands that those differences be acknowledged and respected and fosters solidarity among the disabled. It challenges the able-bodied paradigm of humanity and creates the possibility of a deeper challenge to the idealization of the body and the demand for its control. Invisibly disabled people tend to be drawn to solutions that emphasize difference, because our need to have our struggles acknowledged is great, and we have far less experience than those who are visibly disabled of being symbolic to the able-bodied.

Whether one wants to emphasize sameness or difference in dealing with the problem of being "the other" depends in part on how radically one wants to challenge the value-structure of the dominant group. A very important issue in this category for both women and disabled people is the value of independence from the help of others, so highly esteemed in our patriarchal culture and now being questioned in feminist ethics (see, for example, Sherwin 1984, 1987; Kittay and Meyers 1987) and discussed in the writings of disabled women (see, for example, Fisher and Galler 1981; Davis 1984; Frank 1988). Many disabled people who can see the possibility of living as independently as any able-bodied person, or who have achieved this goal after long struggle, value their independence above everything. Dependence on the help of others is humiliating in a society which prizes independence. In addition, this issue holds special complications for disabled women; reading the stories of women who became disabled as adults, I was struck by their struggle with shame and loss of self-esteem at being transformed from people who took physical care of others (husbands and children) to people who were physically dependent. All this suggests that disabled people need every bit of independence we can get. Yet there are disabled people who will always need a lot of help from other individuals just to survive (those who have very little control of movement, for example), and to the extent that everyone considers independence necessary to respect and self-esteem, those people will be condemned to be de-valued. In addition, some disabled people spend tremendous energy being independent in ways that might be considered trivial in a culture less insistent on self-reliance; if our culture valued *interdependence* more highly, they could use that energy for more satisfying activities.

In her excellent discussion of the issue of dependency and independence, Barbara Hillyer Davis argues that women with disabilities and those who care for them can work out a model of *reciprocity* for all of us, if we are willing to learn from them. "Reciprocity involves the difficulty of recognizing each other's needs, relying on the other, asking and receiving help, delegating responsibility, giving and receiving empathy, respecting boundaries" (Davis 1984, 4). I hope that disabled and able-bodied feminists will join in questioning our cultural obsession with independence and ultimately replacing it with such a model of reciprocity. If *all* the disabled are to be fully integrated into society without symbolizing failure, then we have to change social values to recognize the value of depending on others and being depended upon. This would also reduce the fear and shame associated with dependency in old age—a condition most of us will reach.

Whether one wants to emphasize sameness or difference in dealing with the problems of being "other" is also related to whether one sees anything valuable to be preserved by maintaining, either temporarily or in the long run, some separateness of the oppressed group. Is there a special culture of the oppressed group or the seeds of a special culture which could be developed in a supportive context of solidarity? Do members of the oppressed group have accumulated knowledge or ways of knowing which might be lost if assimilation takes place without the dominant culture being transformed?

It would be hard to claim that disabled people as a whole have an alternative culture or even the seeds of one. One sub-group, the deaf, has a separate culture from the hearing, and they are fighting for its recognition and preservation, as well as for their right to continue making their own culture (Sacks 1988). Disabled people do have both knowledge and ways of knowing that are not available to the able-bodied. Although ultimately I hope that disabled people's knowledge will be integrated into the culture as a whole, I suspect that a culture which fears and denigrates the real body would rather silence this knowledge than make the changes necessary to absorb it. It may have to be nurtured and cultivated separately while the able-bodied culture is transformed enough to receive and integrate it.

THE KNOWLEDGE OF DISABLED PEOPLE AND HOW IT IS SILENCED

In my second year of illness, I was reading an article about the psychological and philosophical relationship of mind to body. When the author painted a rosy picture of the experience of being embodied, I was outraged at the presumption of the writer to speak for everyone from a healthy body. I decided I didn't want to hear *anything* about the body from anyone who was not physically disabled. Before that moment, it had not occurred to me that there was a world of experience from which I was shut out while I was able-bodied.

Not only do physically disabled people have experiences which are not available to the able-bodied, they are in a better position to transcend cultural mythologies about the body, because they *cannot* do things that the able-bodied feel they *must* do in order to be happy, "normal" and sane. For example, paraplegics and quadriplegics have revolutionary things to teach about the possibilities of sexuality which contradict patriarchal culture's obsession with the genitals (Bullard and Knight 1981). Some people can have orgasms in any part of their bodies where they feel touch. One man said he never knew how good sex could be until he lost the feeling in his genitals. Few able-bodied people know these things, and, to my knowledge, no one has explored their implications for the able-bodied.

If disabled people were truly heard, an explosion of knowledge of the human body and psyche would take place. We have access to realms of experience that our culture has not tapped (even for medical science, which takes relatively little interest in people's *experience* of their bodies). Like women's particular knowledge, which comes from access to experiences most men do not have, disabled people's knowledge is dismissed as trivial, complaining, mundane (or bizarre), *less than* that of the dominant group.

The cognitive authority (Addelson 1983) of medicine plays an important role in distorting and silencing the knowledge of the disabled. Medical professionals have been given the power to describe and validate everyone's experience of the body. If you go to doctors with symptoms they cannot observe directly or verify independently of what you tell them, such as pain or weakness or numbness or dizziness or difficulty concentrating, and if they cannot find an objectively observable cause of those symptoms, you are likely to be told that there is "nothing wrong with you," no matter how you feel. Unless you are very lucky in your doctors, no matter how trustworthy and responsible you were considered to be *before* you started saying you were ill, your experience will be invalidated.[13] *Other* people are the authorities on the reality of your experience of your body.

When you are very ill, you desperately need medical validation of your experience, not only for economic reasons (insurance claims, pensions, welfare and disability benefits all depend upon official diagnosis), but also for social and psychological reasons. People with unrecognized illnesses are often abandoned by their friends and families.[14] Because almost everyone accepts the cognitive authority of medicine, the person whose bodily experience is radically different from medical descriptions of her/his condition is invalidated as a knower. Either you decide to hide your experience, or you are socially isolated with it by being labelled mentally ill[15] or dishonest. In both cases you are silenced.

Even when your experience is recognized by medicine, it is often re-described in ways that are inaccurate from your standpoint. The objectively observable condition of your body may be used to determine the severity of your pain, for instance, regardless of your own reports of it. For example, until recently, relatively few doctors were willing to acknowledge that severe phantom limb pain can persist for months or even years after an amputation. The accumulated experience of doctors who were themselves amputees has begun to legitimize the other patients' reports (Madruga 1979).

When you are forced to realize that other people have more social authority than you do to describe your experience of your own body, your confidence in yourself and your relationship to reality is radically undermined. What can you know if you cannot know that you are experiencing suffering or joy; what can you communicate to people who don't believe you know even this?[16] Most people will censor what they tell or say nothing rather than expose themselves repeatedly to such deeply felt invalidation. They are silenced by fear and confusion. The process is familiar from our understanding of how women are silenced in and by patriarchal culture.

One final caution: As with women's "special knowledge," there is a danger of sentimentalizing disabled people's knowledge and abilities and keeping us "other" by doing so. We need to bring this knowledge into the culture and to transform the culture and society so that everyone can receive and make use of it, so that it can be fully integrated, along with disabled people, into a shared social life.

Conclusion

I have tried to introduce the reader to the rich variety of intellectual and political issues that are raised by experiences of physical disability. Confronting these issues has increased my appreciation of the insights that feminist theory already offers into cultural attitudes about the body and the many forms of social oppression. Feminists have been challenging medicine's authority for many years now, but not, I think, as radically as we would if we knew what disabled people have to tell. I look forward to the development of a full feminist theory of disability.[17] We need a theory of disability for the liberation of both disabled and able-bodied people, since the theory of disability is also the theory of the oppression of the body by a society and its culture.

NOTES

Many thanks to Kathy Gose, Joyce Frazee, Mary Barnes, Barbara Beach, Elliott Gose and Gordon Renwick for helping me to think about these questions, and to Maureen Ashfield for helping me to research them.

1. Itzhak Perlman, when asked in a CBC interview about the problems of the disabled, said disabled people have two problems: the fact that the world is not made for people with any weaknesses but for supermen and the attitudes of able-bodied people.

2. An excellent description of this last issue as it confronts the deaf is found in Sacks 1988.

3. See Matthews 1983; Hannaford 1985; Rooney and Israel 1985; Browne, Connors, and Stern 1985; Deegan and Brooks 1985; Saxton and Howe 1987; and, for a doctor's theories, Kleinman 1988.

4. We also need a feminist theory of mental disability, but I will not be discussing mental disability in this essay.

5. In a recent article in *Signs*, Linda Alcoff argues that we should define "woman" thus: "woman is a position from which a feminist politics can emerge rather than a set of attributes that are 'objectively identifiable.' " (Alcoff 1988, 435). I think a similar approach may be the best one for defining "disability."

6. For example, pelvic inflammatory disease causes severe prolonged disability in some women. These women often have to endure medical diagnoses of psychological illness and the skepticism of family and friends, in addition to having to live with chronic severe pain. See Moore 1985.

7. Feminism has challenged the distribution of responsibility for providing such resources as childcare and protection from family violence. Increasingly many people who once thought of these as family or personal concerns now think of them as social responsibilities.

8. Some people save me that trouble by *telling me* I am fine and walking away. Of course, people also encounter difficulties with answering "How are you?" during and after crises, such as separation from a partner, death of a loved one, or a nervous breakdown. There is a temporary alienation from what is considered ordinary shared experience. In disability, the alienation lasts longer, often for a lifetime, and, in my experience, it is more profound.

9. The idealization of the body is clearly related in complex ways to the economic processes of a consumer society. Since it pre-dated capitalism, we know that capitalism did not cause it, but it is undeniable that idealization now generates tremendous profits and that the quest for profit demands the reinforcement of idealization and the constant development of new ideals.

10. Susan Griffin, in a characteristically honest and insightful passage, describes an encounter with the fear that makes it hard to identify with disabled people. See Griffin 1982, 648–649.

11. Thanks to Joyce Frazee for pointing this out to me.

12. When Simone de Beauvoir uses this term to elucidate men's view of women (and women's view of ourselves), she emphasizes that Man is considered essential, Woman inessential; Man is the Subject, Woman the Other (de Beauvoir 1952, xvi). Susan Griffin expands upon this idea by showing how we project rejected aspects of ourselves onto groups of people who are designated the Other (Griffin 1981).

13. Many women with M. S. have lived through this nightmare in the early stages of their illness. Although this happens to men too, women's experience of the body, like women's experience generally, is more likely to be invalidated (Hannaford 1985).

14. Accounts of the experience of relatively unknown, newly discovered, or hard-to-diagnose diseases and conditions confirm this. See, for example, Jeffreys 1982, for the story of an experience of chronic fatigue immune dysfunction syndrome, which is more common in women than in men.

15. Frequently people with undiagnosed illnesses are sent by their doctors to psychiatrists, who cannot help and may send them back to their doctors saying they must be physically ill. This can leave patients in a dangerous medical and social limbo. Sometimes they commit suicide because of it (Ramsay 1986). Psychiatrists who know enough about living with physical illness or disability to help someone cope with it are rare.

16. For more discussion of this subject, see Zaner 1983 and Rawlinson 1983.

17. At this stage of the disability rights movement, it is impossible to anticipate everything that a full feminist theory will include, just as it would have been impossible to predict in 1970 the present state of feminist theory of mothering. Nevertheless, we can see that besides dealing more fully with the issues I have raised here, an adequate feminist theory of disability will examine all the ways in which disability is socially constructed; it will explain the interaction of disability with gender, race and class position; it will examine every aspect of the cognitive authority of medicine and science over our experiences of our bodies; it will discuss the relationship of technology to disability; it will question the belief that disabled lives are not worth living or preserving when it is implied in our theorizing about abortion and euthanasia; it will give us a detailed vision of the full integration of disabled people in society, and it will propose practical political strategies for the liberation of disabled people and the liberation of the able-bodied from the social oppression of their bodies.

REFERENCES

Addelson, Kathryn P. 1983. The man of professional wisdom. In *Discovering reality*. Sandra Harding and Merrill B. Hintikka, eds. Boston: D. Reidel.

Alcoff, Linda. 1988. Cultural feminism versus poststructuralism: The identity crisis in feminist theory. *Signs: Journal of Women in Culture and Society* 13(3):405–436.

Beauvoir, Simone de. 1952. *The second sex*. New York: Alfred A. Knopf.

Browne, Susan E., Debra Connors, and Nanci Stern, eds. 1985. *With the power of each breath—A disabled women's anthology*. Pittsburgh: Cleis Press.

Bullard, David G., and Susan E. Knight, eds. 1981. *Sexuality and physical disability*. St. Louis: C. V. Mosby.

Bury, M. R. 1979. Disablement in society: Towards an integrated perspective. *International Journal of Rehabilitation Research* 2(1):33–40.

Campling, Jo, ed. 1981. *Images of ourselves—Women with disabilities talking*. London: Routledge and Kegan Paul.

Davis, Barbara Hillyer. 1984. Women, disability and feminism: Notes toward a new theory. *Frontiers: A Journal of Women Studies* VIII(1): 1–5.

Davis, Melanie, and Catherine Marshall. 1987. Female and disabled: Challenged women in education. *National Women's Studies Association Perspectives* 5:39–41.

Deegan, Mary Jo, and Nancy A. Brooks, eds. 1985. *Women and disability—The double handicap*. New Brunswick: Transaction Books.

Dinnerstein, Dorothy. 1976. *The mermaid and the minotaur: Sexual arrangements and human malaise*. New York: Harper and Row.

Ehrenreich, Barbara, and Dierdre English. 1979. *For her own good: 150 years of the experts' advice to women*. New York: Anchor.

Fine, Michelle, and Adrienne Asch, eds. 1988. *Women with disabilities: Essays in psychology, culture and politics*. Philadelphia: Temple University Press.

Finger, Anne. 1983. Disability and reproductive rights. *off our backs* 13(9):18–19.

Fisher, Bernice, and Roberta Galler. 1981. Conversation between two friends about feminism and disability. *off our backs* 11 (5):14–15.

Frank, Gelya. 1988. On embodiment: A case study of congenital limb deficiency in American culture. In *Women with disabilities*. Michelle Fine and Adrienne Asch, eds. Philadelphia: Temple University Press.

Griffin, Susan. 1981. *Pornography and silence: Culture's revenge against nature*. New York: Harper and Row.

Griffin, Susan. 1982. The way of all ideology. *Signs: Journal of Women in Culture and Society* 8(3):641–660.

Halpern, Sue M. 1988. Portrait of the artist. Review of *Under the eye of the clock* by Christopher Nolan. *The New York Review of Books*, June 30:3–4.

Hannaford, Susan. 1985. *Living outside inside. A disabled woman's experience. Towards a social and political perspective*. Berkeley: Canterbury Press.

Jeffreys, Toni. 1982. *The mile-high staircase*. Sydney: Hodder and Stoughton Ltd.

Kittay, Eva Feder, and Diana T. Meyers, eds. 1987. *Women and moral theory*. Totowa, NJ: Rowman and Littlefield.

Kleinman, Arthur. 1988. *The illness narratives: Suffering, healing, and the human condition*. New York: Basic Books.

Lessing, Jill. 1981. Denial and disability. *off our backs* 11(5):21.

Madruga, Lenor. 1979. *One step at a time*. Toronto: McGraw-Hill.

Matthews, Gwyneth Ferguson. 1983. *Voices from the shadows: Women with disabilities speak out*. Toronto: Women's Educational Press.

Moore, Maureen. 1985. Coping with pelvic inflammatory disease. In *Women and Disability*. Frances Rooney and Pat Israel, eds. *Resources for Feminist Research* 14(1).

Newsweek. 1988. Reading God's mind. June 13:56–59.

Ramsay, A. Melvin. 1986. *Postviral fatigue syndrome, the saga of Royal Free disease*. London: Gower Medical Publishing.

Rawlinson, Mary C. 1983. The facticity of illness and the appropriation of health. In *Phenomenology in a pluralistic context*. William L. McBride and Calvin O. Schrag, eds. Albany: SUNY Press.

Rich, Adrienne. 1976. *Of woman born: Motherhood as experience and institution*. New York: W. W. Norton.

Rooney, Frances, and Pat Israel, eds. 1985. *Women and disability. Resources for Feminist Research* 14(1).

Sacks, Oliver. 1988. The revolution of the deaf. *The New York Review of Books*, June 2:23–28.

Saxton, Marsha, and Florence Howe, eds. 1987. *With wings: An anthology of literature by and about women with disabilities*. New York: The Feminist Press.

Shaul, Susan L., and Jane Elder Bogle. 1981. Body image and the woman with a disability. In *Sexuality and physical disability*. David G. Bullard and Susan E. Knight, eds. St. Louis: C. V. Mosby.

Sherwin, Susan. 1984. A feminist approach to ethics. *Dalhousie Review* 64(4):704–713.

Sherwin, Susan. 1987. Feminist ethics and in vitro fertilization. In *Science, morality and feminist theory*. Marsha Hanen and Kai Nielsen, eds. Calgary: The University of Calgary Press.

Sontag, Susan. 1977. *Illness as metaphor*. New York: Random House.

U.N. Decade of Disabled Persons 1983–1992. 1983. *World programme of action concerning disabled persons*. New York: United Nations.

Whitbeck, Caroline. 1983. Afterword to the maternal instinct. In *Mothering: Essays in feminist theory*. Joyce Trebilcot, ed. Totowa: Rowman and Allanheld.

Zaner, Richard M. 1983. Flirtations or engagement? Prolegomenon to a philosophy of medicine. In *Phenomenology in a pluralistic context*. William L. McBride and Calvin O. Schrag, eds. Albany: SUNY Press.

If Age Becomes a Standard for Rationing Health Care . . .

NORA KIZER BELL ❖ ❖ ❖

Daniel Callahan, the influential Director of the Hastings Center, has boldly and re-peatedly advanced the provocative thesis that age be a limiting factor in decisions to allocate certain kinds of health services to the elderly. However, when one looks at available data, one discovers that there are many more elderly women than there are elderly men, and these older women are poorer, more apt to live alone, and less likely to have informal social and personal supports than their male counterparts. Older women, therefore, will make the heaviest demand on health care resources. If age becomes a standard for limiting the provision of health care, the limits that will be set will affect women more drastically than they affect men. This essay examines the implications for elderly women of using age as such a limiting factor.

In two recent and controversial books, *Setting Limits* (1987) and *What Kind of Life: The Limits of Medical Progress* (1990), Daniel Callahan of the Hastings Center has put forth a provocative thesis: that "intergenerational equity" might require us to rethink some of the traditional goals of medicine as they affect care that is provided to the elderly. Specifically, Callahan suggests that the increasing numbers of the elderly, coupled with medicine's increased technological capabilities, create the potential within medicine for "an unending medical struggle against aging and death" that is, perhaps, not properly one of medicine's "deepest ends" or goals.

In his view, we have reached a crisis in medicine—about the meaning and nature of health, as well as about the proper role that an open-ended pursuit of health should play in the future. "We have come ever more to desire what we cannot any longer have in unlimited measure—a healthier, extended life—and cannot even afford to pursue much longer without harm to our personal lives and our social institutions" (Callahan 1990, 11).

Others advance a similar claim: put bluntly, society is going to have to make some hard choices. Many believe that one of those choices should be to limit the public provision of expensive, life-extending medical treatment for persons beyond age seventy or eighty. The claim is that in an era of scarce resources and spiraling health care costs—when important social goods are competing with expanding health care needs—persons can no longer expect to pursue medical advances "wher-ever they lead us."

On its face, this thesis is one for which I have a great deal of sympathy. I have

been present in the ICU when a ninety-two-year-old woman with terminal met-
astatic cancer is intubated repeatedly each time she extubates herself. I have argued
in favor of the "validity" of giving effect to a living will that was executed in a
state other than the one in which the elderly patient finds herself hospitalized. I,
myself, have argued that the prolongation of life, or the forestalling of death, can
be a "false goal" of medicine. I agree that one's quality of life is not necessarily a
function of the length of one's life, and I, too, worry about "creeping medical
immortality."

But I am more worried about society's setting *involuntary* limits. If age becomes
a limiting factor in the provision of medical treatment, apart from the obvious
consequences to which many before me have taken objection, there is yet another
consequence that I feel must not be overlooked. The limits that will be set will
be limits that affect women more drastically than they affect men because the so-
called "frontier" of old age extends indefinitely for many more women than it does
men.

My objective in writing this essay, therefore, is to examine the implications of
such a thesis for elderly women.

RECONSTRUCTING THE ENDS OF AGING

To propose using age as a specific criterion for the allocation and limitation of
health care is to suggest that upon reaching the end of a "natural life span" further
medical intervention should be acknowledged as inappropriate.

This, however, seems to imply a conception of life and the natural end of one's
life in old age different from what we have normally taken it to be, a conception
that focuses on the fact that one's life *on the whole* has had numerous and bountiful
experiences whose richness in old age now suggests completeness. Such a conception of life makes no evaluative claims about the experiences by which one's life
is so defined. Rather, on this so-called *biographical* definition of life there simply
comes a time when the biography is complete, even though there might be many
more pages one could write.

> For the lifelong reader there will still be many old books not read, and a
> constant stream of new books to be read. For the painter, there will be an infinite
> number of further possibilities, as there will be for one who enjoys investing in
> the stock market, understanding nature, watching scientific and other knowledge
> being discovered, growing a garden, observing the sunset, enjoying music, and
> taking walks. In that sense, however, life's possibilities will never be ex-
> hausted. . . . Yet even if we will lose such possibilities by death in old age, we
> will on the whole already have had ample time to know the pleasures of such
> things. (Callahan 1987, 67)

As Callahan argues in *What Kind of Life*, recognizing the necessity of setting
limits on the provision of health care acknowledges acceptance of a full ("but not
necessarily biologically maximum") life span, the appropriateness of death from

"conditions whose eradication would require an unreasonable expenditure of resources, and a circumscribed place for the pursuit of health as a societal good"
(Callahan 1990, 151).

On such a view, the end of the aging process is not properly spent, therefore,
"warring" against the diseases that accompany longevity. Rather, death at the end
of a long and full life is fitting and orderly. Furthermore, the natural end to a long
and full life is a "tolerable death": (1) a death that occurs when one has accomplished most of what life has to offer, (2) a death that occurs when one has fulfilled
one's obligations to all those to whom one has responsibilities, and (3) a death
that no longer offends or engenders rage and despair at human finitude (Callahan
1987, 66).

The goal of geriatric medicine, therefore, is not to seek new ways to predict
or prevent late-onset genetic disease, it is not to define "premature" death as a
function of state-of-the-art medicine at any given moment, it is not to seek "just
a little longer life," it is not to practice opportunistic medicine or to imagine
medicine as providing the fountain of youth. Rather, so that one may experience
the natural end of life, the goal is to put aside the allures that medicine offers for
staving off old age. Hence, society should seek to impose limits on health care for
the elderly so that the richness and fullness of old age aren't lost, and so that old
age isn't vilified by our fight against it.

> It is a tragedy when life ends prematurely even though it is possible to save
> that life, and when old age is full of burdens even though resources are available
> to relieve them. It is an outrage when, through selfishness, discrimination, or
> culpable indifference, the elderly are denied what they need and deserve. But it
> is only a sadness, an ineradicable part of life itself, when after a long and full life
> a person ages and dies. . . . It is wise to want to banish the tragedy and the
> outrage, but not the sadness. (Callahan 1987, 204)

In fact, Callahan acknowledges that the notion of a decent biographical life
span may be different for different persons and that we may have obligations to
have helped with preventive medicine early in an individual's life—with immu-
nizations and with decent primary care. Yet, he argues, we are not obliged "to
follow the culture of modernized aging wherever it might lead, especially when we
come to know what it will cost, and how little in improved happiness we might
get anyway" (Callahan 1990, 153). Society, he concludes, would be perfectly
justified in setting an age limit on the public provision of expensive, life-extending,
curative health care.

TOLERABLE OR TRAGIC DEATHS?

The elderly are currently the heaviest users of health services, and the great
bulk of those services is spent in "forestalling death" and in "warehousing" persons
until their deaths. These facts represent part of the challenge society would face
in setting limits. When one looks closely at the data, however, what one very

quickly discovers is that there are many more elderly women than there are elderly men, and these older women are poorer, more apt to live alone, and less likely to have informal social and personal supports than their male counterparts. Furthermore, a disproportionate number of nursing home patients are women. Older women, therefore, are more likely to make the heaviest demand on health care resources.[1]

What would it mean in practice, then, to have a health policy for the aged of the kind outlined above?

Unfortunately, serious problems underlie using age as a criterion for rationing health care, problems that, despite the insistence that the elderly would never be denied compassionate and thoughtful care, redound negatively against such a thesis. I want to argue that setting limits according to the rationale outlined above may in some cases still be properly described as a "tragedy" and an "outrage."

None of the arguments for rationing by age take note of the implications for women of employing such a criterion, or of the special plight of women among the aged (except to mention that women are burdened more than men in being caregivers for sick and aging parents). None of the arguments about the limits of society's obligations to the aged acknowledges historical failures of the health care system to note gender differences in medical research, diagnosis, and treatment. None of the arguments addresses the question of whether there might be differences in the definition of "natural life span" or one's perception of a "tolerable death" that are gender-relative. None of the arguments takes note of the fact that the limits they suggest imposing may have tragic consequences for women.

On my view, however, these are the very consequences of age-based rationing that need to be examined more carefully. In what follows, I would like to offer such an examination by looking more closely at Callahan's three-part definition of what counts as a tolerable death.

First: *A tolerable death is one that occurs when an individual has accomplished most of what life has to offer.*

Such a biographical definition of life fails to take adequate note of the differences in the biographies of men and women. To believe that it is desirable to adopt the use of an age standard suggests that a woman's life should be viewed as completed earlier in her biological chronology than it actually is, that is, when procreation, childrearing, housekeeping, and the maintaining of conjugal relationships are complete. The argument in favor of believing that there is an appropriate time in a person's biography for claiming that her life could be considered full strikes me as advancing recognized forms of male bias: both a general *devaluation of women's concerns* and *an indifference to a woman's "life possibilities" apart from her abasement into more servile positions.* (That is not to say that I couldn't agree that one's life from a certain point forward might not be worth living or might itself be intolerable.)

Why shouldn't one believe, as James Childress (1984) has suggested, that the use of an age standard seems to symbolize a willingness on our part to abandon older female persons and exclude them from communal care?[2] Furthermore, as Childress seems to believe, the use of an age criterion for determining how to allocate health care resources seems to manifest society's perception that youth is valuable and advanced age, particularly advanced female age, has less worth. The testimony of older persons, especially older women, who profess to believe that they are willing, and maybe even morally obliged, to let a younger person (say, a child or a grandchild) live in their stead is less evidence in favor of accepting the argument than it is evidence confirming society's devaluation of older persons and advancing age. Besides, willingness on the part of some older persons to elect to forego certain resources or experiences in favor of giving them to younger persons does not imply that a standard for accomplishing that should be *imposed*. Unless Childress's claim about the use of an age criterion is true—that is, unless we really do believe that youth is more valuable—why should it be obvious that we should prefer to limit resources to older persons in favor of allocating to younger persons? Why shouldn't we believe that electing such a standard makes women's deaths premature? Why isn't it obvious that women's old age *is* full of burdens? Is it obvious that there aren't resources available to relieve them?

A biographical definition of life also seems to measure a person's life by the notion of a "range of experiences" without taking note of any qualitative measure of those experiences. This understanding of measuring one's life seems counter-intuitive. It doesn't seem enough to say that the range of a person's experiences, or the range of her exposure to resources, is greater by virtue of her having lived longer. Surely the *quality* of those experiences or of those resources colors them in a way that cannot be ignored. For that reason, it seems culpable indifference to fail to count the quality of those experiences as significant. Insofar as women have historically been disadvantaged with respect to their achievements, their interests, their economic, social, and political status, and their sexuality, many would argue that the quality of their life experiences has been so low that with respect to the first criterion of what counts as a tolerable death, such a definition begs the question.

This brings me to the second part of the definition of what counts as a tolerable death:

A tolerable death is one that occurs when one has fulfilled one's obligations to all those to whom one has responsibilities.

Women are beginning to enter the paid labor force in substantial numbers, but in spite of their economic emergence, women continue to be in disadvantaged positions in the marketplace both in terms of the wages they command and the jobs open to them. As human capital, women are valued less highly than men (Bergmann 1986). This can be viewed as a natural consequence of the fact that "[i]n the past, women's place in the economy was an assignment to sole responsibility for the care of the children, and to housework and other works that could efficiently be combined in the home with child care. Men were given sole responsibility for earning money, and exempted from taking a share in 'women's work' " (Bergmann 1986, 7). The importance assigned to earning money, among other things, helped contribute to devaluing "women's work." Reskin and Hartmann (1986) and others delineate some of the kinds of work that have been so devalued: *caring work* (child care and nursing care, for example), *consumption work* (all those tasks involved in purchasing goods and services), *kin work* (tasks involved in keeping up with family birthdays, weddings, funerals, and simply "keeping in touch"), *invisible work* (housework, cooking, sewing, washing, ironing, for example). A further indication of the lack of value attached to such work is found in the fact that government and industry have been slow to move to "industrialize" child care and housework, making it even harder for women (especially single mothers) to compete effectively in the job market (Bergmann 1986, 275–98).[3]

Because of the value attached to providing for another financially, women's responsibilities to others continue in large part to be described as consisting in caring work, kin work, consumption work and other forms of so-called invisible work. It is easy to imagine someone arguing that a woman who is single, or who outlives her spouse, or whose children are independent has outlived her usefulness and her obligations. Furthermore, because women live longer than men and have been in the work force a shorter period of time than men, and hence have contributed less to public funds and have limited provisions of their own for their old age, women could also be perceived as undeservedly requiring more in the way of others' responsibilities *to* them. As the largest and poorest population of the elderly, it is women who will make the heaviest demands on public monies for health care. It is the older woman who will have the greatest need for increased social and nonfinancial forms of support. It is she who will be society's greatest burden, and it is she for whom limits will be set.

It is this larger social and moral context to which I want to appeal in evaluating the thesis that age be a standard for rationing care. Using age as a standard for rationing is much more complex than it appears on its face. For his part, Callahan acknowledges that an age standard has "symbolic significance" when its use is colored by its context, or by the rationale articulated for its use (1987, 169). He also acknowledges that death is a tragedy and an outrage if it comes on the heels of one's having been denied what one needs through discrimination or indifference (1987, 204).

A death is tolerable when it no longer offends or engenders rage and despair.

Of course, many who advocate an upper age limit on providing health services don't necessarily desire to deal women out. If anything, their arguments are ones that I have heard many so-called senior citizens express almost as eloquently themselves. And I do agree that we have to be sensible about utilizing medical resources, especially in cases where they aren't likely to benefit the recipient or alter an inevitably bad outcome. I acknowledge that we are fast approaching a time in our history when the largest segment of our population, our largest special interest lobby, if you will, is the aging and the elderly. However, I can't agree that employing age as a standard in rationing would transform its present use into a use that "affirms" and does not denigrate old age (Callahan 1987, 170).

I want to argue that there is tremendous symbolic significance for women in adopting an age standard, a significance that derives from and is colored by woman's social and moral history. Honoring a "natural life span" could mean believing that a natural life normally ends in the mid-seventies (the life expectancy for males), and in accepting that age standard, Callahan-style policy makers might adopt measures that preclude women from receiving essential services at the ends of our (longer) lives.

Among the items left over from the "old" anti-ageism agenda (Butler 1975), the widespread problem of elder abuse and neglect should generate outrage. A

University of Massachusetts study suggests that there are six times as many cases of abuse of the elderly as are actually reported (Elder Abuse 1988). Abuse, neglect, and exploitation include failing to provide the ill and the fragile with minimal medical care, medication, and hospitalization. Why don't the proponents of such sweeping policy change give this problem more prominence?

Again because of their numbers, women constitute the majority of those affected by abuse and neglect. When I worry about setting limits, I worry about the attitudes engendered by promulgation of the belief that there is an age beyond which one is getting more than her fair share. I worry about the fact that so-called entitlement policies—that would focus on providing health care to "disadvantaged groups" who have been deprived of benefits available to the population as a whole—don't mention women except as their health care affects the health status of their offspring (Callahan 1990, 197).

Arguments for rationing on the basis of age seem to rest on the presumption that there is little value in providing certain health services to persons who have reached the end of full and natural lives. I protest that presumption because "natural life span" and "tolerable death" are not gender neutral. Providing health services to the very old has been devalued, in part because medical intervention can dehumanize the natural end to one's natural life span. I wonder if that absence of value is not also due in large measure to the fact that there are few male competitors for these services. Couldn't we believe that, like other items in women's social history, when men move to evaluate something that is peculiarly the province of women, it then becomes devalued?

Given this social and moral context, woman's old age is not affirmed by setting limits; it is debased. Given this context, the deaths of older women *will* engender rage and despair. Given this context, appealing to an age standard will make the deaths of women premature in the fullest sense of the word. Not only will their deaths be sad, they will be a tragedy and an outrage.

NOTES

I am especially grateful to my colleague Ferdinand Schoeman for the many helpful suggestions he made about various aspects of this discussion.

1. Older women now outnumber older men three to two. This represents a dramatic increase from 1960, when the ratio of elderly men to elderly women was five to four. Furthermore, the ratio changes markedly with increased age. The 1984 census found only 40 men for every 100 women at age 85, but 81 men for every 100 women between the ages of 65 and 69. By the year 2050, the projected life expectancy for females will reach 83.6 years as contrasted with a life expectancy for males of 79.8 years. The gender ratios are important for the further reason that they indicate that more women than men will be living alone in old age. Although more than one-third of all elderly disabled men living in their communities were cared for by their wives, only one in ten elderly disabled women were cared for by their husbands (Special Committee on Aging 1985).

An obvious concern, and the concern that underlies Callahan's interest in examining medicine's goals for an aging society, is that the projected increase in the size of the older population implies correlative increases in the demand for health care resources and the provision of services to the elderly. In addition, elderly persons are more likely than other adults to be poor. However, the economic statistics are especially grim for elderly women. According to a study published in 1985 by the United States Senate's Special Committee on Aging, of those persons between the ages of 65 and 69, white males had a median income of $12,180 per year as compared to a median income of $5,599 for elderly women. Because they live longer than their male counterparts, elderly women average a longer period of retirement than elderly men and must, therefore, rely on private and public sources of income longer than elderly men. Not surprisingly, nearly three-quarters of the population of the elderly poor are women (1985, 2).

Although at present only about five percent of the elderly live in nursing homes, close to 75 percent of all nursing home residents have no spouse and are institutionalized because they have health problems that significantly limit their ability to care for themselves. Not surprisingly, a disproportionate number (74.6 percent) of nursing home patients are very old, white, female, and without spouse (Special Committee on Aging 1985). The economic implications of an aging population are obvious. If limits are not set, Callahan predicts that health care expenditures for the elderly will exceed $200 billion by the year 2000. By 2040, he predicts that pension and health programs will account for 14.5 percent of the GNP and 60.4 percent of the federal budget, respectively (1987, 228).

2. Childress does not make this argument with respect to older women in particular. He makes it with respect to all older persons.

3. Furthermore, some social changes designed to benefit women economically have actually worked to their detriment. "No-fault divorce looked like a civilized way for equal adults to deal with marital incompatibility. [Yet] its implementation has cut adrift millions of middle-aged and elderly housewives who had every right to believe they had been guaranteed a comfortable home for life. Well meaning efforts to reform welfare failed miserably to lead single mothers out of poverty" (Bergmann 1986, 300).

REFERENCES

Aging America: Trends and projections. 1983. US Senate Special Committee on Aging (in conjunction with AARP). Washington, DC.

America in transition: An aging society. 1985. US Senate Special Committee on Aging. Washington, DC. 99-B.

A profile of older americans—1986. American Association of Retired Persons. Washington, DC.

Bergmann, Barbara. 1986. *The economic emergence of women.* New York: Basic Books.

Butler, R. N. 1975. *Why survive? Being old in America.* New York: Harper and Row.

Callahan, Daniel. 1987. *Setting limits: Medical goals in an aging society.* New York: Simon and Schuster.

Callahan, Daniel. 1990. *What kind of life: The limits of medical progress.* New York: Simon and Schuster.

Childress, James F. 1984. Ensuring care, respect, and fairness for the elderly. *The Hastings Center Report* 14(5): 27–31.

Day, Alice T. 1984. Who cares? Demographic trends challenge family care for the elderly. *Populations Trends and Public Policy.* Washington, DC: Population Reference Bureau, Inc.

Elder abuse reports are growing in SC. 1988. *The State.* Columbia, SC. June 5.

Long term care: A review of the evidence. 1986. University of Minnesota, School of Public Health: Division of Health Services.

May, William. 1982. Who cares for the elderly? *The Hastings Center Report* 12(6): 31–37.
Projections of the population of the US by age, sex and race: 1983–2080. Washington, DC: US
    Bureau of the Census. Series P-25, 952.
Reskin, Barbara, and H. Hartmann, eds. 1986. *Women's work, men's work.* Washington,
    DC: National Academy Press.
Waldo, Daniel, and H. Lazenby. 1984. Demographic characteristics and health care use
    and expenditures by the aged in the US: 1977–1984. *Health Care Financing Review*
    6(1).

THE ROLE OF CARING
IN HEALTH CARE

The Role of Caring in a
Theory of Nursing Ethics

SARA T. FRY ❖ ❖ ❖

The development of nursing ethics as a field of inquiry has largely relied on theories of medical ethics that use autonomy, beneficence, and/or justice as foundational ethical principles. Such theories espouse a masculine approach to moral decision making and ethical analysis. This essay challenges the presumption of medical ethics and its associated system of moral justification as an appropriate model for nursing ethics. It argues that the value foundations of nursing ethics are located within the existential phenomenon of human caring within the nurse/patient relationship instead of in models of patient good or rights-based notions of autonomy as articulated in prominent theories of medical ethics. Models of caring are analyzed and a moral-point-of-view (MPV) theory with caring as a fundamental value is proposed for the development of a theory of nursing ethics. This type of theory is supportive to feminist medical ethics because it focuses on the subscription to, and not merely the acceptance of, a particular view of morality.

INTRODUCTION

During the past ten years, a number of books on ethics in nursing practice have appeared (Benjamin and Curtis 1986; Davis and Aroskar 1983; Jameton 1984; Muyskens 1982; Thompson and Thompson 1985; Veatch and Fry 1987). Unlike earlier writings that viewed ethics in nursing as primarily feminine etiquette (Aikens 1916; Gladwin 1937; Robb 1900), these books view nursing ethics as a subset of contemporary medical ethics. Accordingly, they apply medical ethics to the practice of nursing using frameworks from bioethical theory (Beauchamp and Childress 1983), theologically-based contract theory (Veatch 1981), pluralistic secular-based theory of human rights (Engelhardt 1986), and a well-known, liberal theory of justice (Rawls 1971).

This influence on the development of nursing ethics has been quite extensive. Current nursing ethics discussions tend to revolve around deontological versus utilitarian theories, the weight of medical ethical principles and rules in nurses' decision making, and the relative importance of nursing's contract with society

Hypatia vol. 4, no. 2 (Summer 1989) © by Sara T. Fry

and individual patients. Empirical studies in nursing ethics have almost exclusively used justice-based theories of moral reasoning from cognitive psychology to interpret their findings on nurses' moral behavior, moral judgment, and moral reasoning (Crisham 1981; Ketefian 1981a, 1981b, 1985; Munhall 1980; Murphy 1976). In addition, medical ethical frameworks guide the majority of normative discussions of ethics in nursing (Cooper 1988; Silva 1984; Stenberg 1978). The result is a trend in nursing ethics that does not take into consideration the role of nurses in health care, the social significance of nursing in contemporary society, or the value standards for nursing practice. By focusing on the terms of justification, gender-biased considerations of justice, and the language of principles and rules, nursing ethics has seemingly adopted the "language of the father," to use Noddings's apt terminology (1984, 1).

This essay challenges the presumption of medical ethics, especially a "masculine" medical ethics, as an appropriate model for nursing ethics. By a "masculine" medical ethics, I mean ethical theorizing and associated argumentation that proceeds as if it were governed by an implicit, logical necessity between hierarchically arranged levels of ethical principles, rules, and actions. Often called "the engineering model" of medical ethics (Caplan 1982, 1983), this type of theorizing has been criticized by bioethicists for a number of years (Ackerman 1980, 1983; Basson 1983; Toulmin 1981). Medical ethics based on this type of theorizing often relies on a lexical ordering of principles (Toulmin 1981) or the context of justification for ethical decision making rather than the context within which such decision making takes place (Noddings 1984) or the kinds of reasons that are regarded appropriate to the making of moral judgments (Frankena 1983).

Drawing on the results of empirical studies on physician and nurse decision making as well as philosophical discussions of nursing ethics, I show that the theoretical and methodologic foundations of nursing ethics have been largely derived from "masculine" forms of medical ethics. I argue that caring ought to be the foundational value for any theory of nursing ethics. In addition, caring must be grounded within a moral-point-of-view of persons rather than any idealized conception of moral action, moral behavior, or system of moral justification.

If successful, my argument might be significant in two respects. First, it just might be supportive to a feminist medical ethic. While we might agree that medical ethics, in general, ought to be capable of being practiced by both males and females, surely feminist medical ethics necessarily must be capable of being practiced by females. Since the nursing profession, the largest group of health care providers in the United States, has already articulated caring as an important value (Fry 1988; Gadow 1985; Watson 1985) and nursing is usually practiced by females, this means that caring and the type of functions that are usually associated with the practice of nursing are related to one another—at least in the minds of a significant portion of individuals in the health care arena. Hence, the connections between the value of caring and feminism cannot be easily denied. Since the phenomenon of human caring need not be gender related, any claim to feminist medical ethics must demonstrate that it has broader applications than either just to medical practice or just to females. After all, patients are cared for by individuals other than physicians, and those who do this caring are not always females. A nursing ethic with caring as a foundational value might be an important asset to the perceived need to articulate a feminist medical ethic.

Second, since articulation of the phenomenon of human caring has already challenged justice-based theories of moral development and moral judgment (Gilligan 1982, 1987) and theories of ethics and moral education (Noddings 1984), a theory of nursing ethics with a moral-point-of-view of caring as a central value might also challenge any theory of medical ethics that utilizes traditional ethical principles or that depends on the context of justification for determining what is morally right and/or wrong in medical practice. Given the present dissatisfaction with traditional foundations of biomedical ethics, moral-point-of-view theories as well as a caring-based ethic might prove very attractive as the discipline of bioethics moves into the twenty-first century and faces new tests for its moral foundations and traditional arguments.

TRADITIONAL VALUE FOUNDATIONS OF NURSING ETHICS

Several interesting approaches have been used to identify the moral foundations of nursing and the central value(s) of the nursing ethic. For example, empirical studies of the clinical decision making of nurses have pinpointed autonomy as a fundamental value affecting moral dimensions of nursing practice (Alexander, Weisman, and Chase 1982; Prescott, Dennis, and Jacox 1987). The results of one other study have suggested that subjective values, such as producing the greatest good for the greatest number, are foundational to nurses' ethical decision making (Self 1987). Unfortunately, the results of these studies were interpreted in terms of these values as predetermined ideologies for nursing practice. In other words, autonomy and producing good were categories that the researchers expected to find because autonomy and producing good are prominent features of medical ethics. What was assumed to be the case in medical ethics was assumed to be the case in nursing ethics, as well.

This should not surprise us. Both of these values—autonomy and producing good—*are* prominent features of theories of medical ethics. Engelhardt (1986), for example, posits autonomy as the foundational value of secular bioethics while Pellegrino and Thomasma (1981, 1988) urge the restoration of beneficence as the fundamental principle of medical ethics. As used in these theories, autonomy and producing good constitute idealized value components of a social ethic for the practice of medicine and function within a structured framework of ethical principles and rules for physician decision making. Both theories rely on traditional interpretations of their central principles and utilize traditional patterns of moral justification as articulated by leading bioethicists. The same views of autonomy and beneficence have even been claimed by some nurses as the moral basis for needed social reform on the institutional setting in which nursing is practiced (Yarling and McElmurry 1986). However, there is no good reason to assume that autonomy and producing good are, de facto, the appropriate value foundations for the practice of nursing simply because they are accepted for the practice of medicine. While no one would dispute that autonomy and producing good are related to the practice of nursing, neither of these values, derived from theories of medical ethics, has been convincingly argued to be the primary moral foundation(s) of the nursing ethic.

Other approaches to identifying the moral foundations of nursing or the fundamental value of the nursing ethic have been both analytical and normative. For example, Stenberg (1979) analyzes value concepts of several theoretical frameworks in medical ethics for their relevance to the practice of nursing. She analyzes the concepts of code, contract, and context as discussed in the works of May (1975) and Fletcher (1966) and finds them inadequate bases for the nursing ethic. However, the concept of covenant as discussed in the medical ethical works of Ramsey (1970) and May (1975) is adequate as an "inclusive and satisfying model for nursing ethics" (Stenberg 1979, 21). Viewing covenant as the foundational value for such health worker actions as fidelity, promise-keeping, and truth-telling in patient care, Stenberg adopts it without alteration. Because covenant is a moral foundation for the physician/patient relationship, Stenberg considers it valid for the nurse/patient relationship, as well. This tendency to adopt medical ethical frameworks as valid moral foundations for the practice of nursing is repeated in more recent analyses of the moral foundations of the nursing ethic (Bishop and Scudder 1987; Cooper 1988).

Again, what is appropriate to the practice of medicine or is argued as a moral foundation for the physician/patient relationship is not necessarily the case for the practice of nursing or the nurse/patient relationship.

THE MORAL VALUE OF CARING AS A FOUNDATION FOR NURSING ETHICS

Forgoing recourse to medical ethics, a few nurses have attempted to articulate other foundational values for the moral practice of nursing. Sally Gadow (1985), for example, argues that the value of caring provides a foundation for a nursing ethic that will protect and enhance the human dignity of patients receiving health care. Viewing caring in the nurse/patient relationship as a commitment to certain ends for the patient, Gadow analyzes existential caring as demonstrated in the nursing actions of truth-telling and touch. Through truth-telling, the nurse assists the patient to assess the subjective as well as objective realities in illness and to make choices based on the unique meaning of the illness experience. Through touch, the nurse assists the patient in overcoming the objectness that often characterizes a patient's experience in the health care setting. To touch the patient is to affirm the patient as a person rather than an object and to communicate the value of caring as the basis for nursing actions. This approach identifies a moral foundation for nursing ethics based on the reality of the nurse/patient encounter in health care. It has also been supported by others who wish to articulate caring as a foundation of the nurse/patient relationship and its meaning (Griffin 1983; Huggins and Scalzi 1988; Packard and Ferrara 1988).

Building on the ideas of Gadow, Jean Watson (1985) proposes a slightly different view of caring as the foundation of "nursing as a human science" (13). Viewing nursing as a means to the preservation of humanity within society, Watson posits caring as a human value that involves "a will and a commitment to care, knowledge, caring actions, and consequences" (1985, 29). Such a view of caring requires a commitment toward protecting human dignity and preserving humanity on the part of the nurse. Caring becomes a professional ideal when the notion of caring transcends the act of caring between nurse and patient to influence collective acts of the nursing profession with important implications for human civilization. Like Gadow, Watson views caring as a moral ideal that is rooted in our notions of human dignity. However, unlike Gadow, Watson's human caring constitutes a philosophy of action with many unexplained metaphysical and spiritual dimensions. As such, her view of caring supports her abstract philosophy of nursing but does *not* adequately support caring as a moral value that ought to be a foundation for the nursing ethic. The value of caring remains an ideal rather than an operationalized aspect of nursing judgments and/or actions.

Like Gadow (1985) and Watson (1985), Griffin (1983) posits caring as a central value in the nurse/patient relationship. She considers caring to be, first, a mode of being. A natural state of human existence, it is one way that individuals relate to the world and to other human beings. This is not unlike Heidegger's (1962) notion of care as a fundamental way that humans exist in the world and Noddings's (1984) view of caring as a natural sentiment of being human. As a mode of being, caring is natural—a feeling or an internal sense made universal in the whole species; it is neither moral nor non-moral.

Second, caring is considered a precondition for the care of specific entities— other things, others, or oneself (Griffin 1983). This means that a conceptual *idea* about caring exists as a structural feature of human growth and development prior to the point at which the process of caring actually commences.

Third, caring is identified with social and moral ideals. For example, Watson views caring as occurring in society in order to serve human needs such as protection from the elements or the need for love. Gadow views caring as a means to protect the human dignity of patients while their health care needs are met. Thus, caring, a phenomenon of human existence, gains moral significance because it is consistently reinforced as an ideal by those who have responsibility to serve the needs of others (Griffin 1983). Since the practice of nursing is socially mandated to assist the health needs of individuals (American Nurses' Association 1980) and the nurse/patient relationship has undeniably moral dimensions, caring becomes strongly linked to the social and moral ideals of nursing as a profession.

THREE MODELS OF CARING RELEVANT TO NURSING ETHICS

Given these attributes of caring as defined by accounts of the nurse/patient relationship, at least three models are relevant for a theory of nursing ethics which posits caring as a foundational value.

NODDINGS'S MODEL OF CARING

The first model is found in the work of Nel Noddings (1984) and is theoretically based on ethics and social psychology. Building on the work of Carol Gilligan (1977, 1979, 1982), Noddings has combined knowledge of ethics with perspectives on moral development in women. She states her purpose to be "feminine in the deep classical sense, rooted in receptivity, relatedness, and responsiveness" (Noddings 1984, 2), yet she is careful to develop her notion of caring to be applicable to both females and males.

Caring is a feminine value in that the attitude of caring expresses our earliest memories of being cared for—one's store of memories of both caring and being cared for is associated with the mother figure. However, caring is also masculine in that it involves behaviors that have moral content and that can be adopted and embraced by men, even though it is not in their natural tendencies to adopt such notions. In defining care, Noddings states, " . . . to care may mean to be charged with the protection, welfare, or maintenance of something or someone" (1984, 9). Rather than an attitude that begins with moral reasoning, it represents the attitude of being moral or the "longing for goodness" (Noddings 1984, 2). Rather than an outcome of behavior, Noddings's view of caring *is* ethics itself. As such, it is not necessarily gender-dependent but is gender-relevant.

Central to this view of caring are the notions of receptivity, relatedness, and responsiveness: the acceptance or confirmation by the one-caring of one who is the cared-for (receptivity), the relation of the one-caring to one who is cared-for as a fact of human existence (relatedness), and commitment from one-caring to one who is cared-for (responsiveness). Ethical caring is simply the relation in which we meet another morally. Motivated by the ideal of caring in which we are a partner in human relationships, we are guided not by ethical principles but by the strength of the ideal of caring itself, claims Noddings. Thus, instead of the notions inherent in conditions for traditional moral justification (Beauchamp 1982), Noddings's ethic of caring depends on "the maintenance of conditions that will permit caring to flourish" (1984, 5). It is a person-to-person encounter that ultimately results in joy as a basic human affect within relationships bound by ethical caring.

Scholarship on the caring phenomenon, in general, has been strongly influenced by Noddings's model of caring. Her view has stressed the ethics and morality of caring from a perspective that is definitely gender-related although Noddings herself would undoubtedly deny that she is advocating a "feminist model." Yet, the model's relevance to the practice of nursing remains largely unexplored. For those who recognize the limitations of the bioethical model of ethical decision-making, however, Noddings's model is a rich ground for the future discussion of nursing ethics. It may also prove to be an acceptable model for the descriptive study of ethical decision making in nursing practice. While its focus on the ethic of caring as feminine might not be attractive to nurses who are not also female, its foundations in the notions of receptivity, relatedness, and responsiveness be-

tween the one-caring and the one who is cared-for make it a viable framework for
the realistic nature of the nurse/patient relationship.

PELLEGRINO'S MORAL OBLIGATION MODEL OF CARING

Edmund Pellegrino, a humanist and physician, has written extensively on caring
as a derivative value of the physician's obligation to do good (1985; Pellegrino and
Thomasma 1988). When discussing the role of the physician to the patient, Pellegrino notes that there are at least four senses in which the word "care" is understood by the practice of medicine (1985). The first sense is "care as compassion"
or being concerned for another person. This is a feeling, a sharing of someone's
experience of illness and pain, or just being touched by the plight of another person.
To care in this sense, according to Pellegrino, is "to see the person who is ill" as
more than the object of our ministrations (1985, 11). He or she is "a fellow human
whose experiences we cannot penetrate fully but which we can be touched by
simply because we share the same humanity" (Pellegrino 1985, 11).

The second sense of caring is "doing for others" what they cannot do for
themselves (1985). This entails assisting others with the activities of daily living
that are compromised by illness (for example, feeding, bathing, clothing, and
meeting personal needs). Pellegrino recognizes that physicians do little of this type
of caring but that nurses and nurses' assistants do a great deal.

The third sense of caring discussed by Pellegrino is caring for the medical
problem experienced by the patient (1985). It includes: (1) inviting the patient
to transfer responsibility and anxiety about what is wrong to the physician, (2)
assuring that knowledge and skill will be directed to the patient's problem, and
(3) recognizing that the patient's anxiety needs a specialized type of caring that is
presumed available from a physician.

Pellegrino's fourth sense of caring is to "take care" (1985, 12). This means to
carry out all the necessary procedures (personal and technical) in patient care with
conscientious attention to detail and with perfection. He finds this a corollary of
the third sense of care but argues that it is differentiated from the third sense by
its emphasis on the craftsmanship of medicine. Together, the third and fourth
senses of caring comprise what most physicians understand as *competence*.

Pellegrino does not find these four senses of caring separable in clinical practice.
Care that satisfies the four senses that he has defined is called "integral care" (1985).
This type of care is, for Pellegrino, a moral obligation of health professionals. It
is not an option that can be exercised or interpreted "in terms of some idiosyncratic
definition of professional responsibility" (1985, 13). The moral obligation to care
in this manner is created by the special human relationship that brings together
the one who is ill and the one who offers to help (1985).

In assessing whether the caring model is foundational for medical practice,
Pellegrino reexamines the roles of physicians to their patients and concludes that
"to care for the patient in the full and integral sense, requires a reconstruction of
medical ethics" (1985, 17). What is needed, he claims, is an ethic that attends
to the concept of care in its broadest sense and that makes caring a strong moral

obligation between patient and professional. Instead of a relationship of curing between physician and patient, a relation of caring is needed to express the nature of the obligation between physician and patient.

Underlying Pellegrino's notion of care is the good of the individual, a complex notion that has at least three components. For Pellegrino, "a morally good clinical decision should attend to all three senses of patient good and satisfactorily resolve conflicts among them" (1985, 20).

The first sense of good is "biomedical good"—the good a medical intervention can offer by modifying the natural history of disease in a patient. It takes into consideration the craftsmanship of physicians (and presumably, nurses), of science, and the medical indication for treatment (1985, 21).

The second sense of good is the patient's concept of his or her own good. It takes into consideration what patients consider worthwhile, or in their best interests, and can be designated to surrogate decision makers (1985, 21).

The third sense of patient good is "the good most proper to being human" (1985, 22). For Pellegrino, this is the capacity to make choices, to set up a life plan, and to determine one's goals for a satisfactory life. It is whatever fulfills our potentialities as individuals of a rational nature, respects patient dignity, and expresses human freedom.

In comparing these three senses of patient good to one another and to our ideas of social good, Pellegrino argues that patient good is prior to any other notion of good within the practice of medicine. Within a human obligation model of caring, patient good ultimately guides a physician's decision making where a patient's health and illness are concerned. Hence, while the senses of caring engender desirable physician behaviors with the patient, the physician's decision making is primarily guided by the notions of patient good. In the final analysis, Pellegrino's "integral caring" is reduced to a derivative value of patient good. It succumbs to typical medical ethical frameworks by utilizing a more general (and traditional) value as the foundational value for a theory of medical ethics. Rather than a theory of caring, Pellegrino actually proposes a theory of patient good that simply uses caring to operationalize patient good.

While Pellegrino's ideas about caring, in general, fit in with the practical sense of nursing practice, caring's subordinate role within his theory of medical ethics makes it problematic for nursing ethics. For nursing, caring seems to be more than a mere behavior between nurse and patient and might not always be derived from a notion of patient good. For example, even when the good of the patient is undecided or unknown, the nurse carries out interventions designed to care for the patient (as in emergency situations). Conversely, even when the patient's good has been made evident, nursing interventions may be carried out that do not, in fact, contribute to this sense of patient good (for example, when the physician's interpretation of the patient's good is not accepted by those planning and administering nursing care for the patient). The value of caring, for the nurse, extends beyond the notion of patient good as conceived by Pellegrino because nurse caring relates to the patient's status as a human being (Gadow 1985; Griffin 1983). For this reason, Pellegrino's moral obligation model of caring is not truly appropriate to the practice of nursing.

FRANKENA'S MORAL-POINT-OF-VIEW THEORY ON CARING

The third and final model of caring relevant to the development of nursing ethics is the moral-point-of-view (MPV) version. It is largely discussed by William Frankena in his critique of other MPV theories (1983) and entails adopting a certain point of view by defining its moral principle or central moral value. The result is a type of ethical theory (MPVT) for which Frankena seems to be a major spokesman.

In essence, one takes a moral-point-of-view by (1) subscribing to a particular substantive moral principle (or value) and (2) taking a general approach, perspective, stance or vantage point from which to proceed. While most MPV theories contain views about moral judgments and principles, about the differences between them and nonmoral principles, and views about the general nature of their justification, taking the MPV, by itself, simply means to adopt a moral principle (or value) and one's methodology to argue for that principle. It entails endorsing a general outlook or method by someone seeking to reach conclusions in a particular field (Frankena 1983).

According to Frankena, various moral principles have served as the central principles (or values) of MPV theories. Mill, for example, accepts a principle of utility that is pivotal to his MPV theory—that of utilitarianism (1863). Mill starts with a particular outlook (his moral point of view) and adopts the principle of utility as *the* moral principle that indicates the kinds of facts that one would make moral judgments about. Frankena, however, argues for taking the MPV more fully than simply accepting a certain view of morality. For him, taking the MPV entails not only acceptance of a particular view of morality but entering the moral arena oneself, "using moral considerations of the kind defined as a basis for evaluative judgments" (Frankena 1983, 70). It means subscribing to a particular view of morality and living that morality in one's life rather than merely accepting a certain view of morality and the conditions for the separation of the moral from the nonmoral.

This is a significant move for Frankena as it establishes the crucial difference between his conception of taking the MPV and the approaches of others who espouse MPVs and their related theories. Like Hume (1751), who espouses sympathy as his "sentiment of humanity," Frankena believes that there is always something that "moves us to approve or disapprove of persons" (1983, 70). This something is an attitude or precondition that is ultimately the source or motivating factor of anyone who takes the MPV. In other words, the setting forth of any particular fact is not so much the reason for deciding what is good and right in taking the MPV as is what generates the setting forth of that particular fact (and not some other fact).

For Frankena, this attitude or precondition concerns the fundamental status of persons and their human dignity. While he never explicitly defines what this attitude or precondition is for his own MPV, he eventually claims that this attitude generates the MPV of Caring or, as he puts it, "a Non-Indifference about what happens to persons and conscious sentient beings *as such*" (1983, 71). Frankena's substantive moral value is the value of caring and takes the form of Kantian respect-for-persons or Christian love. It includes making normative judgments and a concern for being rational in one's judgments but does *not* entail the acceptance or use of any particular test of justifiability, validity, or truth. A judgment based on caring is assumed to be morally justifiable because it "would be agreed to by all who genuinely take the MPV and are clear, logical, and fully knowledgeable about relevant kinds of facts (empirical, metaphysical, or whatever)" (1983, 72).

Frankena's view on caring is quite different from the view of Pellegrino. Where Pellegrino's notion of patient good provides the basis for the physician's evaluative judgments, Frankena posits caring as the basis of human normative judgments, in general. His focus on caring is direct and involves taking the MPV toward caring as a fundamental moral value or principle for normative judgments involving persons rather than the indirect focus on caring (through patient good) that is characteristic of Pellegrino's medical ethics. Like Noddings, Frankena eschews the structures of moral justification that typify traditional medical ethical theorizing and the separation of the conditions for justification from the context of ethical decision making with persons. Where much of moral philosophy takes the MPV by simply acting on principle or out of duty, Frankena's MPV requires a human response from the one taking the MPV in the form of respect-for-persons or Christian love. It requires an identifiable form of response from the one-caring to the one cared-for, to use Noddings's terminology.

Unfortunately, Frankena makes no attempt to define exactly what he interprets as respect-for-persons and certainly does not discuss his principle of caring in terms relevant to feminist philosophy. However, he does indicate that adopting the MPV of caring is made from an undefined preconditional attitude toward personhood and human dignity. This is not unlike Noddings's notions of receptivity, relatedness, and responsiveness which anchor her view of ethical caring. While it would not be appropriate to interpret Frankena's view of caring as identical or even similar to Noddings's view, certainly his method of arriving at caring as a lived principle for a system of morality (taking the MPV) bears some relevance to Noddings's views and a feminist approach to medical ethics.

CONCLUSIONS

Given the models of caring proposed by Noddings (1984), Pellegrino (1985), and Frankena (1983), and the views on caring that have been developed by nurses (Gadow 1985; Griffin 1983; Watson 1988), several recommendations for the future development of a theory of nursing ethics and any system of feminist medical ethics seem relevant.

First, theories of medical ethics as currently proposed do not seem appropriate to the development of a theory of nursing ethics. The context of nursing practice requires a moral view of persons rather than a theory of moral action or moral behavior or a system of moral justification. Present theories of medical ethics have a tendency to support theoretical and methodological views of ethical argumentation and moral justification that do not fit the practical sense of nurses' decision making in patient care and, as a result, tend to deplete the moral agency of nursing practice rather than enhance it. Any theory of nursing ethics will need to consider the nature of the nurse/patient relationship within health care contexts and adopt a moral-point-of-view that focuses directly on this relationship rather than on theoretical interpretations of physician decision making and their associated claims to moral justification for this decision making. The same might be said for any theory of feminist medical ethics, depending on how the nature of the relationship between the one-caring and the one who is cared-for is perceived.

Second, the value of caring ought to be central to any theory of nursing ethics and any theory of feminist medical ethics, as well. Given the need for nursing care within our society, nursing's perceived social mandate to provide the "diagnosis and treatment of human responses to actual or potential health problems" (American Nurses' Association 1980, 9), and the nature of the nurse/patient relationship, nursing has a significant opportunity to influence the quality of patient care through the acceptance and use of its theories. The profession of nursing has already made substantial commitment to the role of caring in several conceptions of nursing ethics and nursing science. In addition, there appears to be an important link between the value of caring and nursing's views toward persons and human dignity. As proposed by Frankena, there is good reason to subscribe to a MPV that is rooted in an attitude of respect toward persons. If a theory of nursing ethics is to have any purpose, it must necessarily make evident a view of morality that not only truly represents the social role of nursing, as a profession, in the provision of health care but that also promises a moral role for nursing in the care and nurture of individuals who have health care needs. For theory to achieve this purpose, its view of morality ought to turn on a philosophical view that posits caring as a foundational value rather than a derivative value. The same might also be said for any theory of feminist medical ethics that uses caring as a gender-relevant (but not gender-dependent) moral principle or value.

Third, taking the moral-point-of-view and developing a MPV theory need not necessarily include the acceptance or use of any particular test of moral justification. This means that any theory of nursing ethics need not endorse typical frameworks of justification contained in theories of medical ethics for moral judgments made within its parameters to be regarded as true, valid, or rationally justified. It is true that such judgments must be justified within the MPV and pertain to the sorts of facts considered relevant according to the MPV theory. However, the MPV of the theory of nursing ethics itself is not defined by reference to such a system of justification. This means that feminist models of moral decision making with similar views about moral justification may have particular relevance to the development of nursing ethics and vice versa.

To the extent that any theory of nursing ethics takes seriously the claims of MPV theorizing and the role of caring as a central value within its framework, there is reason to believe that medical ethics will benefit, for such a theory cannot develop apart from the practice of medical ethics or from the evolution of bioethics as an applied ethics discipline. Likewise, claims to feminist medical ethics cannot be made apart from all health care practices (medicine as well as nursing) and necessarily draw on the development of moral thought within bioethical theorizing. Perhaps the links between all three types of theorizing are more important than currently realized.

REFERENCES

Ackerman, Terrance F. 1980. What bioethics should be. *Journal of Medicine and Philosophy* 5:260–275.

Ackerman, Terrance F. 1983. Experimentalism in bioethics research. *Journal of Medicine and Philosophy* 8:169–180.

Aikens, Charlotte A. 1916. *Studies in ethics for nurses*. Philadelphia: W. B. Saunders Company.

Alexander, Cheryl S., Carol S. Weisman, and Gary A. Chase. 1982. Determinants of staff nurses' perceptions of autonomy within different clinical contexts. *Nursing Research* 31 (1):48–52.

American Nurses' Association. 1980. *Nursing: A social policy statement*. Kansas City: The Association.

Basson, Marc D. 1983. Bioethical decision making: A reply to Ackerman. *Journal of Medicine and Philosophy* 8:181–185.

Beauchamp, Tom L., and James F. Childress. 1983. *Principles of biomedical ethics* (2nd ed.). New York: Oxford University Press.

Benjamin, Martin, and Joy Curtis. 1986. *Ethics in nursing*. New York: Oxford University Press.

Bishop, Anne H., and John R. Scudder, Jr. 1987. Nursing ethics in an age of controversy. *Advances in Nursing Science* 9 (3):34–43.

Caplan, Arthur. 1982. Applying morality to advances in biomedicine: Can and should this be done? In *New knowledge in the biomedical sciences*. William B. Bondeson, H. Tristram Engelhardt, Stuart F. Spiker, and John M. White, eds. Boston: D. Reidel.

Caplan, Arthur. 1983. Can applied ethics be effective in health care and should it strive to be? *Ethics* 93:311–319.

Cooper, C. Carolyn. 1988. Covenantal relationships: Grounding for the nursing ethic. *Advances in Nursing Science* 10 (4):48–59.

Crisham, Patricia. 1981. Measuring moral judgment in nursing dilemmas. *Nursing Research* 30:104–110.

Davis, Anne J., and Mila A. Aroskar. 1983. *Ethical dilemmas and nursing practice*. Norwalk, Conn.: Appleton-Century-Crofts.

Engelhardt, H. Tristram, Jr. 1986. *The foundations of bioethics*. New York: Oxford University Press.

Fletcher, Joseph. 1966. *Situation ethics: The new morality*. Philadelphia: Westminister Press.

Frankena, William K. 1983. Moral-point-of-view theories. In *Ethical theory in the last quarter of the twentieth century*. Norman E. Bowie, ed. Indianapolis: Hackett Publishing Company.

Fry, Sara T. 1988. The ethic of caring: Can it survive in nursing? *Nursing Outlook* 36 (1):48.

Gadow, Sally. 1985. Nurse and patient: The caring relationship. In *Caring, curing, coping: Nurse, physician, patient relationships*. Anne H. Bishop and John R. Scudder, Jr., eds. Birmingham, Ala.: University of Alabama Press.

Gilligan, Carol. 1977. In a different voice: Women's conception of self and of morality. *Harvard Educational Review* 47:481–517.

Gilligan, Carol. 1979. Woman's place in man's life cycle. *Harvard Educational Review* 49:431–446.

Gilligan, Carol. 1982. *In a different voice.* Cambridge, Mass.: Harvard University Press.

Gilligan, Carol. 1987. Gender difference and morality: The empirical base. In *Women and moral theory.* E. R. Kittay and D. T. Meyers, eds. Totowa, N.J.: Rowman & Littlefield.

Gladwin, Mary E. 1937. *Ethics: A texbook for nurses.* Philadelphia: W. B. Saunders Company.

Griffin, Anne P. 1983. A philosophical analysis of caring in nursing. *Journal of Advanced Nursing* 8:289–295.

Heidegger, Martin. [1927] 1962. *Being and time.* J. Macquarrie and E. Robinson, trans. New York: Harper & Row.

Huggins, Elizabeth A., and Cynthia C. Sclazi. 1988. Limitations and alternatives: Ethical practice theory in nursing. *Advances in Nursing Science* 10 (4):43–47.

Hume, David. [1751] 1957. *An inquiry concerning the principles of morals.* Indianapolis: Bobbs-Merrill Company.

Jameton, Andrew. 1984. *Nursing practice: The ethical issues.* Englewood Cliffs, N.J.: Prentice-Hall.

Kant, Immanuel. [1785] 1964. *Groundwork of the metaphysic of morals.* H. J. Paton, trans. New York: Harper & Row.

Ketefian, Shake. 1981a. Critical thinking, educational preparation, and development of moral judgment among selected groups of practicing nurses. *Nursing Research* 30:98–103.

Ketefian, Shake. 1981b. Moral reasoning and moral behavior among selected groups of practicing nurses. *Nursing Research* 30:171–176.

Ketefian, Shake. 1985. Professional and bureaucratic role conceptions and moral behavior among nurses. *Nursing Research* 32:248–253.

May, William F. 1975. Code, covenant, contract, or philanthropy. *Hastings Center Report* 5(1):29–38.

Mill, John S. [1863] 1971. *Utilitarianism.* S. Gorovitz, ed. Indianapolis: Bobbs-Merrill Co., Inc.

Munhall, Patricia. 1980. Moral reasoning levels of nursing students and faculty in a baccalaureate nursing program. *Image* 12(3):57–61.

Murphy, Catherine C. 1976. *Levels of moral reasoning in a selected group of nursing practitioners.* New York, Teachers College, Columbia University (unpublished doctoral dissertation).

Muyskens, James L. 1982. *Moral problems in nursing: A philosophical investigation.* Totowa, N.J.: Rowman & Littlefield.

Noddings, Nel. 1984. *Caring: A feminine approach to ethics & moral education.* Berkeley, CA: University of California Press.

Packard, John S., and Mary Ferrara. 1988. In search of the moral foundation of nursing. *Advances in Nursing Science* 10 (4):60–71.

Pellegrino, Edmund D. 1985. The caring ethic: The relation of physician to patient. In *Caring, curing, coping: Nurse, physician, patient relationships.* Anne H. Bishop and John R. Scudder, Jr., eds. Birmingham, Ala.: University of Alabama Press.

Pellegrino, Edmund D., and David C. Thomasma. 1988. *For the patient's good.* New York: Oxford University Press.

Prescott, Patricia A., Karen E. Dennis, and Ada K. Jacox. 1987. Clinical decision making of staff nurses. *Image* 19(2):56–62.

Ramsey, Paul. 1970. *The patient as person.* New Haven: Yale University Press.

Rawls, John. 1971. *A theory of justice.* Cambridge, Mass.: Harvard University Press.

Robb, Isabel H. 1900. *Nursing ethics: For hospital and private use.* Cleveland: E. C. Loeckert.

Self, Donnie J. 1987. A study of the foundations of ethical decision-making of nurses. *Theoretical Medicine* 8:85–95.

Silva, Mary C. 1984. Ethics, scarce resources, and the nurse executive: Perspectives on distributive justice. *Nursing Economics* 2:11–18.

Stenberg, Marjorie J. 1979. The search for a conceptual framework as a philosophic basis for nursing ethics: An examination of code, contract, context, and covenant. *Military Medicine* 144:9–22.

Thompson, Joyce B., and Henry O. Thompson. 1985. *Bioethical decision making for nurses.* Norwalk, Conn.: Appleton-Century-Crofts.

Toulmin, Stephen. 1981. The tyranny of principles. *The Hastings Center Report* 11 (6):31–39.

Veatch, Robert M. 1981. *A theory of medical ethics.* New York: Basic Books.

Veatch, Robert M., and Sara T. Fry. 1987. *Case studies in nursing ethics.* Philadelphia: J. B. Lippincott Company.

Watson, Jean. 1985. *Nursing: Human science and human care.* Norwalk, Conn.: Appleton-Century-Crofts.

Yarling, Roland B., and Beverly J. McElmurry. 1986. The moral foundation of nursing. *Advances in Nursing Science* 8 (2):63–73.

A Comment on Fry's "The Role of Caring in a Theory of Nursing Ethics"

JEANNINE ROSS BOYER and
JAMES LINDEMANN NELSON

Our response to Sara Fry's essay focuses on the difficulty of understanding her insistence on the fundamental character of caring in a theory of nursing ethics. We discuss a number of problems her text throws in the way of making sense of this idea, and outline our own proposal for how caring's role may be reasonably understood: not as an alternative object of value, competing with autonomy or patient good, but rather as an alternative way of responding toward that which is of value.

Sara T. Fry takes on two significant tasks: to reveal the masculine bias in standard nursing ethics theory, and to sketch the outline of an alternative view, sensitive to the influence of the sex-gender system in nursing, appreciative of the standpoint and experiences of women. She convincingly shows that contemporary work in nursing ethics, in the main, takes little note of the crucial fact that nursing is overwhelmingly a female profession; hence, mainstream treatments couch their discussion of the profession's moral dimension in terms taken virtually directly from the "standard" repertoire—contract theory, consequentialism versus nonconsequentialism, and other familiar, somewhat shopworn, notions. We very much appreciate this part of Fry's work, as it underscores by implication, but powerfully enough for that, just how invisible gender remains to nonfeminist theorists: if thoughtful scholars can miss the significance of gender differences when addressing a field as massively gender stratified as nursing, then the obscuring forces are powerful indeed.

In her second task, Fry meets with less success. When she tries to construct the foundations of a feminist nursing ethics—another endeavor much to be praised—we find that her constructive remarks have their own obscurities. Although some of these may be due to our deficiencies as readers of her text, her argument presents many interpretive puzzles. Here we attempt to put scattered pieces together—perhaps trimming a bit here and there and occasionally cutting new pieces to get a better fit. Although other parts of her essay also confuse us, we will focus our remarks on what she says about the *fundamental* character of caring in a feminist theory of nursing ethics. This idea is obviously central to her discussion, and a topic of great interest for both feminist ethical theory and feminist applied ethics. But it requires considerable work to sort out just what it is for a value to be "fundamental" in Fry's sense.

Consider her comments on Pellegrino's concept of "integral caring." On Fry's account, his model won't do for a theory of nursing ethics because the caring of which he speaks turns out to be merely a "derivative value," intended only to operationalize "patient good" (Fry, p. 100 above). She is unsatisfied because caring is more than a "mere behavior" between nurse and patient, and because nurse caring might not always be derived from a notion of patient good.

Insisting that caring is more than mere behavior is important, as doing so underscores the sense in which caring is a *particular* way of acting and hints that this sense may be morally significant, and neglected in mainstream ethics. For example, while mothers typically respond to a child's needs with a variety of attitudes and motivations, one can imagine a mother helping a child largely because of her conviction that duty demands it. But suppose Mom lays aside her writing to listen to Jamie's lengthy, rather self-involved narrative less out of duty than out of love for the child. It seems quite plausible that the more "caring" way in which the mother of this second image responds conveys a significant good of its own.[1] This sort of good seems fairly characteristic of the kind of nurturing work—including nursing—women have been assigned, and its worth has been inadequately explored. Unfortunately, Fry's paper does little to remedy that neglect. What she criticizes in Pellegrino is his failure to make caring fundamental, his willingness to subordinate it to a notion of patient good.

But unless something fairly significant is made out of caring as a particular kind of ethical response, it seems difficult to avoid seeing it as in some sense derivative. Caring, after all, seems necessarily to be caring about something, and to take at least some of its value from the object to which it is directed. (One could, for example, display "receptivity, relatedness, and responsiveness" toward the practice of wife-beating.)

What perhaps needs to be clarified is that caring does not parallel "autonomy" in the principle of "respect for autonomy"; it does not parallel "utility" in the principle "maximize overall utility." What it more nearly corresponds to (and provides an alternative to) are the ideas of "respect" and "maximization," the ways in which we comport ourselves regarding that which we value.

Now, putting the point thus baldly is no doubt too atomistic. Just as the object of a response can color our moral assessment of the response, so too the character of the response can affect our evaluation of its object. Further, for the kind of reasons alluded to in the story of Mom and Jamie, we're quite willing to accord an intrinsic significance to the caring response itself. But none of this seems to interest Fry. She prefers to criticize Pellegrino by maintaining that nurse caring may at times not be guided by his sense of patient's good (Fry, p. 100). Now, this seems dubious as a description of admirable nursing practice, especially when one recalls just how commodious is Pellegrino's notion of patient good—it embraces biomedical good, patients' conception of their own good, and the good that pertains to our nature as persons. One might well wonder, if you're not caring for a patient's good in one of these senses, just what are you caring for?

It is surely true that nursing involves cases where patients' subjective determination of their own good—one of Pellegrino's senses—may need to be challenged. For example, nurses who work in sexually transmitted disease clinics sometimes face the "worried well," who repeatedly present themselves for HIV testing; it may not always be an appropriate form of care to continually give them what they ask for. And there are even cases where a nurse may have to set aside, or at least subordinate, concern for one patient's good in all three senses: a public health nurse caring for a new mother and infant may be concerned enough about the baby's failure to thrive, or worried sufficiently about the infant's being exposed to sexual abuse, to override the protests of her other patient—the mother—and inform social services. But in neither of these cases is the nurse's caring directed to some end other than those delineated by Pellegrino. In the first case, the nurse may take herself to be enhancing the patient's ability to make meaningful choices, thus responding to the second and third of his senses; in the second, she is forced to care for the good of one of her patients to the possible detriment of the other.

Further, some ethicists recently have explored other grounds on which professionals may refuse to treat a patient according to that patient's desires. For example, Tomlinson and Brody have argued that a health care professional may refuse to initiate or continue cardiopulmonary resuscitation, despite the contrary wishes of the patient or patient surrogates.[2] But this kind of refusal to treat is either still based on patient good, or based on values that do not seem to have much to do with caring. In the *Journal of the American Medical Association*, Abigail Zuger reports that a patient rapidly dying from AIDS was, in effect, persuaded not to request a full code because his physician was convinced that his death and suffering would be prolonged by such intervention (Zuger 1989, 2988). If a nurse were to refuse a certain kind of treatment to a patient on this basis, she would not be ignoring patient good, but rather acting out of an understanding of patient good which is not identical to the patient's own assessment of his condition and needs, and hence acts as does the STD clinic nurse in our example.

A nurse might also be motivated to refuse to respond to a patient's request because she is convinced that to do so would be futile, and she objects to what she takes to be a misuse of her skills. But even if this ground for refusal—sometimes referred to as "professional integrity"—is allowed, it doesn't seem to cohere with caring in as natural a way as does the Pellegrino notion of patient good. It lacks the element of other-directedness that Fry's notion of care continually maintains. Of course, it could be argued that this is a flaw in Fry's understanding, that the nurse's need to *care for herself* should be more thoroughly explored, especially given the theoretical reservations that some feminists have had about the propensity of a care morality to reinforce the oppression of women, as well as the stark reality of the ongoing exploitation of nurses. However, at least in the main, the exploitation of nurses seems less a matter of their relationship with patients and more a matter of their relationship with other health care workers and the health care system. Legitimating the nurse's recognition of her own care-worthiness is not likely, therefore, to provide her with a basis for interaction with patients that is not sensitive to patient good.

Fry's own examples don't do any better than ours in showing what kind of caring distinct from patient good is supposed to be going on here. She points out that nurses care for patients whose good they don't know—but this is not the same thing as saying that their care is directed to something other than the patient's good. She points out that nurses and physicians may disagree about patient good, but that surely is not the same as labeling nursing interventions that do not contribute to the patient's good as "caring." Fry tells us that nurse caring relates to the patient's "status as a human being" (Fry, p. 100). But this is painfully obscure. In what way does it relate to the patient's status as a human being? And, even more crucially, how does its relation to the patient's status as a human being prevent caring from becoming a derivative value?

Perhaps some light can be cast on this by comparing her discussion of Pellegrino to her treatment of Frankena, on whose notion of the moral-point-of-view Fry so depends. Frankena speaks of care taking the form of respect for persons, or Christian love, and Fry seems to have no difficulty with this way of putting the matter (Fry, p. 103). But it would seem that the value of respect for persons, or of Christian love, plays a highly analogous role to patient good in Pellegrino's conception. It may well be that Frankena's moral-point-of-view idea contains more suggestive features for a developing feminist ethic than Pellegrino's—it incorporates an insistence on action, rather than simply belief in the acceptance of a theory, and its metaethical commitments seem more open. But while both of these points deserve further scrutiny, neither of them seems to distinguish the two positions in point of the derivativeness or otherwise of the value of caring. Caring, once again, seems a particular way in which one's regard for others is expressed. In our view, it is none the less important or distinctive for that.

In fact, if one returns to Gilligan's work, it seems that the major differences between the women and men she describes can be characterized as much in terms of process as in terms of what is valued. Recall Amy and Jake's response to Kohlberg's "Heinz dilemma," in which a woman will die unless her husband obtains a cure from a druggist who is charging an exorbitant, unaffordable fee (Gilligan 1982, 27–32). It is far from evident that Amy's hesitation over the option of stealing the drug comes from a belief that life is less important than property; looking at her response in that way was precisely Kohlberg's mistake. Much of what seems distinctive in her response is a concern for the maintenance of relationships, and that concern feeds a scope and a flexibility in her thinking, as well as a refusal to be beguiled by the artificial limits of Kohlberg's way of putting the case. These features of her moral response are surely virtues which tend to be overlooked by mainstream accounts of ethics, and if they are more characteristic of women than of men, then that is all the more reason why a feminist ethics of a woman-dominated field ought to make much of them.

Reflecting on Amy and Jake may suggest a solution to the puzzle Fry's text presents about the way in which caring is fundamental. A value may be fundamental in the sense that other values get their significance from the way they help or hinder it. But another sense in which a value can be fundamental is that it expresses a basic tendency toward action—not simply, as Frankena puts it, a nonindifference to others, but a positive and responsive nonindifference: a disposition to foster the other which may logically entail a prior knowledge of the other's good, but, considered psychologically, precedes it. Jake knew, logically enough, that the value of human life overrides that of property, and if the moral life is a mathematical exercise with human values serving as the "values of the variables," then his response was just right. But the moral life isn't like that at all, and Amy's stance of "empathetic nonindifference"—of caring enough to regard the characters in the Heinz hypothetical as though they were actually people with pasts and ongoing stories—is much preferable. None of this excuses caring from needing something to care for, and hence being a bit of a logical parasite. But it does indicate what point there is to insisting, despite its logically derivative character, that a fundamental moral stance of caring for persons, rather than, say, maintaining respect for principles, is a morally important idea.

It remains unclear how this way of understanding the fundamental role of caring in a theory of nursing ethics squares with the notion of human dignity, or with the role of values such as respect for persons or Christian love in a moral-point-of-view theory; perhaps Fry is groping after something quite different from what we are suggesting here.

But it does seem to us that she is both clear and correct about the idea of caring being a rich one for the development of a gender-sensitive nursing ethic. Attention to it may well highlight the special moral strengths of women (and men) who are members of the "caring professions," and seeing these strengths more clearly may, as Fry hopes, enhance theory and practice in other areas as well. And, as we noted earlier, attention to care possesses another, quite crucial advantage: it can alert us to its *dangers*. The exploitation of nurses by the health care system must be a major issue in any reasonable nursing ethic, as the exploitation of women by the patriarchy must be a chief concern in any reasonable general ethic. A focus on the role of caring in women's lives can aid in both understanding and challenging these deeply entrenched patterns.

NOTES

Our thanks to Hilde Lindemann Nelson for her careful reading of an earlier draft. This comment was originally published in *Hypatia* 5(3): 153–158 (1990).

1. See chapter 7, concerning the intrinsic value of the altruistic emotions, in Lawrence Blum (1980).

2. See, for example, Tomlinson and Brody (1988), 43–46.

REFERENCES

Blum, Lawrence A. 1980. *Friendship, altruism and morality*. Boston: Routledge and Kegan Paul.

Gilligan, Carol. 1982. *In a different voice.* Cambridge, Mass.: Harvard University Press.
Tomlinson, Tom, and Howard Brody. 1988. Ethics and communications in do-not-resuscitate orders. *New England Journal of Medicine* 318: 43–46.
Zuger, Abigail. 1989. High hopes. *Journal of the American Medical Association* 262 (21): 2988.

Ethics of Caring and the Institutional Ethics Committee

BETTY A. SICHEL ❖ ❖ ❖

Institutional ethics committees (IECs) in health care facilities now create moral policy, provide moral education, and consult with physicians and other health care workers. After sketching reasons for the development of IECs, this essay first examines the predominant moral standards it is often assumed IECs are now using, these standards being neo-Kantian principles of justice and utilitarian principles of the greatest good. Then, it is argued that a feminine ethics of care, as posited by Carol Gilligan and Nel Noddings, is an unacknowledged basis for IEC discussions and decisions. Further, it is suggested that feminine ethics of care can and should provide underlying theoretical tools and standards for IECs.

Institutional ethics committees[1] may be ideal vehicles for the ethical decision making and standards advocated in the feminine ethics of Nel Noddings (1984) and women's moral reasoning of Carol Gilligan (1982). If it accepts a Gilligan-Noddings theoretical framework, an institutional ethics committee (IEC) can be a communicative network with everyone concerned with the moral dilemma, can contribute to problem resolution, and can even frame policy. The ethical standards of a Gilligan-Noddings theory would include caring-for, compassion, concern, responsiveness,[2] and sensitivity to context. At present, however, studies of institutional ethics committees[3] rarely mention any of these standards as the basis for the goals, functions, and processes of these committees.[4] After briefly discussing the inception of IECs, their goals, structure, and functions, and the ethical standards they use, I examine how theories derived from Gilligan's and Noddings's work can provide a different theoretical framework for these committees.

HISTORICAL PERSPECTIVE: WHY INSTITUTIONAL ETHICS COMMITTEES

The impetus to form IECs in part derived from the consequences of a cluster of legal cases and federal mandates. Three of these indicate why health care professionals were motivated to establish IECs:

(i) *The New Jersey Supreme Court decision in the Karen Ann Quinlan case* (Weir 1977): Karen Quinlan, a comatose patient, was on a respirator. Though she was incompetent and irreversibly brain damaged (in a persistent vegetative state), Karen Quinlan was not brain-dead. Her father, a religious man, petitioned the Superior Court of New Jersey to have the respirator removed. The court justified its decision not to authorize removal of the respirator in a number of ways, e.g., citing expert medical testimony against removing the respirator, noting that the rapid advancement of medical knowledge made it impossible to foresee what future knowledge would mean for the patient's health, recognizing the absence of medical tradition to warrant the act, and referring to legal precedent. When Karen Quinlan's father then appealed the case to the Supreme Court of New Jersey, that court reversed the first decision and authorized the removal of the respirator[5] on the basis of an individual's right of privacy (Weir 1977).

The specific features of this case and both court decisions are unimportant here. However, one aspect of the decision drastically changed the character of medical institutional ethics. The Supreme Court judge stated that such institutions should seek the prior approval of an "ethics committee" for decisions regarding dilemmas like the Quinlan case. As noted by Fost and Cranford (1985, 2688), the expression "hospital ethics committee" in this decision "was a misnomer" since what the court "clearly intended was a neurological consultation committee: a group of persons expert in the medical, and particularly neurological prognosis of the patient." The court assumed that an ethical dilemma could be settled with the empirical facts of the case. The judge's decision in retrospect can be interpreted as positivistic since it assumed that facts would speak for themselves to reveal ethical choices; that expert medical knowledge alone could determine what decision should be made in a medical case. Though they realized that the judge had pinpointed a method and structure to resolve unusually difficult medical ethical dilemmas, some health care workers also recognized that expert knowledge alone would not suffice. Thus, they implicitly rejected a positivistic approach.

(ii) *The Baby Doe case*: The consequences of this 1982 Bloomington, Indiana, case frightened health care professionals and provided further impetus for the formation of IECs.[6] When Baby Doe was born with Down Syndrome and a malformed esophagus, the parents, agreeing with one of two conflicting medical opinions, decided that no operation should be performed and that the baby should just be kept comfortable. The hospital administration went to court to reverse the parents' decision. The legal efforts of the hospital failed when Baby Doe died. However, the case created considerable public outcry that included numerous newspaper and magazine articles and editorials. One ominous consequence of this case was intervention by the federal government. The resulting federal regulations on neonatal care were struck down in court for procedural reasons. Even though ensuing federal regulations were far less pernicious, administrators of health care facilities clearly saw the specter of massive federal intervention into medical policy and decision making. The question asked by health care professionals was, how can we avoid federal intervention? The American Academy of Pediatrics, in its desire to avoid "compulsory hospital notices, hotlines, and Baby Doe Squads" (Kuhse and Singer 1982, 177), promulgated policy on critically ill newborns. This policy included recommendations about the formation of IECs.

(iii) *The mandating of Institutional Review Boards (IRBs) to review experimentation with human beings in health care facilities*: Biomedical research in hospitals and other health care institutions often created a wide variety of ethical problems. When patients were used as subjects in these experiments, problems might include what comprised informed consent and what sorts of experiments should not be conducted even if subjects gave informed consent. For example, if one group of patients were to be given a medication that might alleviate symptoms of life-threatening illness and another sample with the same illness were given a placebo, should the experiment be permitted even if all patients give informed consent? The federal government was not concerned with the answer to this question, but with the method for making the decision.

In 1966, the federal government mandated the establishment of IRBs to evaluate the acceptability of biomedical research with patients of health care institutions and prescribed minimum guidelines for the membership of the boards (Glantz 1984). With this mandating, health care workers realized that there was considerable precedent for federal government intervention. Even if IRBs are now considered beneficial, the mandating of these boards was a further reason for health care professionals to seek other internal means to resolve day-to-day difficult and sensitive ethical dilemmas in all clinical situations. In addition, the relative success of IRBs suggested a general structure and method by which health care institutions could make ethical policy, provide consultative services, make ethical decisions, and offer educational services.

In addition to court cases and government intervention, other conditions during the late 1970s and early 1980s contributed to the belief that IECs could resolve new, unique, and complex health care ethical dilemmas. First, new medical technology created ethical situations with few if any precedents (Rosner 1985). Second, patients and their families no longer accepted passive roles but demanded active parts in making decisions about medical treatment. The rights movement resulted in the belief that each human being was an autonomous agent capable of making informed decisions regarding his or her own life and medical care. Even when patients such as infants, minor children, individuals with dementia senility, and the comatose were incompetent to make decisions, physicians felt constrained and without the right to make the ultimate decision about medical treatment. The question raised was, who had the right to make these decisions?

A change in the ethical climate of society is a fifth reason for the development of IECs. Just as with every other profession, there have been questions about the ethical behavior of physicians, e.g., questions about physicians receiving excessive Medicare and Medicaid payments and questions about how some families obtain infants without "normal" adoption procedures. Furthermore, malpractice suits against hospitals and physicians have caused health care professionals and institutions considerable concern about how they might protect themselves.

INSTITUTIONAL ETHICS COMMITTEES: PRESENT STATUS

This brief background sketch indicates that, in the late 1970s and early 1980s, the time was ripe for a new structure for making medical ethical decisions; an autonomous physician no longer could make all medical and ethical judgments for his or her patients. The structure chosen went beyond what was recommended by the court in the Quinlan case. IECs were formed; their purpose, according to Fost and Cranford (1985, 2688), is the "improvement of intrainstitutional or extrainstitutional public relations, education, development of policy and guidelines, a consultation for active decisions." No matter what articles about IECs state, a primary purpose for these committees is to protect health care institutions and personnel against malpractice claims. Therefore, committees usually include an attorney with expert knowledge of legal precedents in health care cases, e.g., such matters as the rights of families of patients to decide that a do-not-resuscitate (DNR) order be issued; instances of withdrawal of life support systems; questions about what treatment and care is considered a "life support system"; and court decisions overriding religious freedom especially in the case of minors. Even if protection against malpractice suits is mentioned as only one of a spectrum of purposes, legal ramifications still seem a major concern.

The emphasis on the legal consequences of health care policy and medical decisions may be one reason for arguing that a principled ethic of justice and rights underlies deliberations of IECs. A second reason that a theory of rights, principles, and justice seems basic to the deliberations of IECs is that certain policies and decisions involve questions of competition, prioritization, and scarce resources. Such a committee might justify the unequal allocation of scarce resources, provided that ethical principles govern the procedures, deliberation, and decisions on the distribution of these resources and the making of medical policy about such distribution.

As an example of scarce resource allocation, let us look at a case described by Macklin (1987, 155–156). All 15 beds in an intensive care unit (ICU) are taken. One patient is "an intravenous drug abuser with a diagnosis of acquired immune deficiency syndrome (AIDS) who . . . [is] considered terminally ill." Another is a brain-dead nineteen-year-old man whose family insists that every means be used to keep him alive. If a 63-year-old physics professor with a heart attack is brought to the emergency room, what decision should be made about who has priority for an ICU bed? Who has the right to this scarce resource? Should one of the patients in the ICU be transferred to a regular medical care floor? Should priority be given to the physicist? On what ethical basis should this decision be made? Should a theory of rights and justice or a form of utilitarian consequentialism be used to make the necessary choice? A theory of utilitarian consequentialism would ensure the maximization of the good, the greatest good for the greatest number. The saving of the physics professor's life by giving him the scarce resource, a bed in the ICU, the utilitarian might argue, would maximize the good since the physicist could subsequently contribute much greater good to human life than the brain-dead teenager or the terminally ill AIDS patient.

Deliberations and decisions might also be based on deontological theories, on neo-Kantian ethics, e.g., the principles of John Rawls's theory of justice as fairness. Rawls provides philosophical justification for the lexical or serial ordering of competing moral principles. Rather than accepting intuitively chosen principles, Rawls argues:

We can suppose that any principle in the (lexical) order is to be maximized subject to the condition that the preceding principles are fully satisfied. As an important case I shall . . . propose an ordering of this kind by ranking the principle of equal liberty prior to the principle regulating economic and social inequalities. This means, in effect, that the basic structure of society is to arrange the inequalities of wealth and authority in ways consistent with the equal liberties required by the preceding principle. (Rawls 1971, 43)

Just as Rawls gives priority to equal liberty, those deliberating on medical ethics policy might argue that certain principles have priority. The question to be answered by an IEC that accepts the notion of lexical ordering, would be which principles have priority, not the question of whether there should be such priority.

In still another sense, the decisions of IECs can be seen through a Rawlsean framework. When an IEC formulates medical policy, the committee is following a Rawlsean distinction between justifying rules or policy and justifying actions under rules (Rawls 1955). In the case of justifying rules or policy, the problem is how one justifies principles or general rules that would then be standards for making moral judgments. Though a moral principle or general moral rule could apply to a large class of moral dilemmas, it is logically possible for a moral rule to apply to a class of one or zero. For example, an IEC might stipulate policy for procedures in the adoption of newborns in the hospital and for physician involvement in these practices. Though there is policy for medical personnel to use in making decisions in potential adoption cases, there is no need for an adoption case ever to occur.

In the case of justifying actions under a rule, according to Rawls, an agent faced with a concrete moral dilemma uses appropriate moral rules or principles to resolve the dilemma. This is not a matter of automatically applying a set of rules to the moral dilemma and thereby having a simple formula to solve all moral dilemmas within an appropriate class. Even if a moral principle or rule exists, considerable reasoning will be necessary. The agent will have to decide the parameters of the problem, how the moral dilemma relates to the larger experiential situation, what moral principle or rule applies to the dilemma, and how hypothetical judgments relate to action and consequences.

For example, an IEC may have developed policy confirming a competent patient's right of informed consent prior to treatment or intrusive procedures. In a concrete moral dilemma, however, there often is a grey area between competency and incompetency. If a patient is unquestionably incompetent to make an informed decision, e.g., in the case of a comatose patient, who has the right to make decisions for the patient?

AN ETHICS OF CARE AND IECs

A different vantage point can reveal that many IECs can and do operate differently and tacitly seem to make use of the theories of Gilligan and Noddings. With a theory of universal and abstract principles, e.g., as articulated by Rawls, moral agents are not particular, concrete individuals with their own unique life histories, desires, and emotions. Further, neither these dimensions nor relationships with others, neither friendships nor community, should affect moral judgments. Instead, the moral agent is like a placemark, a variable in an algebraic equation, no better and no worse than any other person in that given moral situation. The criteria of deontological moral theory require that moral agents put themselves into the role of all relevant others, all of whom should be given equivalent weight.

Women's moral language of response and caring starts from a very different perspective: Moral dilemmas are particular, unique situations in which all parties retain their individual identities, their life histories, emotions, feelings, and re-lationships. Caring and relationship occur between particular concrete individuals. Moral situations exist within a particular historical and sociological context; they are bound by time and place. Women's morality emphasizes concrete situations, networks of relationships, caring, interpersonal communication, not hurting others, and responsiveness.

Nel Noddings's feminine ethical theory distinguishes between "caring for" and "caring about." Caring about something can distance the agent from the object of caring and involves impersonality, the cause and institution, numerous others never seen or known, the scientific experiment and the mathematical problem. Caring for focusses on emotions, feelings, and attitudes; yet, as with Hume (1967) and others, reasoning and intellectual processes are at the service of sentiment and emotion. The change of venue advocated by Noddings does not wholly ignore the theoretical contributions of traditional ethics, but assumes that only certain aspects of these ethics can inform and enrich the moral life of the one who cares for. The interpretation of Noddings's theory as accepting dimensions of traditional ethics may at first seem at odds with the stance she takes. For two reasons however, Noddings's theory can accommodate certain features of traditional theories, first, by virtue of a number of characteristics of public life and second, due to features of traditional theories that can interlock with her theory.

(i) *Ethical theories and forms of public life.* Noddings's feminine ethical theory refers to the individual moral agent, the one-caring, the one who cares for another. The theory can affect how hospital and nursing home workers resolve moral di-lemmas and how they care for another. However, the institution itself might very well not subscribe to this feminine ethic of caring. In other words, some health care professionals within the institutions would subscribe to an ethic of caring and would care for others, but the institution itself would subscribe to a different ethic. The institutional use of ethical principles of justice would not undermine Noddings's theory; but would embed it within a wider social, political, and legal context. In a sense, this is the continual struggle of morality, that a person's moral beliefs conflict with those of other individuals, institutions, or groups.[7] Individuals at times may change the quality of relationships within a group or institution through their adherence to an ethical theory other than the one underlying the institution.

(ii) *Traditional ethical theories and Noddings's theory.* Noddings's theory does not entirely stray from certain ideas in traditional ethical theories. Noddings accepts the idea that someone using an ethics of caring, someone caring for another, must often reason to make judgments to know what is right or wrong in order to care for another. We can find theoretical structures for this reasoning in recent works on feminist epistemology and feminist ways of knowing, and even in a wide range of traditional philosophical theories. Some of these ideas are hidden in the crevices of commonly accepted ethical theories,[8] and others are found in such resources as literature (Nussbaum 1983). Noddings would avoid the abstract principles of traditional theories. She would walk a narrow ridge to avoid the excessive abstractness and generalizations of traditional views and simultaneously would sidestep a profusion of unorganized, anarchic, fragmented facts.

AN ETHICS OF CARE AND IEC PRACTICE

When we examine the procedures, deliberations, goals, and functions of IECs, we realize that a rights and justice model is not necessarily appropriate, even though an IEC must often consider legal dimensions or precedents. In a number of ways, the workings of some IECs can be seen to be consistent with the feminine ethics of Noddings and women's moral reasoning of Gilligan. As in other caring relationships, the relationship between the one-caring, in this case the IEC, and the cared-for, the patient, requires a delicate balance. If the cared-for is a fully competent adult and thus able to make a decision, at what point does the one-caring intrude and override the cared-for's choice? Should an IEC ever override the cared-for's choice?

(i) *A Jehovah's Witness case.* A particularly difficult case is the cared-for who is a Jehovah's Witness.[9] IECs often develop policy regarding the refusal of a member of Jehovah's Witnesses to have blood transfusions. This policy may stipulate such items as when a person is fully competent and capable of making an informed consent, and what decisions medical personnel can make when an incapacitated Jehovah's Witness requires emergency care. The moral dilemma of Jehovah's Witnesses' patients who refuse blood transfusions is not settled because the patient has legal rights or because there is legal precedent and hospital policy. There may be problems such as whether family members apply undue pressure on the patient to refuse the transfusion or questions about when a patient is incapacitated. Medical professions may have a different type of moral dilemma in that they personally cannot accept the consequences of a patient's refusing a blood transfusion. Health care professionals may thus consult with an IEC about a particular patient.

In this consultation, an IEC is not an extraneous or artificial one-caring, but rather the committee joins an already established communicative network of ones who care for the patient. When a fully competent patient makes a decision to reject a blood transfusion, she probably has considered her membership in a caring network and has questioned what is required to continue to belong to that network. The patient judges on the basis of the values, beliefs, and the way of life that are accepted by herself and numerous other cherished members of the communicative network, in this case, other Jehovah's Witnesses. An IEC may accept this patient's decision not merely because of legal precedents and the patient's rights, but also because the committee puts aside its values and beliefs and becomes a member of the patient's primary caring network. By doing this, the IEC recognizes what it means to care-for and be cared-for within the patient's own primary network.

Through the choices and caring-for others of this IEC, the quality of relationships in both the Jehovah's Witness local community and in the IEC itself has been strengthened and changed.

Macklin (1987, 21–22) terms this type of problem a procedural problem. In an ethics of caring, who decides for an incompetent patient may be part of the ethical dilemma. For example, according to legal precedent, in the case of an elderly incompetent person, the spouse would usually decide; if there is no spouse or the spouse is incompetent, the oldest child would make the decision. Since Gilligan, in women's moral language of care, stresses the importance of communicative networks for the resolution of a moral dilemma, one person making a moral decision for an incompetent patient might destroy a primary communicative network. Thus, the decision of who is involved in making the decision, whether it is the entire familial network or only one person, is itself a critical component of a moral dilemma.

(ii) *A fictionalized case handled by an IEC.* The responsible physician at Big City Hospital brings a case to the hospital's IEC. The case concerns an 87-year-old man who lives by himself in a two-family home where his youngest daughter and her family live in the upper floor apartment. The living conditions are ideal. For the father can take care of himself, go to the senior citizens center, play cards with his cronies, make his own tea and linger over his newspaper, invite his friends to visit, have his other children and grandchildren visit him in his apartment, have privacy, take walks, etc. At the same time, his youngest daughter and her family can keep an eye on him and he can enjoy the intimacy of their relationship with him. One day he is brought to the hospital with chest pains and then admitted since the medical team is not certain of diagnosis. From the time Mr. A. enters the hospital, he keeps repeating things like, "I do not want to be connected to any of those fancy devices." "I do not want to be kept alive if I am a vegetable." "Don't let me suffer." "I've had a good life and now it is probably time to go." Members of the medical team describe him as a feisty, self-willed, confident person. He may not have had a college education, but he does have what is traditionally known as common sense.

By the time the IEC begins to consider the case, Mr. A. is in a coma. In addition to the heart condition, there are other more life-threatening conditions including pancreatic cancer. Mr. A. is now considered terminally ill. The responsible physician asks whether the patient's earlier comments warrant the issuance of a DNR order. In other words, should the earlier comments be interpreted as informed consent? The youngest daughter, who lives with the father in the two-family house, agrees with the physician, that a DNR order should be issued. However, the youngest daughter is a minority of one. The remaining children are horrified at the suggestion of issuing a DNR order. The IEC agrees with the physician and youngest daughter that the patient, when competent, gave permission for a DNR order. They argue that no matter what medical treatment and care may be given, Mr. A. will never have the human relationships with family and friends that had made life so valuable for him. He is irrevocably separated from his caring network. His network of caring others can care for him, but he can never again care for the other members of the network.

According to a theory of rights and justice, the committee's deliberations about this case might be considered completed; but with an ethics of caring, this cannot be the end of this case. The IEC also considers what the issuing of a DNR order against the wishes of the majority of the family will mean. It will not result in a malpractice suit against the physician or hospital, but serious damage may very well be done to a caring network. The other siblings may reject the youngest daughter or may argue among themselves as to why they had not been more strenuous in their objections. In order to avoid a serious rupture in a caring network, the IEC suggests that two of its members, a social worker and a cleric, should meet with the family to discuss the problem of the DNR order. At the meeting, these members of the IEC ask the family about their father, about his values and beliefs, about the father's conversations with them concerning their mother's suffering and treatment at the time of her death. In the end, after great emotional turmoil, thought, memories, and tears, the children themselves state that the DNR order should be issued. In this face-to-face relationship with the family, the IEC has indeed become the one-caring for a family. They encourage family members to recognize what they have to do if they are to continue to be the ones caring for their father. In all of this, the IEC members have been compassionate, collaborative, communicative, and sensitive. They have acted according to an ethic of care and compassion.

These examples by themselves do not *prove* that ethical theories derived from the work of Gilligan and Noddings can or should underlie the procedures, deliberations, and decisions of IECs. The examples do forcefully sustain two assertions made in this essay. First, the deliberations and methods of some IECs can presently be interpreted as consistent with an ethics of care and second, that such an ethics ought in the future to contribute to the strengthening of the quality of the decision-making process of IECs.

NOTES

1. In addition to the expression "institutional ethics committee," these committees are often known as medical ethics committees, clinical ethics committees, or hospital ethics committees. The institutional ethics committee should not be confused with an institutional review board that decides on the safety, efficacy, and ethics of experiments with human subjects.

2. The term "responsiveness" is not used by Gilligan. Throughout *In a Different Voice*, she uses the term "responsibility." However, since responsibility has traditionally been aligned with deontological theories, theories of rights and justice, I modify her term "responsibility" to "responsiveness." See Lyons 1983; Sichel 1985.

3. For a bibliography of studies of IECs or hospital ethics committees, see Macklin and Kupfer 1988, A5–A9.

4. Dugan (1987) attempts to understand the feminine voice in the ethical decision making of medical ethics committees, but does not recognize the theoretical components of that voice. He describes the model as the one "utilized by hospital Medical Ethics Committees" and as consistent with an integration of the "masculine and feminine voices." However,

the model presented by Dugan could be interpreted as John Dewey's method of reflective thinking.

5. It is noted that the Supreme Court did not authorize the removal of all life-support apparatus. Karen Quinlan continued to receive nourishment through various devices. For the distinction between life-support systems and normal care in this case, see Rachels 1986, p. 101.

6. Two other cases are frequently mentioned as triggers for institutional ethics committees. These were the Baby Jane Doe case in New York State and the case of the People v. Barber and Nejdl. For these and similar cases, see Kuhse and Singer 1982; Macklin 1987, 113–129.

7. For a discussion of these two moralities and the conflicts between the two, see Hampshire 1983, esp. pp. 101–125, 140–169.

8. One example can be found in the Socratic dialogues. Classical scholars traditionally have stressed Socrates' search for an abstract, universal meaning of an ethical term and the *aporia* ending of the early dialogues. What has received limited attention is the particularity of Socrates and an interlocutor's dialogue. Both Socrates and each interlocutor are actual persons with unique life histories. Furthermore, the early dialogues cannot be understood without understanding their particularity. Thus, in a variety of ways, these dialogues could yield ideas to strengthen feminist ethics.

9. According to most legal decisions, a fully competent adult who explicitly refuses a blood transfusion in a life threatening situation on religious grounds has a right to make this decision even if it results in his or her death. The patient according to this view has a right guaranteed by the First Amendment to the Constitution. There have been dissenters to this interpretation of the Constitution in that some legal opinions have asserted that even with a fully competent adult, there can be conflicting rights and that the religious right to choose not to have a blood transfusion is not absolute.

REFERENCES

Dugan, Daniel O. 1987. Masculine and feminine voices: Making ethical decisions in the care of the dying. *The Journal of Medical Humanities and Bioethics* 8: 129–140.

Fost, Norman, and Ronald E. Cranford. 1985. Hospital ethics committees. *Journal of the American Medical Association* 253: 2687–2692.

Gilligan, Carol. 1982. *In a different voice*. Cambridge, Mass.: Harvard University Press.

Glantz, Leonard H. 1984. Contrasting institutional review boards with institutional ethics committees. In *Institutional ethics committees and health care decision making*. Ronald E. Cranford and A. Edward Doudera, eds. Ann Arbor, Mich.: Health Administration Press.

Hampshire, Stuart. 1983. *Morality and conflict*. Cambridge, Mass.: Harvard University Press.

Kuhse, Helga, and Peter Singer. 1985. *Should the baby live?* Oxford: Oxford University Press.

Lyons, Nona Plessner. 1983. Two perspectives on self, relationship, and morality. *Harvard Educational Review* 53: 125–145.

Macklin, Ruth. 1987. *Mortal choices*. New York: Pantheon Books.

Macklin, Ruth, and Robin B. Kupfer. 1988. *Hospital ethics committees: Manual for a training program*. New York: Albert Einstein College of Medicine.

Noddings, Nel. 1984. *Caring: A feminine approach to ethics & moral education*. Berkeley, Calif.: University of California Press.

Nussbaum, Martha Craven. 1983. Flawed crystals: James's *The Golden Bowl* and literature as moral philosophy. *New Literary History* 15: 25–50.

Paget, Marianne A. 1988. *The unity of mistakes*. Philadelphia: Temple University Press.

Rachels, James. 1986. *The end of life*. Oxford: Oxford University Press.

Rawls, John. 1971. *A theory of justice*. Cambridge, Mass.: Harvard University Press.

Rawls, John. 1955. Two concepts of rules. *Philosophical Review* 64: 3–32.

Rosner, Fred. 1985. Hospital medical ethics committees: A review of their development. *Journal of the American Medical Association* 253: 2693.

Sichel, Betty A. 1985. Women's moral development in search of philosophical assumptions. *The Journal of Moral Education* 14: 149–161.

Weir, Robert F., ed. 1977. *Ethical issues in death and dying*. New York: Columbia University Press.

WOMEN AND CLINICAL
EXPERIMENTS

Re-visioning Clinical Research: Gender and the Ethics of Experimental Design

SUE V. ROSSER ❖ ❖ ❖

Since modern medicine is based substantially in clinical medical research, the flaws and ethical problems that arise in this research as it is conceived and practiced in the United States are likely to be reflected to some extent in current medicine and its practice. This paper explores some of the ways in which clinical research has suffered from an androcentric focus in its choice and definition of problems studied, approaches and methods used in design and interpretation of experiments, and theories and conclusions drawn from the research. Some examples of re-visioned research hint at solutions to the ethical dilemmas created by this biased focus; an increased number of feminists involved in clinical research may provide avenues for additional changes that would lead to improved health care for all.

INTRODUCTION

Since the practice of modern medicine depends heavily on clinical research, flaws and ethical problems in this research are likely to result in poorer health care and inequity in the medical treatment of disadvantaged groups. The first purpose of this essay is to explore some ways in which clinical research has been impaired and compromised by an androcentric focus in its choice and definition of problems studied, approaches and methods used, and theories and conclusions drawn.[1] Second, I shall describe some attempts to correct this biased focus and envision further improvement through feminist perspectives and approaches.

In scientific research, it is rarely admitted that data have been gathered and interpreted from a particular perspective. Since scientific research centers on the physical and natural world, it is presumed "objective"; therefore, the term "perspective" does not apply to it. However, the decisions, either conscious or unconscious, regarding what questions are asked, who is allowed to do the asking,

Hypatia vol. 4, no. 2 (Summer 1989) © by Sue V. Rosser

what information is collected, and who interprets that information create a particular vantage point from which the knowledge or truth is perceived.

Historians of science, particularly Thomas Kuhn (1970) and his followers, have pointed out that scientific theories are not objective and value-free but are paradigms that reflect the historical and social context in which they are conceived. In our culture, the institutionalized power, authority, and domination of men frequently result in acceptance of the male world view or androcentrism as the norm. Recognizing the influence of this androcentric perspective is particularly difficult for scientists because of their traditional belief in the objectivity of science which makes it difficult for them to admit that they actually hold any perspectives which may influence their data, approaches, and theories.

Feminist philosophers of science (Fee 1981, 1982; Haraway 1978; Hein 1981; Keller 1982) have described the specific ways in which the very objectivity said to be characteristic of scientific knowledge and the dichotomy between subject and object are, in fact, male ways of relating to the world, which specifically exclude women. Research has also become a masculine province in its choice and definition of problems studied, methods and experimental subjects used, and interpretation and application of experimental results.

Revealing the distortions in clinical research that emanate from the androcentric biases uncovers points at which a feminist ethics might influence this research. Feminist scientists (Bleier 1984; Birke 1986; Holmes 1981) and philosophers (Fee 1983) have called for more people-oriented and patient-centered research which would be likely to provide better health care for all.

Choice and Definition of Problems Studied

With the expense of sophisticated equipment, maintenance of laboratory animals and facilities, and salaries for qualified technicians and researchers, virtually no medical research is undertaken today without federal or foundation support. Gone are the days when individuals had laboratories in their homes or made significant discoveries working in isolation using homemade equipment. In fiscal 1987, the National Institutes of Health (NIH) funded approximately $6.1 billion of research (*Science and Government Report* 1988). Private foundations and state governments funded a smaller portion of the research (*NSF Science and Engineering Indicators* 1987).

The choice of problems for study in medical research is substantially determined by a national agenda that defines what is worthy of study, i.e. funding. As Marxist (Zimmerman 1980), African-American (McLeod 1987) and feminist critics (Hubbard 1983) of scientific research have pointed out, the scientific research that is undertaken reflects the societal bias towards the powerful who are overwhelmingly white, middle/upper class, and male in the United States. Obviously, the members of Congress who appropriate the funds for NIH and other federal agencies are overwhelmingly white, middle/upper class, and male; they are more likely to vote funds for research which they view as beneficial to health needs, as defined from their perspective.

It may be argued that actual priorities for medical research and allocations of funds are not set by members of Congress but by leaders in medical research who are employees of NIH or other federal agencies or who are brought in as consultants. Unfortunately the same descriptors—white, middle/upper class, and male—must be used to characterize the individuals in the theoretical and decision-making positions within the medical hierarchy and scientific establishment.

Women are lacking even at the level of the peer review committee, which is how NIH determines which of the competitive proposals submitted by researchers in a given area are funded. In the ten year interval 1975–1984, women went from 16.9 percent of NIH peer review committee members to only 17.9 percent; during this time, the total number of members nearly doubled from 733 to 1,264 (Filner 1986). Because the percentage of women post-doctoral fellows increased by 32 percent during the same time period, it seems likely that qualified women were available, but not used.

I believe that the results of having a huge preponderance of male leaders setting the priorities for medical research have definite effects on the choice and definition of problems for research:

1) Hypotheses are not formulated to focus on gender as a crucial part of the question being asked. Since it is clear that many diseases have different frequencies (heart disease, lupus), symptoms (gonorrhea), or complications (most sexually transmitted diseases) in the two sexes, scientists should routinely consider and test for differences or lack of differences based on gender in any hypothesis being tested. For example, when exploring the metabolism of a particular drug, one should routinely run tests in both males and females. Two dramatic, widely publicized recent examples demonstrate that sex differences are *not* routinely considered as part of the question asked. In a longitudinal study of the effects of cholesterol-lowering drugs, gender differences were not tested since the drug was tested on 3,806 men and no women (Hamilton 1985). In a similar test of the effects of aspirin on cardiovascular disease, which is now used widely by the pharmaceutical industry to support "taking one aspirin each day to prevent heart attacks," no females were included (Steering Committee of the Physicians Health Study Research Group 1988).

2) Some diseases which affect both sexes are defined as male diseases. Heart disease is the best example of a disease that has been so designated because of the fact that heart disease occurs more frequently in men at younger ages than women. Therefore, most of the funding for heart disease has been appropriated for research on predisposing factors for the disease (such as cholesterol level, lack of exercise, stress, smoking, and weight) using white, middle-aged, middle-class males.

This "male disease" designation has resulted in very little research being directed towards high risk groups of women. Heart disease is a leading cause of death in older women (Kirschstein 1985) who live an average of eight years longer than men (Boston Women's Health Book Collective 1984). It is also frequent in poor black women who have had several children (Manley et al. 1985). Virtually no research has explored predisposing factors for these groups who fall outside the disease definition established from an androcentric perspective. Recent data indicate that the designation of AIDS as a disease of male homosexuals and drug users has led researchers and health care practitioners to fail to understand the etiology and diagnosis of AIDS in women (Norwood 1988).

3) Research on conditions specific to females receives low priority, funding, and prestige. Some examples include dysmenorrhea, incontinency in older women, and nutrition in post-menopausal women. Effects of exercise level and duration upon alleviation of menstrual discomfort and amount of exposure to VDTs that results in the "cluster pregnancies" of women giving birth to deformed babies in certain industries have also received low priority. In contrast, significant amounts of time and money are expended upon clinical research on women's bodies in connection with other aspects of reproduction. In this century up until the 1970s considerable attention was devoted to the development of contraceptive devices for females rather than for males (Cowan 1980; Dreifus 1978). Furthermore, substantial clinical research has resulted in increasing medicalization and control of pregnancy, labor, and childbirth. Feminists have critiqued (Ehrenreich and English 1978; Holmes 1981) the conversion of a normal, natural process controlled by women into a clinical, and often surgical, procedure controlled by men. More recently, the new reproductive technologies such as amniocentesis, in vitro fertilization, and artificial insemination have become a major focus as means are sought to overcome infertility. Feminists (Arditti et al. 1984; Corea and Ince 1987; Corea et al. 1987) have warned of the extent to which these technologies place pressure upon women to produce the "perfect" child while placing control in the hands of the male medical establishment.

These examples suggest that considerable resources and attention are devoted to women's health issues when those issues are directly related to men's interest in controlling production of children. Contraceptive research may permit men to have sexual pleasure without the production of children; research on infertility, pregnancy, and childbirth has allowed men to assert more control over the production of more "perfect" children and over an aspect of women's lives over which they previously held less power.

4) Suggestions of fruitful questions for research based on the personal experience of women have also been ignored. In the health care area, women have often reported (and accepted among themselves) experiences that could not be documented by scientific experiments or were not accepted as valid by the researchers of the day. For decades, dysmenorrhea was attributed by most health care researchers and practitioners to psychological or social factors despite the reports from an overwhelming number of women that these were monthly experiences in their lives. Only after prostaglandins were "discovered" was there widespread acceptance among the male medical establishment that this experience reported by women had a biological component (Kirschstein 1985).

These four types of bias raise ethical issues: Health care practitioners must treat the majority of the population, which is female, based on information gathered from clinical research in which drugs may not have been tested on females, in

*painful menstration

which the etiology of the disease in women has not been studied and in which women's experience has been ignored.

Approaches and Methods

1) The scientific community has often failed to include females in animal studies in basic research as well as in clinical research unless the research centered on controlling the production of children. The reasons for the exclusion (cleaner data from males due to lack of interference from estrus or menstrual cycles, fear of inducing fetal deformities in pregnant subjects, and higher incidence of some diseases in males) are practical when viewed from a financial standpoint. However, the exclusion results in drugs that have not been adequately tested in women subjects before being marketed and in lack of information about the etiology of some diseases in women.

2) Using the male as the experimental subject not only ignores the fact that females may respond differently to the variable tested, it may also lead to less accurate models even in the male. Models which *more accurately* simulate functioning complex biological systems may be derived from using female rats as subjects in experiments. Women scientists such as Joan Hoffman have questioned the tradition of using male rats or primates as subjects. With the exception of insulin and the hormones of the female reproductive cycle, traditional endocrinological theory assumed that most of the 20-odd human hormones are kept constant in level in both males and females. Thus, the male of the species, whether rodent or primate, was chosen as the experimental subject because of his noncyclicity. However, new techniques of measuring blood hormone levels have demonstrated episodic, rather than steady, patterns of secretion of virtually all hormones in both males and females. As Hoffman points out, the rhythmic cycle of hormone secretion as also portrayed in the cycling female rat appears to be a more accurate model for the secretion of most hormones (Hoffman 1982).

3) When women have been used as experimental subjects, often they are treated as not fully human. In his attempts to investigate side effects (Goldzieher et al. 1971a) such as nervousness and depression (Goldzieher et al. 1971b) attributable to oral contraceptives, Goldzieher gave dummy pills to 76 women who sought treatment at a San Antonio clinic to prevent further pregnancies. None of the women were told that they were participating in research or receiving placebos (Veatch 1971; Cowan 1980). The women in Goldzieher's study were primarily poor, multiparous,* Mexican Americans. Research that raises similar issues about the ethics of informed consent was carried out on poor Puerto Rican women during the initial phases of testing the effectiveness of the pill as a contraceptive (Zimmerman 1980).

Frequently it is difficult to determine whether these women are treated as less than human because of their gender or whether race and class are more significant variables. From the Tuskegee syphilis experiment in which the effects of untreated syphilis were studied in 399 men over a period of forty years (Jones 1981), it is clear that men who are black and poor may not receive appropriate treatment or information about the experiment in which they are participating. Feminist scholars

* tending towards multiple births

(Dill 1983; Ruzek 1988) have begun to explore the extent to which gender, race and class become complex, interlocking political variables that may affect access to and quality of health care.

4) Current clinical research sets up a distance between the observer and the human object being studied. Several feminist philosophers (Keller 1985; Hein 1981; Haraway 1978; Harding 1986) have characterized this distancing as an androcentric approach. Distance between the observer and experimental subject may be more comfortable for men who are reared to feel more comfortable with autonomy and distance (Keller 1985) than for women who tend to value relationship and inter-dependency (Gilligan 1982).

5) Using only the methods traditional to a particular discipline may result in limited approaches that fail to reveal sufficient information about the problem being explored. This may be a particular difficulty for research surrounding medical problems of pregnancy, childbirth, menstruation, and menopause for which the methods of one discipline are clearly inadequate.

Methods which cross disciplinary boundaries or include combinations of methods traditionally used in separate fields may provide more appropriate approaches. For example, if the topic of research is occupational exposures that present a risk to the pregnant woman working in a plant where toxic chemicals are manufactured, a combination of methods traditionally used in social science research with methods frequently used in biology and chemistry may be the best approach. Checking the chromosomes of any miscarried fetuses, chemical analysis of placentae after birth, Apgar scores of the babies at birth, and blood samples of the newborns to determine trace amounts of the toxic chemicals would be appropriate biological and chemical methods used to gather data about the problem. In-depth interviews with women to discuss how they are feeling and any irregularities they detect during each month of the pregnancy, or evaluation using weekly written questionnaires regarding the pregnancy progress are methods more traditionally used in the social sciences for problems of this sort.

Jean Hamilton has called for interactive models that draw on both the social and natural sciences to explain complex problems:

> Particularly for understanding human, gender-related health, we need more in-teractive and contextual models that address the actual complexity of the phe-nomenon that is the subject of explanation. One example is the need for more phenomenological definitions of symptoms, along with increased recognition that psychology, behavioral studies, and sociology are among the 'basic sciences' for health research. Research on heart disease is one example of a field where it is recognized that both psychological stress and behaviors such as eating and cigarette smoking influence the onset and natural course of a disease process. (1985, IV-62)

Perhaps more women holding decision-making positions in designing and funding clinical research would result in more interdisciplinary research to study issues of women's health care such as menstruation, pregnancy, childbirth, lactation, and menopause. Those complex phenomena fall outside the range of methods of study provided by a sole discipline. The interdisciplinary approaches developed to solve these problems might then be applied to other complex problems to benefit all health care consumers, both male and female.

THEORIES AND CONCLUSIONS DRAWN FROM THE RESEARCH

The rationale which is traditionally presented in support of the "objective" methods is that they prevent bias. Emphasis upon traditional disciplinary approaches that are quantitative and maintain the distance between observer and experimental subject supposedly removes the bias of the researcher. Ironically, to the extent that these "objective" approaches are in fact synonymous with a masculine approach to the world, they may introduce bias. Specifically, androcentric bias may permeate the theories and conclusions drawn from the research in several ways:

1) First, theories may be presented in androcentric language. Much feminist scholarship has focussed on problems of sexism in language and the extent to which patriarchal language has excluded and limited women. (Thorne 1979; Lakoff 1975; Kramarae and Treichler 1986). Sexist language is a symptom of underlying sexism, but language also shapes our concepts and provides the framework through which we express our ideas. The awareness of sexism and the limitations of a patriarchal language that feminist researchers have might allow them to describe their observations in less gender-biased terms.

An awareness of language should aid experimenters in avoiding the use of terms such as "tomboyism" (Money and Erhardt 1972), "aggression" and "hysteria," which reflect assumptions about sex-appropriate behavior (Hamilton 1985) that permeate behavioral descriptions in clinical research. Once the bias in the terminology is exposed, the next step is to ask whether that terminology leads to a constraint or bias in the theory itself.

2) An androcentric perspective may lead to formulating theories and conclusions drawn from medical research to support the status quo of inequality for women and other oppressed groups. Building upon their awareness of these biases, women scientists have critiqued the studies of brain-hormone interaction (Bleier 1984) for their biological determinism used to justify women's socially inferior position. Bleier has repeatedly warned against extrapolating from one species to another in biochemical as well as behavioral traits. Perhaps male researchers are less likely to see flaws in and question biologically deterministic theories that provide scientific justification for men's superior status in society because they as men gain social power and status from such theories. Researchers from outside the mainstream (women for example) are much more likely to be critical of such theories since they lose power from those theories. In order to eliminate bias, the community of scientists undertaking clinical research needs to include individuals from backgrounds of as much variety and diversity as possible with regard to race, class, gender, and sexual preference (Rosser 1988). Only then is it less likely that the perspective of one group will bias research design, approaches, subjects, and interpretations.

Some changes in clinical research have come about because of the recognition of flaws and ethical problems for women discussed in this paper. Some of the changes are the result of critiques made by feminists and women scientists; some of the changes have been initiated by men.

The rise of the women's health movement in the 1970s encouraged women to question established medical authority, take responsibility for their own bodies (Boston Women's Health Book Collective 1984; Cowan 1980) and express new demands for clinical research and for access to health care. Feminist demands have led to increased availability of health related information to women consumers. Litigation and federal affirmative action programs have resulted in an increase from about 6% to about 40% of women medical students from 1960 to the present (Altekruse and Rosser in press). Consumer complaints and suggestions have fostered minor reforms in obstetrical care. The decor, ambiance, and regimens of birthing facilities have improved to provide personal and psychological support for the mother and to promote infant-parent bonding. However, concurrent with modest obstetrical modifications in hospitals, nurse midwives in most states have felt the backlash of professional efforts to control their practice and licensure status (Altekruse and Rosser in press). Efforts to increase the understanding of the biology of birth and translate that knowledge into clinical care expressed as acceptable infant mortality rates remain inadequate.

2) Guidelines have been developed that require any research project that is federally funded to ensure humane treatment of human subjects and fully informed consent. The impetus for the formation of the National Commission for the Protection of Human Subjects of Biomedical and Behavioral Research was the revelation of the abuses of human subjects during the Nuremberg war crimes trials and the Tuskegee syphilis experiments (Belmont Report 1975). However, the attention drawn by men such as Veatch (1971) to unethical issues surrounding the testing of oral contraceptives in women helped to ensure that women, especially pregnant women, were given particular consideration in the papers forming the basis of the Belmont Report (Levine 1978).

3) In recent years U.S. government agencies have shown increased sensitivity to clinical research surrounding women's health issues and the difficult ethical issues of including women in pharmacological research. The Public Health Service (PHS) Task Force on Women's Health Issues was commissioned to aid the PHS "as the agency works within its areas of jurisdiction and expertise to improve the health and well-being of women in the United States" (U.S. Department of Health and Human Services 1985). In her insightful commissioned paper "Avoiding Methodological and Policy-Making Biases in Gender-Related Health Research" for the Report to the Task Force, Jean Hamilton makes strong recommendations:

PHS consensus-development conference on "Gender-related Methods for Health Research" (for the development of guidelines) should be held. . . . The feasibility of including women in certain types of research needs to be reexamined. . . . A number of working groups should be formed: A working-group to reconsider the difficult ethical issues of including women in pharmacological research (e.g., extra-protection for women as research subjects, versus other means for informed consent) . . . A working-group to identify and to consider mechanisms to enhance the kind of multi-center, *collaborative* or *clinical research center* studies that would be most efficient in advancing our understanding of women and their health. . . . A working group or committee to consider ways to foster subject-selection in a way that allows for an examination of possible age, sex, and hormonal status effects. (Hamilton 1985, IV, 63–64)

4) Some attempts at patient involvement in research design and implementation have provided a mechanism to shorten the distance between the observer and subjects observed. Elizabeth Fee describes an account of occupational health research in an Italian factory:

Prior to 1969, occupational health research was done by specialists who would be asked by management to investigate a potential problem in the factory. . . . The procedure was rigorously objective, the results were submitted to management. The workers were the individualized and passive objects of this kind of research. In 1969, however, when workers' committees were established in the factories, they refused to allow this type of investigation. . . . Occupational health specialists had to discuss the ideas and procedures of research with workers' assemblies and see their "objective" expertise measured against the "subjective" experience of the workers. The mutual validation of data took place by testing in terms of the workers' experience of reality and not simply by statistical methods; the subjectivity of the workers' experience was involved at each level in the definition of the problem, the method of research, and the evaluation of solutions. Their collective experience was understood to be much more than the statistical combination of individual data; the workers had become the active subjects of research, involved in the production, evaluation, and uses of the knowledge relating to their own experience. (1983, 24)[2]

CONCLUSION

Replacing the androcentrism in the practice of medical research and the androcentric bias in the questions asked, methods used, and theories and conclusions drawn from data gathered with a feminist approach represents a major change with profound ethical implications. Lynda Birke, a feminist scientist, suggests that feminism will change science and medicine from research that is oppressive to women and potentially destructive to all towards liberation and improvement for everyone.

Perhaps this discussion of creating a feminist science seems hopelessly utopian. Perhaps. But feminism is, above all else, about wanting and working for change, change towards a better society in which women of all kinds are not devalued, or oppressed in any way. Working for change has to include changing science, which not only perpetuates our oppression at present, but threatens also to destroy humanity and all the other species with whom we share this earth. (1986, 171)

I have described some hints of the re-visioning of clinical research, prompted by liberation movements of the 1970s and 1980s, that have made health care somewhat less elitist, more humane, and more accessible to all. If a stronger feminist presence were to be felt in design and interpretation of research, who knows what additional improvements might occur? Bound by my own training in traditional science, I wear the blinders provided by the society to individuals of my class, race, and gender in the late 1980s. How can those of us, living with the current reality, visualize the new reality that can come about by the changes we are beginning?

Suzette Haden Elgin in her futuristic novel *Native Tongue* describes the impossibility of envisioning the new reality:

> "Perceive this . . . there was only one reason for the Encoding Project, really, other than just the joy of it. The hypothesis was that if we put the project into effect it would change reality."
>
> "Go on."
>
> "Well . . . you weren't taking that hypothesis seriously. I was."
>
> "We were."
>
> "No. No, you weren't. Because all your plans were based on the old reality. The one before the change."
>
> "But Nazareth, how can you plan for a new reality when you don't have the remotest idea what it would be like?" Aquina demanded indignantly. "That's not possible!"
>
> "Precisely," said Nazareth. "We have no science for that. We have pseudo-sciences, in which we extrapolate for a reality that would be nothing more than a minor variation on the one we have . . . but the science of actual reality change has not yet been even proposed, much less formalized." (1984, 294)

NOTES

1. Numerous feminist scientists (Keller 1982, 1985; Bleier 1984, 1986) and historians and philosophers of science (Hein 1981; Fee 1981, 1982; Haraway 1978) have documented an androcentric bias in scientific research.

2. This example challenges more than the quality of information garnered by objective research methods in which distance is maintained between the observer and the subject. It also raises questions addressed partially by the Belmont Report (1975) regarding the ethics of "double blind" experiments: Why shouldn't individuals whose health may be affected have a right to know what is being done for them and why? Is it ethical to give one group of individuals a placebo if the drug being tested is likely to cure a health problem they have or if withholding the drug will exacerbate the health problem? It also raises the more radical idea of subject involvement in experimental design and interpretation: Shouldn't the subjects be involved in defining what the problem is and the best approaches to solving the problem?

REFERENCES

Altekruse, Joan, and Sue V. Rosser. (In press). Women in the biomedical and health care industry. In *Knowledge explosion: Disciplines and debates*. Dale Spender and Cheris Kramarae, eds. New York: Pergamon Press.

Arditti, Rita, Renate Duelli Klein, and Shelley Minden, eds. 1984. *Test-tube women: What future for motherhood?* London: Pandora Press.

Belmont Report. 1978. Washington, DC: Department of Health, Education and Welfare. (Publication No. OS 78-0012).

Birke, Lynda. 1986. *Women, feminism, and biology*. New York: Methuen.

Bleier, Ruth. 1984. *Science and gender: A critique of biology and its theories on women*. New York: Pergamon Press.

Bleier, Ruth. 1986. Sex differences research: Science or belief? In *Feminist approaches to science*. Ruth Bleier, ed. New York: Pergamon Press.

Boston Women's Health Book Collective. 1984. *The new our bodies, ourselves*. New York: Simon and Schuster.

Corea, Gena, J. Hanmer, B. Hoskins, J. Raymond, R. Duelli Klein, H. B. Holmes, M. Kishwar, R. Rowland, R. Steinbacher, eds. 1987. *Man-made women: How new reproductive technologies affect women*. Bloomington: Indiana University Press.

Corea, Gena, and S. Ince. 1987. Report of a survey of IVF clinics in the USA. In *Made to order: The myth of reproductive and genetic progress*. Patricia Spallone and Deborah L. Steinberg, eds. Oxford: Pergamon Press.

Cowan, Belita. 1980. Ethical problems in government-funded contraceptive research. In *Birth control and controlling birth: Women-centered perspectives*. Helen Holmes, Betty Hoskins, and Michael Gross, eds. Clifton, NJ: Humana Press.

Dill, Bonnie T. 1983. Race, class and gender: Prospects for an all-inclusive sisterhood. *Feminist Studies* 9(1): 131–150.

Dreifus, Claudia. 1978. *Seizing our bodies*. New York: Vintage Books.

Ehrenreich, Barbara, and Deirdre English. 1978. *For her own good*. New York: Anchor Press.

Elgin, Suzette H. 1984. *Native tongue*. New York: Daw Book, Inc.

Fee, Elizabeth. 1981. Is feminism a threat to scientific objectivity? *International Journal of Women's Studies* 4: 213–233.

Fee, Elizabeth. 1982. A feminist critique of scientific objectivity. *Science for the People* 14 (4): 8.

Fee, Elizabeth. 1983. Women's nature and scientific objectivity. In *Woman's nature, rationalizations of inequality*. Marian Lowe and Ruth Hubbard, eds. New York: Pergamon Press.

Filner, Barbara. 1982. President's remarks. *AWIS*: XV (4), July/Aug.

Goldzieher, Joseph W., Louis Moses, Eugene Averkin, Cora Scheel, and Ben Taber. 1971a. A placebo-controlled double-blind crossover investigation of the side effects attributed to oral contraceptives. *Fertility and Sterility* 22 (9): 609–623.

Goldzieher, Joseph W., Louis Moses, Eugene Averkin, Cora Scheel, and Ben Taber. 1971b. Nervousness and depression attributed to oral contraceptives: A double-blind, placebo-controlled study. *American Journal of Obstetrics and Gynecology* 22: 1013–1020.

Hamilton, Jean. 1985. Avoiding methodological biases in gender-related research. In *Women's health report of the Public Health Service Task Force on Women's Health Issues*. Washington, DC: U.S. Dept. of Health and Human Services Public Health Service.

Haraway, Donna. 1978. Animal sociology and a natural economy of the body politic, Part I: A political physiology of dominance; and animal sociology and a natural economy of the body politic, Part II: The past is the contested zone: Human nature and theories of production and reproduction in primate behavior studies. *Signs: Journal of Women in Culture and Society* 4 (1): 21–60.

Harding, Sandra. 1986. *The science question in feminism.* Ithaca, NY: Cornell University Press.

Hein, Hilde. 1981. Women and science: Fitting men to think about nature. *International Journal of Women's Studies* 4: 369–377.

Hoffman, J. C. 1982. Biorhythms in human reproduction: The not-so-steady states. *Signs: Journal of Women in Culture and Society* 7 (4): 829–844.

Holmes, Helen B. 1981. Reproductive technologies: The birth of a women-centered analysis. In *The custom-made child?* Helen B. Holmes et al., eds. Clifton, NJ: Humana Press.

Holmes, Helen B., B. B. Hoskins, and Michael Gross, eds. 1980. *Birth control and controlling birth: Women-centered perspectives.* Clifton, NJ: Humana Press.

Hubbard, Ruth. 1983. Social effects of some contemporary myths about women. In *Woman's nature: Rationalizations of inequality.* Marian Lowe and Ruth Hubbard, eds. New York: Pergamon Press.

Jones, James H. 1981. *Bad blood: The Tuskegee syphilis experiment.* New York: The Free Press.

Keller, Evelyn. 1982. Feminism and science. *Signs: Journal of Women in Culture and Society* 7 (3): 589–602.

Keller, Evelyn. 1985. *Reflections on gender and science.* New Haven: Yale University Press.

Kirschstein, Ruth L. 1985. *Women's health: Report of the Public Health Service Task Force on Women's Health Issues.* Vol. 2. Washington, DC: U.S. Department of Health and Human Services Public Health Service.

Kramarae, Cheris, and Paula Treichler. 1986. *A feminist dictionary.* London: Pandora Press.

Kuhn, Thomas S. 1970. *The structure of scientific revolutions.* (2nd ed.). Chicago: The University of Chicago Press.

Lakoff, Robin. 1975. *Language and woman's place.* New York: Harper and Row Publishers, Inc.

Levine, Robert J. 1978. The nature and definition of informed consent. *The Belmont Report: Ethical principles and guidelines for the protection of human subjects of research.* Appendix 1. (DHEW Publication No. OS 78-0013) 3-1-91.

Levine, Robert J. 1986. *Ethics and regulation of clinical research.* (2nd ed.). Baltimore: Urban and Schwarzenberg.

McLeod, S. 1987. *Scientific colonialism: A cross-cultural comparison.* Washington, DC: Smithsonian Institution Press.

Manley, Audrey, Jane Lin-Fu, Magdalena Miranda, Alan Noonan, and Tanya Parker. 1985. Special health concerns of ethnic minority women in women's health. *Report of the Public Health Service Task Force on Women's Health Issues.* Washington, DC: U.S. Department of Health and Human Services.

Money, John, and Anke Erhardt. 1972. *Man and woman, boy and girl.* Baltimore: Johns Hopkins University Press.

National Science Foundation. 1986. *Report on women and minorities in science and engineering.* Washington, DC: National Science Foundation.

National Science Foundation science and engineering indicators. 1987. Washington, DC (NSB-1, Appendix Table 4-10).

Norwood, Chris. 1988. Alarming rise in deaths. *Ms.* July, 65–67.

Rosser, Sue V. 1988. Good science: Can it ever be gender-free? *Women's Studies International Forum* 11 (1): 13–19.

Ruzek, Sheryl. 1988. Women's health: Sisterhood is powerful, but so are race and class. Keynote address delivered at Southeast Women's Studies Association Annual Conference, February 27 at University of North Carolina—Chapel Hill.

Science and government report. 1988. Washington, DC March 1, 18(4): 1. Steering Committee of the Physician's Health Study Research Group. 1988. Special report: Preliminary report of findings from the aspirin component of the ongoing physician's health study. *New England Journal of Medicine* 318 (4): 262–264.

Thorne, Barrie. 1979. Claiming verbal space: Women, speech and language in college classrooms. Paper presented at the Research Conference on Educational Environments and the Undergraduate Woman, September 13–15, Wellesley, MA: Wellesley College.

U.S. Department of Health and Human Services. 1985. *Women's health: Report of the Public Health Service Task Force on Women's Issues.* Vol. 2. Washington, DC: Public Health Service.

Veatch, Robert M. 1971. Experimental pregnancy. *Hastings Center Report* 1: 2–3.

Zimmerman, B., et al. 1980. People's science. In *Science and Liberation.* Rita Arditti, Pat Brennan, and Steven Cavrak, eds. Boston: South End Press.

An Ethical Problem Concerning Recent Therapeutic Research on Breast Cancer

DON MARQUIS ❖ ❖ ❖

The surgical treatment of breast cancer has changed in recent years. Analysis of the research that led to these changes yields apparently good arguments for all of the following: (1) The research yielded very great benefits for women. (2) There was no other way of obtaining these benefits. (3) This research violated the fundamental rights of the women who were research subjects. This sets a problem for ethics at many levels.

Breast cancer is a scourge among women. One in fourteen will get breast cancer during her lifetime. Each year 100,000 cases of breast cancer are diagnosed in the United States and 30,000 deaths are attributed to the disease (DeVita et al. 1985, 1119). Even though surgery for early breast cancer is often curative, women with breast cancer are often forced into continued contact with the medical profession. Chemotherapy or hormonal therapy after apparently successful surgery is often advisable. Chemotherapy for breast cancer where there is clinical evidence of spread beyond adjoining lymph nodes is not curative, but can produce remission. Sometimes multiple remissions can be produced with successive, different chemotherapeutic regimens. Radiation therapy for advanced disease is often beneficial.

Doctors have at least three moral duties to women with breast cancer. One obligation is to offer their patients what is, in their professional judgment, the best treatment or treatments. This duty clearly entails a corresponding patient right: a right to best medical care by one's doctor. This has been called "the therapeutic obligation" (Marquis 1983, 42; Gifford 1986, 348).

Respect for a patient's right of informed consent is another duty of doctors. All persons have the right to refuse invasive medical treatment. Although there are disagreements concerning the basis of this right, one secure foundation appears to be the right of all competent adults to refuse the voluntary touching or invasion of their bodies. Not only medical intrusion, but also domestic violence, rape, and physical sexual harassment fall within the scope of this fundamental and indisputable right.

This right is particularly important in the context of breast cancer. Except in unusual situations the right to refuse medical care is only of theoretical importance when treatment is curative and refusal means death or serious disability. However, a clinical oncologist may be able to offer a woman with breast cancer a choice of chemotherapies in which different probabilities of response are balanced against different toxicities associated with the treatments. In the case of surgery for breast cancer, there has been controversy concerning which surgical procedure produces the best probability of disease-free survival. When there are different degrees of disfiguration associated with the surgeries and no consensus among medical researchers concerning which surgery is best, the right of informed choice among alternatives is of great importance.

This right imposes some positive obligations on doctors. The right to informed consent is meaningless unless a physician explains fairly and with as little bias as possible the treatment options that are available. Accordingly, this right entails a doctor's positive duty to provide a good deal of information. Risks and benefits must be covered. Perhaps the evidence supporting each alternative must be discussed. Arguably, a doctor even has an obligation to present the opinions of other specialists who hold different views concerning recommended treatment. The point of all of this is clear: since a woman has the right to control her own body, she has the right, not just to refuse to sign some consent form, but to as meaningful and as informed a choice as possible concerning her treatment for breast cancer (Katz 1978; Robinson 1972).

Doctors' third moral duty is to pursue an active program of research into the causes, prevention, treatment, and cure of breast cancer. In contrast to the therapeutic obligation, this is not an obligation of each individual doctor. Not all doctors have the duty to engage in research. However, the medical profession as a whole, with society's cooperation, has an obligation to pursue this task. The well-being of all women is the moral basis for this social duty. This will be referred to as "the research obligation."

Recent research into the surgical treatment of breast cancer involves consideration of all three duties because the research necessarily involved women who were actually being treated for breast cancer. Whether observance of all three of these duties was possible in recent breast cancer research raises issues of fundamental importance for feminists.

MASTECTOMY AND CONVENTIONAL RANDOMIZATION

For many years in this country the Halsted radical mastectomy was the standard treatment for early breast cancer. This surgery involved removal of the entire breast surrounding the malignant lump, removal of the lymph nodes under the arm on that side, and removal of the pectoral muscles underneath the cancerous breast. This disfiguring surgery could lead to swelling of the upper arm and to difficulties with moving that arm. Such radical surgery was justified on the grounds that cancer cells might have started to spread through the lymphatic system from the original lump. Hence, removal of as much tissue as possible was necessary in order to maximize the chances of "getting it all."

For various reasons during the 1960s, controversy developed within the medical community concerning whether the length of survival without clinical evidence of recurrence of the cancer (called "disease-free survival") would be as good with less extensive surgery. In particular, the issue concerned whether simple mastectomy, in which only the breast containing the tumor was removed but in which the pectoral muscles immediately under the breast were preserved, yielded a disease-free survival rate that was as good as that of the Halsted radical mastectomy. In 1971, Bernard Fisher and his colleagues began a study to resolve this issue (Fisher et al. 1985b). Fisher's study was a randomized clinical trial. A diagram will aid in understanding its nature (see Figure 1).

Patients who participated in this study had potentially curable breast cancer[1] (Step 1), were asked by their doctors to be in this study (Step 2), and consented to participate (Step 3). Patients consented to have the surgery that they received determined by a randomizing device (Step 4). This means that whether a particular patient in the study received a radical mastectomy or a simple mastectomy was neither chosen by her doctor, nor chosen by the patient. It was determined by some randomizing device, such as the flip of a fair coin.

Many surgeons would be much more comfortable (as physicians) participating in a nonrandomized study in which the outcomes of patients whose surgeons believed radical mastectomy would be best were compared to the outcomes of patients whose surgeons believed simple mastectomy would be best (Taylor 1984, 1365). And undoubtedly many patients would have been more comfortable participating in a study in which they had chosen either the more or less extensive surgery after a chance to weigh and to discuss each alternative. Nevertheless, the community of medical scientists and statisticians believes that neither of these designs would yield reliable results. They believe that this randomized clinical trial of radical vs. simple mastectomy provided the only way of deciding whether disease-free survival after simple mastectomy was as good as disease-free survival after radical mastectomy.

This attitude is not restricted to breast cancer. In the United States randomized clinical trials are ordinarily required by the Food and Drug Administration before a new drug can be released. Differently designed studies can yield data that suggest greater efficacy, of course; however, unless the situation is exceptional, most medical scientists will not regard a claim concerning the effectiveness of treatment in any area of medicine as established unless that claim is confirmed by at least one, and possibly more than one, randomized study (Byar 1979; Sacks, Chalmers, and Smith 1982; Vaisrub 1985; Angell 1984).

The reasons that support this virtual consensus appear compelling. Neglect of the randomized clinical trial requirement in the past has resulted in the use of ineffective treatments (Chalmers 1967; Sacks, Chalmers, and Smith 1982). Furthermore, there seem to be many problems with non-randomized designs for comparing radical and simple mastectomy.

Suppose in the early 1970s one group of patients who received radical mastectomies because their doctors believed that procedure was best for them was compared to another group of patients who received simple mastectomy because their

FIGURE 1

Conventional Randomized Trial
Radical Mastectomy vs. Simple Mastectomy

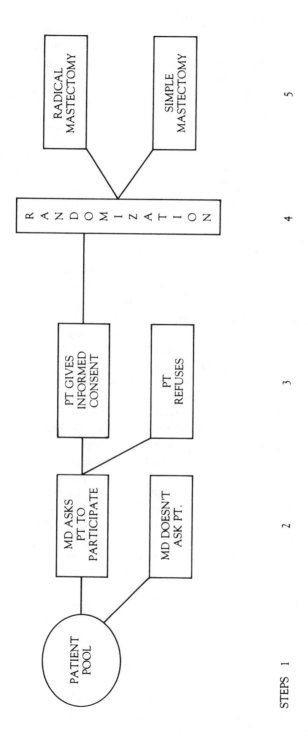

STEPS   1   2   3   4   5

doctors believed that procedure was best for them. Can the disease-free survival of the two groups be compared to *establish* the relative efficacies of the procedures?

This design would yield decisive results only if *all* the factors that are correlated with outcome are evenly distributed between the two groups. This would require heroic and accurate documentation efforts on a huge group of patients (Gifford 1986). It also presupposes that all the factors that are correlated with outcome in women who already have breast cancer are known. *This* presupposition is *known* to be false. Finally, there is some reason for thinking that a worse outcome in the early 1970s would be correlated with being chosen by one's physician for radical rather than simple mastectomy. After all, if a surgeon's clinical judgment suggested that some particular patient had a worse prognosis, he or she would be likely to recommend the more radical surgery. This design, which accords so well with a doctor's therapeutic obligation, would not yield reliable results, which conflicts with doctors' research obligation.

A design comparing patients receiving simple mastectomy to patients receiving radical mastectomy in which the groups are determined by patients' free informed choice is subject to almost the same difficulties. The sample size would have to be huge and the data collecting heroic and accurate. There is some reason to think that patients might choose the more radical surgery because they react to nonverbal communication from their doctors concerning the seriousness of their disease. If this were so, the study would be biased. If many surgeons believed it might be biased (and they would have), then they would continue to do radical mastectomies no matter what the study showed. Accordingly, research designed in this way, although it accords well with a doctor's obligation to respect the right of informed consent, would also not yield results helpful to women.

Compare a randomized design to these other designs. As a result of randomization, *all* factors, known and *unknown*, that might bias the results are themselves randomly distributed. Therefore, the larger the sample of patients studied, the less likely it is that the results will be biased. Statisticians have developed ways of calculating the size of the sample needed to have any specific degree of confidence in the results *without* knowing the biasing factors or the degree of bias. Therefore, there appear to be good reasons for accepting the views of medical researchers that, unless very special circumstances obtain, the randomized clinical trial is the only reliable method we have for establishing that one treatment is better than or as good as another. This is why a randomized study was conducted to answer the question: is radical mastectomy an unnecessarily disfiguring operation?

Not only does Fisher's study design seem superior, it also seems not to have interfered with doctors' other moral duties. If surgeons believe that there is no good medical reason to choose one surgery over another, then they have not violated their therapeutic obligation to their patients by asking them to accept randomization. If a patient's consent to have her treatment determined randomly is as free and informed as possible, then the duty to respect informed consent has not been violated.

This study also fulfilled doctors' research obligations. One thousand seven hundred sixty-five patients were enrolled in this study of radical mastectomy vs. simple mastectomy. Ten year results show *no* better disease-free survival with radical mastectomy than with simple mastectomy (Fisher 1985b). Because many women have been spared unnecessarily deforming surgery this study has been truly beneficial.

Another study was suggested by data that emerged in the 1970s. Some surgeons wondered whether or not good results could be obtained in early breast cancer if only the tumor and a small surrounding margin of breast were removed and the breast was preserved. Although this technically is called "segmental mastectomy," almost everyone, including doctors, calls it "lumpectomy." As a consequence, Fisher and his colleagues began another randomized clinical trial to compare disease-free survival of lumpectomy either with or without radiation therapy to simple mastectomy (Fisher et al. 1985a).

The design of this study was basically the same as the design of the earlier study except that three treatments were compared instead of two. Patients with early breast cancer were asked to give their informed consent to be randomized to receive either lumpectomy with radiation therapy or to receive lumpectomy without radiation therapy or to receive a simple mastectomy.

Enrollment in this study was so slow that the study could not be completed as designed (Fisher et al. 1985a; Ellenberg 1984). It is not difficult to understand why this was so. No doubt women were unwilling to consent to having the issue of whether or not their breasts would be amputated decided by the equivalent of the flip of a coin. Plainly we have the beginnings of a problem. On the one hand, apparently convincing arguments exist for the view that only a randomized study is reliable enough to establish whether or not simple mastectomy is excessively mutilating.[2] On the other hand, such a study could not be completed because, apparently, consent could not be obtained.

THE NATURE OF THE PRERANDOMIZED DESIGN

When Fisher's team realized that their conventionally randomized study could not be completed, they adopted a prerandomized design. A diagram will help explain how prerandomization is different from conventional randomization (see Figure 2). The reason this design is called "prerandomized" is that randomization (Step 3) occurs *before* consent (Step 5). In a conventionally randomized design, by contrast, randomization occurs *after* consent is obtained (compare Figure 1). In this prerandomized design doctors decide which patients shall participate in the study before asking them to participate (Step 2). They then call the statistician to have their patient randomized to a treatment (Step 3) without yet having asked her for consent (Step 5). After doctors learn from the statistician the treatment to which the patient has been assigned by randomization (Step 4), they *then* ask her for consent (Step 5). Prerandomization's proponents believe that prerandomized patients should feel more comfortable consenting to be on the study because they know what treatment they would be getting when they consent. They believe that doctors will feel more comfortable asking patients to participate for the same reason. As a consequence, a prerandomized study is supposed to enroll more rapidly than a conventionally randomized study (Zelen 1979).

FIGURE 2

PRERANDOMIZED CLINICAL TRIAL

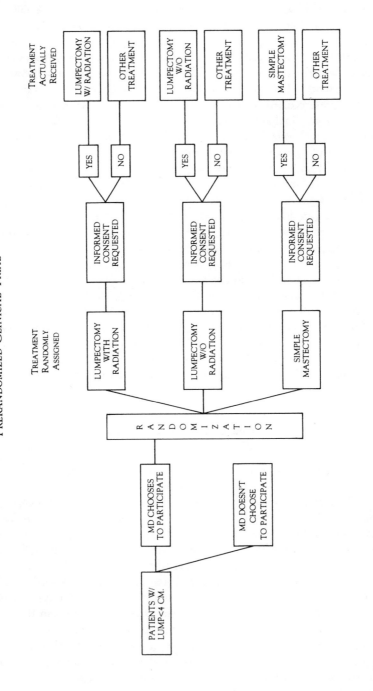

STEPS   1   2   3   4   5   6   7

Of course, patients have the right to decline the treatment to which they were randomized (Step 6). In a study such as this one, surely some will. It seems reasonable to suppose that patients who decline will prefer to receive one of the other treatments on the study. If any patients decline the treatment to which they were randomized, then the group of patients who were *randomly assigned* to a particular treatment (Step 4) will be different from the group of patients who actually *receive* that particular treatment (Step 7). Consider for example a patient randomly assigned to simple mastectomy. The random assignment takes place *before* the doctor discusses the study with the patient. Suppose that patient prefers lumpectomy without radiation therapy. If so when asked for informed consent to participate in the trial by receiving a simple mastectomy, she may decline and may choose lumpectomy without radiation therapy, as she has the right to do. Hence, that patient will be in the group *randomly assigned* to mastectomy, but in the group that *receives* lumpectomy without radiation therapy. Plainly this disparity may occur with any treatment group. Therefore, when the results of a prerandomized study are evaluated, there is a choice that does not exist in a conventionally randomized study. The disease-free survival of patients who actually *receive* each treatment can be compared *or* the disease-free survival of patients who are *randomly assigned* to each treatment can be compared. Which comparison should be made?

Intuitively, it might seem that one should compare the groups actually receiving different treatments. After all, the main purpose of doing this research is to find out whether patients who receive simple mastectomy do better than patients who receive lumpectomy either with or without radiation. In spite of these considerations, there appears to be a decisive argument against this method of evaluation. Membership in the group of patients enrolled in this study who actually *receive* a particular treatment is determined in part by patient choice. The more the treatments to which patients have been randomly assigned are refused, the more patient choice will determine the composition of the treatment groups. The reasons for women's choices may be correlated with the outcome of their diseases. For example, presumably women will be inclined to choose the more mutilating surgery the more serious they believe their disease is. If this belief has any basis in reality, the results of the study will be biased. Indeed, the problem with a prerandomized design in which outcomes of each group *receiving* each treatment are compared is basically the same as the problem with an entirely nonrandomized design in which the groups that are compared are determined entirely by patient choice. And, our earlier discussion showed that this latter design could not yield reliable results.

Therefore in order to preserve the scientific virtues of randomization, the groups randomly assigned to each treatment must be compared even when they include patients who received one of the other treatments. A mastectomy group so constituted will contain women who actually received lumpectomies (see Figure 2). This dilutes the power of the study, that is, the capacity of a given sample size of patients to reflect a difference in treatment efficacy if there really is one. Because of this dilution effect, the larger the percentage of refusals, the larger the sample has to be to retain the power of the study. Even a 15% refusal rate entails that the sample size necessary to complete the study will have to be twice the sample size of the corresponding conventionally randomized study (Ellenberg 1984, 1405).

This characteristic of prerandomized clinical trials makes them less efficient and, consequently, more difficult to complete.[3]

THE ETHICS OF PRERANDOMIZATION

It is easy to understand why surgeons might feel more comfortable asking their patients to participate in a prerandomized study than in a conventionally randomized study. In a prerandomized study they can approach patients with a particular treatment; in a conventionally randomized study, they approach patients with what must seem to be a gambling device. Patients may feel more comfortable consenting to be on a prerandomized study, for when they consent, they know what treatment they would receive. Consenting to conventional randomization is consenting to uncertainty. In short, the doctor-patient interaction in a prerandomized study seems to mimic a purely therapeutic interaction instead of an interaction characterized by chance.

Reflection on the ethics of the doctor-patient interaction in a prerandomized trial suggests a different understanding of the context of prerandomization. Although a surgeon can approach a patient with a particular treatment, this treatment cannot be a therapeutic recommendation. The doctor did not choose that treatment as best for the patient; the surgery "recommended" was determined solely by a randomizing device. A doctor who would like to recommend a particular therapy to a patient because he or she believes it therapeutically superior could not ethically participate in the trial. In such a situation, had the randomizing device selected another treatment, the surgeon would have been in the position of recommending a treatment believed to be inferior. This violates the therapeutic obligation. Accordingly, physicians who are ethical and who participate in a prerandomized trial must destroy in their conversation with patients exactly what may make both doctors and patients comfortable: the appearance of a therapeutic recommendation. Unless doctors do that, patients may easily mistake a recommendation based on chance for a recommendation based on therapeutic judgment.

Of course, each woman facing surgery for breast cancer has the right of informed consent and all that is entailed by that right, whatever her doctor should recommend. In a purely therapeutic context, many women, no doubt, would decide to take their doctors' advice. After all, many chose their doctors because they have confidence in them. In addition, most women who have just learned they have breast cancer feel weak and vulnerable. However, in the context of a prerandomized trial, informed consent becomes even more significant because the physicians who participate in the trial, if ethical, won't have a particular therapeutic recommendation. Women in the study can choose any of the three treatments without the pressure of rejecting an authority figure's therapeutic recommendation. Because the treatment they are offered was actually chosen at random, their physician, if ethical, can have no therapeutic reason for recommending it. Therefore patients on this trial would have a good deal *more* freedom than in the usual purely therapeutic situation to decline the treatment they were offered. They can choose the treatment with which they are most comfortable under the assumption that there is no good reason to believe that any treatment involves a therapeutic disadvantage. All this makes clear that although the prerandomized situation might seem to mimic the purely therapeutic context, randomization must be explicitly recognized by both doctor and patient as central to a *pre*randomized clinical trial.

In view of this, how can one explain how the prerandomized version of the lumpectomy vs. simple mastectomy study actually did enroll enough women to be completed, although the conventionally randomized version did not? One possible explanation is that doctors were more comfortable approaching patients when a prerandomized design for the trial was used because the prerandomized context mimics the purely therapeutic context. The argument in the above paragraph established that physicians in prerandomized trials have a duty to ensure that patients understand that treatment was chosen randomly. Therefore, this explanation succeeds only if physicians violated that duty. Another possible explanation is that women were more willing to participate when they were told outright what treatment they would receive. However, if women were unwilling to accept having the retention of their breast determined by a randomizing device in a conventionally randomized study, it is difficult to understand why they would accept the very same thing in a prerandomized study unless their physicians had failed to explain clearly the nature of the study. Furthermore, a significant percentage of refusals to accept the treatment to which patients are randomly assigned in a prerandomized study requires that the sample size of a prerandomized study be increased as compared with the sample of the corresponding conventionally randomized study. Therefore, the prerandomized study should have been *more* difficult to complete than the conventionally randomized study. Hence, the issue becomes: is there any explanation of the success of the prerandomized mastectomy vs. lumpectomy trial, given the failure of the conventionally randomized version of the trial, that is compatible with the assumption that the trial was conducted ethically?

SOME POSSIBLE EXPLANATIONS

Susan Ellenberg, in a discussion of some ethical concerns regarding prerandomization, has offered what amounts to a *possible* explanation of the success of this prerandomized breast cancer study.

> Knowledge by the physician of the assigned treatment allows conscious or subconscious tailoring of the study presentation to predispose the patient to accept the assigned therapy. If the patient has been assigned to standard therapy, the physician may stress the experimental nature of the new therapy, its potential risks, and the possibility that the new therapy may be worse than the standard one. If the patient has been assigned to the experimental therapy, the physician may stress the unsatisfactory track record of the standard therapy and the promising earlier studies that indicated that the experimental therapy may be an improvement. The physician may gloss over or even omit the information that treatment has been chosen by a random mechanism and imply to the patient

that the assigned therapy has been individually selected for the patient (Ellenberg 1984, 1406–1407).

If doctors in the mastectomy-lumpectomy trial behaved as Ellenberg suggests they may have behaved, then they violated their patients' right of informed consent. Those patients would have been deceitfully manipulated into believing that any treatment to which they were randomly assigned was, in their physicians' view, therapeutically superior. If Ellenberg's possible explanation is the actual explanation of the success of this trial, then the trial was unethical.

Are there other possible explanations for the success of this prerandomized trial? There are some empirical data concerning this study that are illuminating: Taylor (1984) did a study to discover why physicians had not been successful in enrolling patients on the conventionally randomized version of this study. Physicians who returned her questionnaires cited such reasons as (1) the study interfered with the traditional doctor-patient relationship, (2) informed consent was difficult to obtain, (3) physicians had difficulty telling patients they did not know which surgical option was better, (4) some physicians believed they already knew which treatment was better, (5) some physicians believed they would be personally responsible for patients randomized to a treatment that turned out to be worse, and (6) some physicians believed that the research protocol was too inflexible.

Suppose these accounts do explain why the conventionally randomized version of the trial failed. Would prerandomization have caused these physicians' concerns to be reduced if the prerandomized version of the trial were conducted ethically? Let us consider these explanations in order.

Does prerandomization result in less interference with the traditional "doctor knows best" doctor-patient relationship? In both designs the patient's right of informed consent entails that physicians have a duty to admit they don't know which treatment is better. Does prerandomization make informed consent easier to obtain for the ethical physician? Everything a patient must understand for genuine informed consent in a conventionally randomized trial must also be understood in the prerandomized version. Indeed, prerandomization is more difficult to explain. Physicians who have difficulty admitting to patients they do not know which option is better are not aided by prerandomization since they have an obligation to make that admission whichever design is used. Physicians who believe that one treatment is better than the other have a duty not to enroll patients on the trial whether conventionally randomized or prerandomized. If they do, they have violated their therapeutic obligation. A feeling of guilt associated with patients randomized to the treatment eventually shown to be worse could occur in connection with both designs. The research protocol was no more inflexible in the conventionally randomized design than in the prerandomized design. Therefore, if the six reasons offered in the Taylor article are sufficient to explain the failure of the conventionally randomized version of the lumpectomy vs. mastectomy study, they are also sufficient to explain why the prerandomized version would fail if it were ethically conducted. Since the prerandomized version did not fail, if the Taylor explanation is complete, then the prerandomized version of the trial must not have been conducted ethically.

Is there another way of explaining how prerandomization could have been both ethical and successful? Ellenberg (1984, 1408) has suggested that conventional randomization may fail "because patients are reluctant to agree to accept an unknown regimen." If so, prerandomization may improve the acceptance rate, since with this design patients know, when asked, what treatment they will receive.

This explanation, however, does not seem to explain what actually occurred in the lumpectomy vs. mastectomy study. Many conventionally randomized studies are completed in medicine. This suggests that patients *are, in general,* willing to accept an unknown regimen. What would account for the unwillingness of women to accept an unknown regimen in this *particular* study? The obvious answer in this case is that because the surgeries being compared had such different, permanent consequences for one's body, women were unwilling to be randomized to a therapy they viewed as much less desirable in the absence of their physicians' belief that a less desirable treatment offered a therapeutic advantage. Ellenberg's conjecture both "explains too much" and neglects the obvious explanation.

Is there any other possible explanation for the success of this prerandomized study? Appelbaum and his colleagues (1987) have studied informed consent in randomized clinical trials and have identified a "therapeutic misconception": patients will read consent forms, sign them, and still believe that the treatment they are receiving was chosen for them because their doctor thought it best. The therapeutic misconception can easily explain why patients accepted prerandomization. However, whenever the therapeutic misconception is present, obviously genuine informed consent has not been achieved. Hence, Appelbaum's results can explain why prerandomization succeeded in this case only on the condition that doctors' duties to their patients were violated.

Susan Ellenberg has argued that because of the major problems with prerandomization, "prerandomization should be considered a last resort measure" (Ellenberg 1984, 1408). Prerandomization was a last resort measure in the lumpectomy vs. mastectomy study. However, if the analysis up to this point is correct, we cannot explain how the conventionally randomized trial failed while the prerandomized version of the trial both succeeded and was conducted in accordance with generally accepted ethical standards. Put another way, when prerandomization *was* used as a last resort in this case, we cannot explain how it could have been simultaneously both successful and ethical. The absence of such an explanation must be contrasted with the ease of explaining how prerandomization could succeed if not conducted ethically: prerandomized contexts misleadingly mimic purely therapeutic contexts. This supports a considerably stronger conclusion than Ellenberg's: the prerandomized lumpectomy vs. mastectomy study violated generally accepted, and apparently easily defensible, standards of medical ethics.

CONCLUSION

Before concluding that the mastectomy-lumpectomy trial was patently unethical, a look at the results of that trial is in order. The trial established that when both lumpectomy groups were combined, disease-free survival after mastectomy was no better than disease-free survival after lumpectomy. The trial also established that disease-free survival after lumpectomy with radiation was better than after mastectomy (Fisher et al. 1985a). These are wonderful results! It means that most of those 100,000 women each year diagnosed with breast cancer can choose less disfiguring surgery knowing they are not reducing their chances of survival. Furthermore, we have apparently good reasons for believing that there was no other way to get these results. Accordingly, one might want to argue that the beneficial results of this study for women utterly submerge the ethical concerns discussed in this essay.

Tempting as this argument is, it is subject to substantial difficulties. The fundamental right of women to control their own bodies seems fundamental, not only to the ethics of women's health care, but also to the wrongness of rape, domestic violence, and physical sexual harassment. Accordingly, it does not seem to be the sort of right we would want to tamper with under any circumstances in a system of ethics responsive to feminist concerns. In addition, tampering with the right of patients to control their own bodies might be thought to justify medical paternalism for fully competent patients in some cases. Many medical ethicists would regard that price as too great to pay. Finally, most contemporary ethical theorists would defend the view that fundamental rights override social benefits. Indeed, they might argue that what it *means* to say that a right is fundamental is that considerations of social benefit cannot override it.

Analysis of this recent therapeutic research on breast cancer appears to yield the conclusion that obtaining the extraordinarily valuable results of this study *and* protecting the rights of women are incompatible. Since there also appear to be compelling arguments for giving up neither the benefits of this study nor the rights of women, this essay leaves us with a problem, not a solution. Resolution of this problem based upon the resources of feminist ethics or feminist critiques of science or perhaps other approaches to ethical theory requires an analysis far beyond the scope of this essay.

NOTES

Mary Spratt, Ron Stephens, Janet Levy, Jane Henney and Ace Allen made helpful comments on an earlier draft of this essay. Janice Doores and Cynthia Hodges did the word processing. I wish to thank them all.

1. Potentially curable breast cancer is cancer that is not so far advanced that cure is impossible.

2. This point is stated conservatively. The results of a nonrandomized study would probably not have been accepted by surgeons, most of whom were taught the virtues of the Halsted procedure. Furthermore, a nonrandomized study that *falsely* showed that lumpectomy produced as good survival as mastectomy would have tragic consequences for women if accepted.

3. For a more detailed discussion of this efficiency problem see Ellenberg (1984).

REFERENCES

Angell, Marcia. 1984. Patient preferences in randomized clinical trials. *New England Journal of Medicine* 310 (21): 1385–1387.

Appelbaum, Paul S., Loren H. Roth, Charles W. Lidz, Paul Benson, and William Winslade. 1987. False hopes and best data: Consent to research and the therapeutic misconception. *Hastings Center Report* 17 (2): 20–24.

Byar, David P. 1979. The necessity and justification of randomized clinical trials. In *Controversies in cancer: Design of trials and treatment.* Henri J. Tagnon and Maurice Staquet, eds. New York: Masson.

Chalmers, Thomas. 1967. The ethics of randomization as a decision-making technique and the problem of informed consent. *Report of the 14th Conference of Cardiovascular Training Grant Program Directors.* Bethesda, Maryland: National Heart Institute.

DeVita, Vincent T., Jr., Samuel Hellman, and Steven A. Rosenberg. 1985. *Cancer, principles and practice of oncology.* Philadelphia: J. P. Lippincott Company.

Ellenberg, Susan. 1984. Randomization designs in comparative clinical trials. *New England Journal of Medicine* 310 (21): 1404–1408.

Fisher, Bernard, Madeline Bauer, Richard Margolese, et al. 1985a. Five-year results of a randomized clinical trial comparing total mastectomy and segmental mastectomy with or without radiation in the treatment of breast cancer. *New England Journal of Medicine* 312 (11): 665–673.

Fisher, Bernard, Carol Redmond, Edwin R. Fisher, et al. 1985b. Ten-year results of a randomized trial comparing radical mastectomy and total mastectomy with or without radiation. *New England Journal of Medicine* 312 (11): 674–681.

Gifford, Fred. 1986. The conflict between randomized clinical trials and the therapeutic obligation. *The Journal of Medicine and Philosophy* 11 (4): 347–366.

Katz, Jay. 1978. Informed consent in therapeutic relationships: Law and ethics. In *Encyclopedia of bioethics.* Warren T. Reich, ed. Glencoe: The Free Press.

Marquis, Don. 1986. An argument that all prerandomized clinical trials are unethical. *The Journal of Medicine and Philosophy* 11 (4): 367–384.

Marquis, Don. 1983. Leaving therapy to chance: An impasse in the ethics of randomized clinical trials. *Hastings Center Report* 13 (4): 40–47.

Robinson, Spotswood. 1972. *Canterbury vs. Spence.* U.S. Court of Appeals, District of Columbia Circuit. 464 Federal Reporter, 2nd Series, 772.

Sacks, Henry, Thomas Chalmers, and Harry Smith. 1982. Randomized versus historical controls for clinical trials. *The American Journal of Medicine* 72: 233–240.

Taylor, Kathryn M., Richard G. Margolese, and Colin L. Soskolne. 1984. Physicians' reasons for not entering eligible patients in a randomized clinical trial of surgery for breast cancer. *New England Journal of Medicine* 310 (21): 1363–1367.

Vaisrub, N. 1985. Manuscript review from a statistician's viewpoint. *Journal of the American Medical Association* 253 (2): 3145–3147.

Zelen, Marvin. 1979. A new design for randomized trials. *New England Journal of Medicine* 300 (22): 1242–1245.

Zelen, Marvin. 1977. Statistical options in clinical trials. *Seminars in Oncology* 4 (2): 441–446.

Can Clinical Research Be Both Ethical and Scientific?

A Commentary Inspired by Rosser and Marquis

HELEN BEQUAERT HOLMES ❖ ❖ ❖

Problems with clinical research that create conflicts between doctors' therapeutic and research obligations may be fueled by a rigid view of science as determiner of truth, a heavy reliance on statistics, and certain features of randomized clinical trials. I suggest some creative, feminist approaches to such research and explore ways to provide choice for patients and to use values in directing both therapy and science—to enhance the effectiveness of each.

Both Rosser and Marquis point out problems with medical research on human subjects that may result in unfair treatment of women and/or results that have questionable truth value. To me their papers raise the question: can a clinical study be both ethical and scientific at the same time? I shall explore this question from a feminist perspective, using feminist values and recognizing that one major goal of feminism is to eliminate oppression (Sherwin 1989, 70). The oppressed here is the patient: any sick or disabled person. (Even the wealthy sick are oppressed through the pronounced inequality of the doctor-patient relationship.) One paradox is that, although the goal of medical research is to *alleviate* the suffering of this oppressed group, such research sometimes *contributes* to their suffering.

Clinical research may use subjects who have been oppressed in other ways (besides being patients). Inner city teaching hospitals may use poor and minorities; ethnic groups may be selected for use because of a higher genetic or environmental frequency of certain diseases; women may be used in a variety of techniques sometimes called "alternative assisted reproduction." In this final case, wealthy women often finance their doctors' clinical experiments; nevertheless, they are members of at least two oppressed groups: biological females and patients.

In this essay, after defining "ethical" and "scientific," I consider the use of statistics and randomized clinical trials as means of finding "truth." I shall suggest some feminist approaches to questions which these raise and shall propose issues to consider in setting up experimental designs that would be ethically acceptable to feminists.

Hypatia vol. 4, no. 2 (Summer 1989) © by Helen Bequaert Holmes

Some (Arbitrary) Definitions

An *ethical* action, of course, is one done in a right way for a good end. For "right" and "good" we all have common understandings, from classical theories of ethics, or from "principles" found in medical ethics texts, or from values highlighted by feminist ethics theorists, but mostly from simple intuition whereby we usually recognize a "right" action or a "good" person. (But I believe that truly hard cases may have no really ethical solutions.)

To be less vague: drawing upon nonfeminist ethics, I define an action (in this case clinical research) as "ethical" if it is just, is beneficent, and respects autonomy. Drawing upon the insights of feminist ethics, I amplify this definition by proposing that clinical research is ethical if it respects all humans—even if female, poor, or of color—fully, allows them to make informed choices,[1] and at the same time cares for them, recognizes their place in relationships that are vital parts of their lives, and is situation- and context-sensitive. Since authentic ethicists and authentic feminists would behave this way, I consider the adjectives "ethical" and "feminist" equivalent. It was tempting to change the title of this essay, in imitation of Longino (1987) in the first Feminism & Science issue of *Hypatia*, to "Can Clinical Research Be Feminist?"

A *scientific* approach is one that attempts to obtain knowledge of the natural world; arbitrarily I posit that a study is "scientific" if it reveals truth about nature and that it is good for a study to be scientific. Specifically, in the case of medical research, a study should give us accurate information about whether a given drug can cure a given disease, a given surgical treatment can correct a given problem, and so forth.

However, judgments about accuracy and truth present a formidable problem. Only human beings can make such judgments and no humans are free of biases. Let us look at a simple example. A certain chemical solution has been heated to a certain temperature. We may agree that there is a "true" temperature of that solution and that, among arbitrary systems, we shall take centigrade as our scale. However, when my lab partner and I in analytical chemistry read the thermometer, we record different values. I was taught in freshman chemistry to put my eye level with the meniscus of the mercury when reading a thermometer, and she was not. We are both white, middle-class, and female (a common sociological background) and we both want to turn in beautiful graphs on our lab reports and get A's (a common goal), yet we read different temperatures because of little differences in our pasts. Modern automatic devices determine temperature electronically, but human judgment is still involved in setting standards. Scientists accept arbitrary conventions; they then assume (perhaps erroneously) that all other scientists accept the same ones. (I am not raising the question here of whether "temperature" exists only in the human imagination.)

If even a true temperature eludes us, how much more difficult it is to agree whether a given treatment or medication "cures" a disease. With its marvelous mechanisms of recovery, the human body can often heal itself without treatment or in spite of a distinctly harmful treatment. Many sick people survived bleeding by leeches in the 1700s, even though we now know that each lost drop of blood lowered their chance of recovery.

Furthermore, scientists' search for truth is limited by their senses and distorted by their belief systems.[2] However, to proceed I must assume that appropriate studies can help us to fathom the mysteries of nature and to become more effective healers.

STATISTICS

Modern scientists use statisticians as arbiters of truth. In field hospitals during World War II no one experimented to see whether penicillin would work—say, by giving it to only half the gunshot patients. Penicillin obviously stopped infections and saved lives. No statistician was needed to declare significance. But nowadays most new "breakthroughs" in medicine—new drugs, new surgical procedures—may alleviate some symptoms, slow the progress of a disease, stave off the moment of death, or lead to a few more survivors. Is the new treatment better than the old? Is surgery better than a drug? It is not immediately clear.

One must define "success" for each experiment. Does survival count as success if it is survival-confined-to-bed, or survival-with-pain? After success is defined, one must consider what to do with the figures obtained. The researcher goes to the statistician, as to the oracle at Delphi, with the data. After applying the appropriate formula, the statistician tells whether the researcher's "null hypothesis" has not been falsified at the 5% level of significance, and hence is accepted.

Let's use a specific example. One null hypothesis might be that, after breast cancer surgery, radiation plus chemotherapy (therapy A) provides better disease-free survival than chemotherapy alone (therapy B). Of course, if everyone with the first treatment were still alive and half of the second group were dead, there would be no need for statistics (except that statistical testing is expected of every scientist). If tests with the data give a 95% likelihood that therapy A *is* better, the hypothesis is accepted. However there still is a 5% chance that therapy A was really no better than therapy B, in which case a "type two" error has been committed. On the other hand, if the statistics did not quite make the 5% cut-off level, the hypothesis would be rejected: then, if therapy A had actually been better than therapy B, a "type one" error would have been committed (Levine 1988, 190; Ratcliffe and Gonzalez-del-Valle 1988, 386).

The statistical threshold can be crossed by a very slight change in results. On an episode of NOVA, "Do Scientists Cheat?" (NOVA 1988, 6), Dr. Martin Shapiro described a hypothetical experiment with 80 cancer patients, 40 getting treatment, 40 with none (the controls). He displayed results that showed no statistically significant effect of the treatment. However, if one treated patient who died were omitted from the tally, significance would be found. Some very acceptable reasons could be found to decide not to count a particular patient—maybe she did not get quite the full course of the drug? Perhaps her cancer had already begun to metastasize? Perhaps she wasn't in the same age group as the rest? If the treatment *really* works, omitting such a patient would be *ethical*, to avoid committing a type one error, to make a helpful treatment available to future patients. On the other hand, the treatment might NOT really be better. The omission would be unethical if the scientist's motivation was simply to get another published paper (it's almost impossible to publish "non-significant" results) or to continue getting research funds from the pharmaceutical firm that provides the drug.[3]

Ethics and the Randomized Clinical Trial

The United States Food and Drug Administration tries to control the introduction of new drugs, requiring (after animal experimentation) phase I studies on healthy volunteers to determine toxicity, and phase II studies on sick people to determine efficacy (Levine 1988, 6; Silverman 1985, 151). Next, in phase III, should come studies to determine the "truth" about whether a new treatment is actually more effective than the old treatment or better than no treatment at all. The randomized clinical trial (RCT) is considered to be the best way to determine this for medical and surgical treatments.[4] However, since each person (with the possible exception of identical twins) is unique, no method of randomization can be perfect. Each person is physiologically unique—having a unique set of genes, unique life experiences, and unique combinations of previous infections and medical interventions. Thus each collection of people receiving the same treatment in an RCT is heterogenous.

A double-blind study (in which neither patient-subjects nor those who record results know who gets the treatment and who does not) should increase the likelihood that results will be "true," because some biases (that a drug really works, that certain side effects are trivial, etc.) are, in theory, eliminated. Also, a double-blind experiment is supposed to mitigate the "placebo effect." People who receive dummy pills often improve in health—even participants who know that the pill they take has a 50-50 chance of being a dummy. There is a psychological benefit in believing that one is actually being treated. My view, after being given short shrift so often by doctors too busy to listen to all my questions in an annual checkup, is that a patient in an RCT would get such positive emotional vibes in being in the center of attention—with people eagerly recording data about bodily functions—that health would, of course, improve. However, the placebo effect is viewed negatively and sometimes considered dangerous: investigators talk about eliminating it (Levine 1985 and 1988, 204).

Marquis (1989) compares the pre-randomized experimental design (where the cancer patient is told which treatment alternative she'll get before she agrees to participate) with simple randomization (where the patient is told what the different treatments are and agrees to be in a trial, not knowing which she'll get). He points out that, when a large percentage of potential subjects rejects participation in each such type of study, there may be no results to help women in the future. But if physicians who enroll patients in such trials actually have preferred treatments and have not communicated these preferences to their patients, then the therapeutic obligation has vanished. Marquis leaves us with a tangled paradox. Three points may help untangle it.

1) If there were a *very* much better treatment, it would come to light without the randomized trial (a treatment, say, effective on estrogen-dependent cancers as well as others; one effective on metastasized cancers; one effective in low and high dosages, etc.). But when we cannot see for ourselves and must go to Delphi to learn which is better, then there must be little difference between treatments. In such a case, the problems of poor recruitment to the experiment and of pseudo-frankness between doctor and patient would not matter so much.

2) Both the randomized and the pre-randomized designs (with informed consent) should indeed be commended as ways of treating patients as full human persons and unique individuals, but they don't go far enough. Patients should be encouraged to consider (and their choices should be respected) such matters as the following:

> a) Meaning of a worthwhile life. How productive do I want to be in continuing my life? What obligations do I have to people in close relationships? If I become bedridden or crippled, would this be viewed as an opportunity or as an unbearable burden by others?
>
> b) Views on pain and suffering. Is longevity an end in itself? If I have to take huge dosages of pain-killers, has the real me been destroyed? How much longevity counterbalances how much suffering?
>
> c) Altruism. If I participate in an experiment, how much am I willing to suffer to benefit others, if it will not benefit me? Can a belief that I am doing something for others help me to endure pain? Will participation in an experiment give more meaning to my life by giving a special meaning to my death?

Veatch (1987b) has argued:

> A rational person may not want to maximize his or her medical well-being at the expense of something else the person values. . . . Many of the standard concepts of modern medicine are called into question. There is no longer any such thing as a "medically indicated" treatment. (Veatch 1987b, 2)

3) Clinical experiments provide opportunities for doctors to develop into caring persons—perhaps the injection that medicine needs most. They could start by being honest with patients and by admitting their own biases, worries, uncertainties, and lack of knowledge.

Let us look at an imaginary scenario:
A breast cancer patient is told after lumpectomy that there are three therapies being evaluated by medical science. These treatments, she is told, have been chosen by physicians expert in treating cancer, and an experiment to compare them has been designed with the advice of former and current patients (Rosser 1989). She may choose any of the three, a completely free choice. Her doctor explains that all three are helpful in prolonging disease-free survival, but no treatment guarantees it. This experiment has been set up to determine whether one treatment is somewhat better than the other two. She may decide right now to get the decision over with; she may ask her doctor to flip a coin, or she may do some reading and/or talk with people during the next week. If she chooses the last, she is encouraged

to ask questions of members of the local breast cancer support group. The group includes former patients, at least one of whom has had each treatment. The doctor gives her a handout with the phone number of the cancer support group, a list of readings available in the local public library, and a note admitting her to the hospital library where the librarian has a special file of appropriate articles.

The doctor appears relaxed and encourages questions. Should the patient ask what treatment REALLY is best, he or she responds honestly. (An ethical doctor would not agree to participate in the experiment if he or she thought that one of the treatments was seriously inferior.) A response might be, "Frankly, I think that treatment X may be somewhat better because . . . " Or, "I'd prefer you to choose treatment Y because we haven't recently (or the national project hasn't) had many women choose Y—it would provide useful information to help women in the future."

If the patient insists, "You choose for me," the doctor does indeed choose, or says, "I'd prefer you to be in the experiment." He or she then pulls a slip out of an envelope, and says "I've assigned you randomly, and you'll be in the . . . group. Will you accept that?"

The patient would be permitted to change her treatment choice, after further reading or after experiencing side effects, even in the middle of therapy. She may leave suggestions in a suggestion box—anonymously if she wishes—and she is invited to attend meetings of the research team.

In this scenario patients have the opportunity to exercise some control over their therapy; the placebo effect is encouraged and used to promote healing; patients are also allowed to turn back responsibility to the doctor. (In my view, patients should be permitted but never forced to become informed decision-makers, i.e., mini-experts, on every ill that besets their bodies.) But at present this scenario would seldom be feasible. First, it would be difficult to recruit enough subjects to get statistical significance when increments of "success" will likely be tiny. Second, even if doctors were to cooperate, such a trial could be conducted only where there were patient support groups and appropriate library facilities. However, I present it to give specific examples of desirable factors to include when feminists design clinical experiments.

Others' Concerns about RCTs

Although most clinical researchers claim that the randomized clinical trial is "the most reliable method of evaluating the efficacy of therapies" (Byar et al. 1976) or the "gold standard" (Levine 1988, 211), some disagree (Rosner 1987). For example, Weinstein (1974) and others suggest considering individual patient preferences and using adaptive designs that make use of information obtained during the investigation, thereby exposing fewer patients to an inferior treatment.

Veatch (1983 and 1987a) has proposed what he calls the semi-randomized clinical trial which he claims is both scientifically and ethically superior. In this schema, patients are recruited for a trial of, let us say, a new therapy versus the standard therapy. After a randomization procedure, each is assigned to one or the other therapy. At this point patients may reject the assignment, opting for the other treatment. Some patients may prefer standard therapy; others, something new. The patients assigned to the new treatment but choosing the standard are then asked if the researcher may follow the course of their therapy. From this schema, five groups now exist: those who prefer not to be followed; those assigned to standard therapy and accepting it; those assigned to new therapy and accepting it; those assigned to standard who choose new instead, and those assigned to new who choose standard. The results of therapy in the last four groups are then studied over what is probably a course of several years, to determine long-term effects. (In most clinical trials where patients are given a choice to opt out of randomization, they are offered only standard treatment and the results of their treatment are not studied. Or, as described by Marquis (above; also Conn 1974, 1067), they are considered to be in the group to which they were randomized, regardless of treatment.)

Similarities between Veatch's schema and my hypothetical breast-cancer scenario above are obvious. Veatch admits that more subjects will need to be recruited to have large enough groups (statistically speaking) in all categories. However, he claims that this design is superior scientifically because one can make more statistical comparisons: those who choose a therapy vs. those who do not; everyone getting standard therapy vs. everyone getting the new, etc. He points to results from the Boston Inter-Hospital Liver Group's study of therapeutic portacaval anastomosis. Those who were randomized to surgery but insisted on medical treatment did better than those randomized to medical treatment (Veatch 1987a, 133; Conn 1974, 1067). Perhaps some people are in tune with their bodies and use some sort of "sixth sense" in reacting to proposed treatments. Can we use the placebo effect to enhance healing, and let those moved to use the misfortune of their illness to help future patients be the ones who join clinical trials?

Using the typical "principles" language of mainstream bioethics, Veatch gives ethical justification for the semi-randomized clinical trial. Arguments for good experimental design are, he claims, arguments from beneficence, i.e., designs to give more benefits and lower costs to future patients and society.

> Just as the right of patients to consent (based on autonomy) cannot be overridden by consideration of good research design (beneficence), so the right of a least well-off group to be benefitted (based on justice) cannot be overridden on beneficence grounds. (Veatch 1987a, 132)

Veatch has been challenged by other mainstream bioethicists. Lebacqz (1983) claims that a disadvantaged group may be harmed by being allowed to choose a new "treatment," because the language used in experimental design is often deceptive. Something called "therapy" or "treatment" may actually be a "nonvalidated intervention." But, in my view, more harm is done when a patient is *assigned* to such a nonvalidated intervention. Accurate language in consent forms is necessary, whatever the research design (Kopelmann 1983).

According to Gordon and Fletcher (1983, 23) "behavioral and psychologic factors can show strong correlations with the endpoints . . . commonly used to evaluate treatment." Therefore they query, "How can one interpret apparent differences in outcome when the assignment of patients between treatment groups being compared is a consequence of the behavior of either the patient or the physician?" They conclude that semi-randomization is *unjust*, both for Lebacqz's reason (above) and because "semi-randomization in the interest of some penalizes the chances that . . . eventually all will prosper more." But, if Gordon and Fisher permit informed consent, semi-randomization merely allows researchers to collect data on patients who opt out of their assigned treatment—which should *increase* the chances that all will prosper more.

A FEMINIST ANALYSIS

Feminists concerned about proper conduct of clinical trials can adapt and benefit from Veatch's ideas. Let's cleanse his competing-principles language, in which one principle "overrides" another. In this mainstream parlance, "beneficence" as a principle usually ranks lower in the hierarchy because it has a utilitarian taint, whereas "justice" and "autonomy" have higher Kantian credentials.

Now for a feminist wording: A woman coming into the "health" care system is a unique individual psychologically and physically. Part of her identity and thus part of her health and well-being, however, is in her network of close and distant relationships. For example, she may be concerned over the disruption her illness will have on others; she may be worried about infectious transmission to her children or about a genetic susceptibility in her children. Thus a doctor who offers her a true choice about participating in an experiment for the good of future patients respects her complicated network of relationships without needing to understand it. Considering a person as more than just a body is a cornerstone of healing. Experimental results may be better at predicting healing if all participants in all groups in an experiment are free to do what they wish (as much as possible, given their illnesses). All members of each treatment group must benefit in well-being.

Veatch recently (1988, 7), without the usual language of principles, argues in a similar vein. A patient, he says, may have a rational nonmedical reason for choosing one treatment over another, even if doctors do not know which is better, *and* even if the other treatment may provide a statistically significant longer survival than the one chosen by the patient. A patient's choice may be based on "special concerns, interests, fears, or life positions."

However, as feminists we must be sensitive to all forms of oppression, and the semi-randomized design is elitist in some ways. We must accept those people who have blind faith in the medical profession and not try to convert them to our agnosticism. Some people may be too sick, too weary, or too scared to weigh choices. Even the highly educated must not be forced. Processing information may be too difficult for some and too stressful for others. Any feminist theory of clinical experimentation must take into account the various vulnerabilities of patients.

Since science is always biased as practiced (Longino 1987; Ratcliffe and Gonzalez-del-Valle 1988),[5] researchers planning experiments should try to recognize and remove biases where possible and should try to consciously exploit bias toward acceptable values. For example, we can decide to be accountable to women and all sick persons, as Longino suggests:

> If we recognize . . . that knowledge is shaped by the assumptions, values and interests of a culture and that, within limits, one can choose one's culture, . . . we can choose to whom, socially and politically, we are accountable in our pursuit [of scientific understanding]. (Longino 1987, 61)

SOME HARD CASES

So far we have discussed experiments involving rational adults and have pointed out some circumstances in which they should not be expected to be full participants in decision-making. The mentally retarded and patients in comas are never able to be full participants, and a feminist theory must be able to incorporate these persons.

Children are another such group. Let us give a feminist analysis of an experiment currently underway in northeast Thailand, the poorest part of that land (McBride 1988). These children have significantly low levels of zinc and vitamin A in their blood. Each of these deficiencies lowers resistance to disease. Moreover, low levels of zinc impair growth and also prevent vitamin A from functioning—and low levels of vitamin A cause night blindness. The children have been divided into four groups: zinc alone, vitamin A alone, both nutrients, neither nutrient. They will be tested on their susceptibility to infections. "The study may also help resolve the controversy over whether the U.S. diet is adequate in zinc and vitamin A" (McBride 1988, 11).

One unethical aspect of this study is that a vulnerable population of third-world children is used to settle a first-world scientific controversy. Second, it is unlikely that the group with no treatment will benefit in any way. Inclusion of such a group cannot be justified by saying that, if there were no experiment, all children would be untreated. Given what we already know, some treatment for all must be provided so that everyone may benefit from participation.

How would feminists design such an experiment? First, the children themselves should be involved in some way in designing and implementing the experiment. Their creativity could be stimulated, despite poverty and illiteracy. Perhaps each child could choose two friends, each to be in a different group. One group would receive a moderate (non-toxic) amount of zinc with a trace of vitamin A; the second, moderate vitamin A and a trace of zinc; the third, moderate amounts of both zinc and vitamin A. Results from this experiment might answer the question whether one should maximize zinc or vitamin A in a food source to be grown locally. Children in the experiment and children in the future would benefit. All participating children could truthfully be told that the special foods they were getting would help them to see better at dusk. They could even be taught a simple test to use themselves to check their black-and-white vision.

CONCLUSION

Do feminists want clinical experiments? I think we do, although my "yes" is not a hearty one. For example, we want contraceptives that are safer and more effective than ones currently available; differences in both safety and efficacy are likely to be subtle and thus must be tested statistically after well-designed experiments.

I have tried to indicate problems with current randomized clinical trials and to give some specific examples of solutions that might be acceptable to feminists. Rosser (this volume, 134–35) sees some hopeful trends in modern clinical experiments; some mainstream bioethicists such as Veatch (1987b and 1988) urge overt attention to values in "scientific" medicine. Ratcliffe and Gonzalez-del-Valle (1988) claim that truly "rigorous" research

> requires the researcher to have a consciously held, well-thought-out, and coherent ethical framework to guide his or her choices during every phase of the research process. . . . Value-explicit research clearly requires systematic exposure to, reflection upon, and practice in the application of ethical frameworks. (389)

Feminist scientists, physicians, and philosophers need to work together to make scientific medicine both more "scientific" and more "ethical" at the same time. If medicine is to help the people who need it most, science and ethics must merge. Authentic science and authentic ethics may be unattainable absolutes, but for a close approach to those absolutes I believe that each needs the other. Science and ethics, at the least, will have a synergistic effect on each other and should enhance each other's effectiveness.

NOTES

1. An extremely important issue for feminists is informed consent. Although space does not permit such a discussion here, it should be included in any feminist analysis of the ethics of clinical experiments. Feminists need to consider in depth questions about timing and language, about what is true consent, about how much patients need to understand, and about whether demanding consent can be harmful or hazardous to health (Loftus and Fries 1971). Rosner (1987) provides a concise overview of diverse views on these and other issues in informed consent; Kopelmann (1983) discusses informed consent in clinical experiments.

2. One excellent example of belief systems operating in clinical science is the prediction of many in vitro fertilization (IVF) clinic directors that, once the technique is "perfected," the success of IVF will be better than nature (Andrews et al. 1986, 852). Desire to confirm this belief has led to questionable definitions of success, elimination of some patients from statistics, and a selective use of the earlier literature about "natural" rates of conception. See Broad and Wade (1982) for other examples.

3. For a discussion of minor cheating and the fudging of statistics, see Broad and Wade (1983), especially p. 85.

4. See Chalmers (1981), Marquis (1989), or Rosner (1987) for lucid arguments to this effect. For comprehensive discussions of many points about ethics and reliability of RCTs see Levine (1988), Rosner (1987), and Silverman (1985).

5. Longino (1987) cited herein is but one example of the many excellent feminist analyses of the sources and types of distortion and bias in scientific experimentation. The reader is referred to the November 1987 issue of the *Newsletter on Feminism and Philosophy* and its literature overview/bibliography on pages 20–24; also to the two issues of *Hypatia* on Feminism & Science—Volume 2 (3) 1987 and Volume 3 (1) 1988—and the bibliography on pages 145–155 in the latter issue.

REFERENCES

Andrews, Mason C., Suheil J. Muasher, Donald L. Levy, Howard W. Jones, Jr., Jairo E. Garcia, Zev Rosenwaks, Georgeanna S. Jones, and Anibal A. Acosta. 1986. An analysis of the obstetric outcome of 125 consecutive pregnancies conceived in vitro and resulting in 100 deliveries. *American Journal of Obstetrics and Gynecology* 154:848–854.

Broad, William, and Nicholas Wade. 1982. *Betrayers of the truth*. New York: Simon and Schuster.

Byar, David P., Richard M. Simon, William T. Friedewald, James J. Schlesselman, David L. DeMets, Jonas H. Ellenberg, Mitchell H. Gail and James H. Ware. 1976. Randomized clinical trials: Perspectives on some recent ideas. *New England Journal of Medicine* 295:74–80.

Chalmers, T. C. 1981. The clinical trial. *Milbank Memorial Fund Quarterly* 59:325–339.

Conn, Harold O. 1974. Therapeutic portacaval anastomosis: To shunt or not to shunt. *Gastroenterology* 67:1065–1073.

Gordon, Robert S., and John C. Fletcher. 1983. Can strict randomization be ethically acceptable? *Clinical Research* 31 (1):23–25.

Kopelmann, Loretta. 1983. Randomized clinical trials, consent and the therapeutic relationship. *Clinical Research* 31 (1):1–11.

Lebacqz, Karen. 1983. Justice, choice, and the language of research. *Clinical Research* 31 (1):26–27.

Levine, Robert J. 1985. The use of placebos in randomized clinical trials. *IRB* 7 (2):1–4.

Levine, Robert J. 1988. *Ethics and regulation of clinical research*. New Haven: Yale University Press, 2nd ed.

Loftus, Elizabeth F., and James F. Fries. 1979. Informed consent may be hazardous to health. *Science* 204:11.

Longino, Helen E. 1987. Can there be a feminist science? *Hypatia* 2 (3):51–64.

Marquis, Don. 1989. An ethical problem concerning recent therapeutic research on breast cancer. *Hypatia* 4 (2):140–155.

McBride, Judy. 1988. Asian children may quell nutritional controversy. *Agricultural Research* February: 11.

NOVA. 1988, October 25. Do scientists cheat? Boston: WGBS.

Ratcliffe, John W., and Amalia Gonzalez-del-Valle. 1988. Rigor in health-related research: Toward an expanded conceptualization. *International Journal of Health Services* 18 (3):361–392.

Rosner, Fred. 1987. The ethics of randomized clinical trials. *The American Journal of Medicine* 82:283–290.

Rosser, Sue V. 1989. Re-visioning clinical research—gender and the ethics of experimental design. *Hypatia* 4 (2):125–139.

Sherwin, Susan. 1989. Medical and feminist ethics: Two different approaches to contextual ethics. *Hypatia* 4 (2):57–72.

Silverman, William A. 1985. *Human experimentation: A guided step into the unknown.* Oxford: Oxford University Press.

Veatch, Robert M. 1983. Justice and research design: The case for a semi-randomization clinical trial. *Clinical Research* 31 (1):12–22.

Veatch, Robert M. 1987a. *The patient as partner: A theory of human-experimentation ethics.* Bloomington: Indiana University Press.

Veatch, Robert M. 1987b. Emphasis on values prompting a change in medical practice. *Kennedy Institute of Ethics Newsletter* 1 (9):1–2.

Veatch, Robert M. 1988. Should I enroll in a randomized clinical trial? A critical commentary. *IRB* 10 (5):7–8.

Weinstein, Milton C. 1974. Allocation of subjects in medical experiments. *New England Journal of Medicine* 291:1278–1285.

WOMEN AND
NEW REPRODUCTIVE
"CHOICES"

Choice, Gift, or Patriarchal Bargain? Women's Consent to *In Vitro* Fertilization in Male Infertility

JUDITH LORBER ❖ ❖ ❖

This paper explores the reasons why women who are themselves fertile might consent to undergo in vitro fertilization (IVF) with an infertile male partner. The reasons often given are desire to have that particular man's child, or altruism, giving a gift to the partner. Although ethically, the decision should be completely woman's prerogative, because IVF programs usually treat the couple as a unit, she may be offered few other options by the medical staff. In social terms, whether the woman is or is not infertile may be immaterial because in either situation, if she wants to try to have a biological child and maintain the relationship, she may have to make a patriarchal bargain and undergo in vitro fertilization.

> . . . *the whole deceptive problematic of the gift.* . . . *Who could ever think of the gift as a gift-that-takes? Who else but man, precisely the one who would like to take everything?* (Cixous 1976, 888)

Although *in vitro* fertilization (IVF) was originally developed to bypass the blocked or missing fallopian tubes of infertile women, it is now also the treatment of choice in cases of male infertility due to low sperm count, poor sperm motility, or badly shaped sperm. Extra-corporeal fertilization works in male infertility because a *very* small amount of good sperm are needed to fertilize the egg in a petri dish (Gordon 1988). The semen are washed to remove impurities, examined under a microscope to select the best sperm, and can be microinjected into ova in a petri dish. In male infertility, the woman may be physiologically fertile, but nonetheless she would have to undergo hormonal stimulation, sonograms, and intravaginal or intra-abdominal procedures, often under general anesthesia, in order for her ova to be fertilized with her partner's sperm. In most cases, all the man has to do is produce sperm on demand.[1]

Women's consent to undergo IVF has been described by many feminists as not a true choice,[2] given the cultural pressures for women to become mothers, but if they are infertile, it can be understood as a solution to their own physiological problem.[3] Less understandable is the consent of women who are physiologically fertile to undergo IVF to try to have a child with an infertile male partner. The

Hypatia vol.4, no. 3 (Fall 1989). © by Judith Lorber

reason may be the desire to have that particular man's child, or it may be an act of altruism, a gift for the partner. However, despite medical ethics which preclude doing harm, the woman may be given few other options if the medical staff focuses on the couple as a unit. Finally, whether the woman is or is not physiologically infertile may be immaterial because in either situation, she is *socially* infertile. If she wants to try to have a biological child and maintain the relationship, she may have to make a patriarchal bargain and undergo *in vitro* fertilization.

In terms of family dynamics, the closest situations to a woman's consent to IVF when her male partner is infertile are a relative having a child for another woman or donating a kidney for transplantation to a parent, child, or sibling. A few cases of mothers and sisters gestating embryos produced with IVF have been reported (Leeton, King and Harmon 1988; Michelow et al. 1988), but without data on decisions or family conflicts (Roach 1988), which were an important part of the research on live kidney donation by Simmons, Klein Marine and Simmons (1987). Because of the large body of data, this discussion will use the research on live kidney donation as a comparison situation.

I will argue that in male infertility, the two ostensible reasons for the woman's agreeing to IVF, that she wants her partner's biological child or that she altruistically wants to give him a chance to have a biological child, are made suspect by manipulation of the situation by the medical system, by the woman's subordinate status in the marital relationship, and by the unequal burden of childlessness. I conclude that rather than a free choice or a freely given gift, these fertile women undergoing extensive treatment are making a patriarchal bargain (Kandiyoti 1988; Lorber 1987).

USE OF IVF IN MALE INFERTILITY

The first reports of IVF's use in male infertility began appearing in the medical journals in 1984. An early report from England of IVF treatment for low sperm count (oligospermia), low motility (asthenospermia), and abnormal morphology (teratospermia) in 41 couples with an average duration of infertility of 6.5 years had a very high success rate—34 percent (Cohen et al. 1984; see also Cohen et al. 1985). A subsequent communication from Australia was less positive, and warned that " . . . IVF patients experience greater anguish from failed fertilization than from the failure to achieve a pregnancy after embryo transfer" (Yovich et al. 1984, 170; see also Yovich and Stanger 1984, and Yovich, Stanger and Yovich 1985). A pessimistic report from England on the results of IVF treatment in male infertility noted that if such treatment were successful, " . . . it would represent a major, and indeed the only advance in treatment for what seems at present the worst problem in infertility practice" (Hull and Glazener 1984, 231). By 1985, the use of IVF for male infertility was attractive not only because it seemed to be a breakthrough for that specific problem, but because it was the only area that offered a chance to move ahead technologically (Johnston 1987).

The use of IVF in male infertility is now considered one of the most effective treatments (Spark 1988, 339–355), one that, according to the conclusion of a review paper, " . . . opens up an area which will allow the treatment of a substantial population of infertile couples for whom before there was no effective treatment" (Yates and de Kretser 1987, 145).

The extent of male infertility in the population of couples undergoing treatment for infertility has surprised experienced clinicians. At the American Fertility Society's 1987 Annual Meeting, the famed Jones Institute of Reproductive Medicine, in a paper entitled "The Failure of Fertilization in IVF: The 'Occult' Male Factor," reported that of a group of 52 couples in whom no fertilization had occurred, 19.2 percent were initially evaluated as having "oocyte anomalies," 32.6 percent as having "sperm anomalies," and 7.7 percent a combination of both (Oehninger et al. 1988). In 40.4 percent, there was no obvious cause of failed fertilization. After reassessing sperm morphology with new, stricter criteria, they were able to diagnose sperm abnormalities in 61.5 percent of the men, with combined sperm and egg anomalies in 13.4 percent of the couples. The paper concludes, "We therefore emphasize the significance that sperm cell abnormalities may have in failed fertilization and IVF outcome" (Oehninger 1988, 186).

The pervasiveness of male infertility and the difficulty of ameliorating the problem through treatment of the men have made IVF an attractive medical solution. One report of the side effects of IVF considered the effect of invasive procedures on the reproductive system of a physiologically fertile woman. A report from Israel (Ashkenazi et al. 1987) of two cases of tubal adhesions caused by IVF procedures led the authors to note that if male infertility is the only indication for IVF, the side effects of the treatment could prevent the patient from conceiving spontaneously in a further attempt at becoming pregnant with the same or possibly another man. The authors' advice is: "It might be advisable to counsel the couple to attempt AID prior to IVF and, possibly, avoid mechanical infertility" (244).

Despite their final enthusiasm for a possible solution to a stubborn physiological problem, earlier in their review article Yates and de Kretser recommend that because of the low pregnancy rates, couples with less than a history of two years of not being able to conceive should not be subject to the stress and expense of IVF, " . . . unless there is an obvious female factor involved which makes IVF treatment necessary" (1987, 141–142). Nonetheless, the reports in the medical literature indicate that it is being widely recommended to couples where the primary diagnosis is male infertility (Spark 1988, 354–355).

The question to be raised here is, why are physiologically fertile women whose male partners are infertile agreeing to undergo IVF? While the couple may later try artificial insemination by donor or adoption, the issue here is why does a woman who could have a baby with any man's viable sperm go through the emotional stress and physical trauma of IVF at all? Is their action similar to the altruism of the live kidney donor?

GIFTS OF LIFE

In live kidney donation, because of the need for a close tissue match, the donors are usually parents, children, or siblings of the recipient, and the psychosocial and ethical aspects of the situation involve a consideration of family dynamics (Simmons, Klein Marine and Simmons 1987). Recently, kidney transplants from genetically unrelated donors have been successful. It is expected that these donors will be "emotionally related," and so the spouse would be the most likely candidate (Simmons and Abress 1988). Most of the research on live kidney donation has been on genetic relatives, and so they will be the comparison group here. For the person who needs a kidney transplant, a successful donation means freedom from dialysis, and in many cases, survival. About 70 percent retain the kidney, and their subsequent physical and psychological quality of life is good (Simmons, Klein Marine and Simmons 1987, xxii–xxiii). The cost to the donor is loss of a healthy kidney with risk of subsequent failure of the remaining kidney, surgery with general anesthesia, at least a week's hospitalization with consequent loss of stamina, and an extensive abdominal scar. The risk of the operation to a donor's life is calculated at .05 percent and the long-term risk at .07 percent (Simmons, Klein Marine and Simmons 1987, 39, 165–175).

In the case of IVF use for male infertility, a life is not being saved, but if the procedure is successful, a life or lives would be created. However, in contrast to the 70 percent success rate in kidney transplantation, the rates of success when IVF is used for male infertility are lower than when the same procedures are used for female infertility—around 15–20 percent become pregnant and 8–10 percent have a live birth (Yates and de Kretser 1987; Spark 1988, 345). The rates of success depend on the extent to which three common problems are present—low concentrations of sperm, poor motility, and abnormal shape (Kruger et al. 1988). The risks of undergoing IVF for a physiologically healthy woman are infection (Holmes 1988), iatrogenic infertility (Ashkenazi et al. 1987), and psychosis (Bourrit et al. 1988). Given these risks and the low success rates, medical ethics might dictate more reluctance to recommend its use where the woman is not herself physiologically infertile. However, altruism has led healthy people to undergo major surgery to donate kidneys, and physicians might argue that women should have the right to make the choice to try to have their partner's child.

ALTRUISM

In donating kidneys, women are more altruistic than men. According to Simmons, Klein Marine and Simmons, women are less likely to be ambivalent about donating a kidney to a relative than men are (1987, 188–89). Mothers contemplating donating to a child are more likely to be free of ambivalence than fathers (58 percent to 29 percent), and sisters are more likely than brothers to be sure about their decision to donate (56 percent to 28 percent). Daughters asked to donate to a parent are less likely to score high in ambivalence than are sons (11 percent to 27 percent). Immediately after surgery, men have more negative feelings than women do about what they have undergone, and these feelings persist a year later (differences are statistically significant). However, men are more likely to feel better about themselves immediately post-transplant (23 percent to 8 percent of women donors) and one year later (40 percent to 26 percent), indicating that the women's donation may have been taken more for granted as part of their duty *as women.*

The authors summarize the gender differences as follows:

> What these results suggest is that donation is a more momentous event for the male. He is more likely to question whether he wishes to make the sacrifice. If he does make the sacrifice, he reacts more dramatically—either with regret or with a great boost in the self-picture. The female appears to take donation more for granted, neither reacting as negatively nor as likely to perceive the act to be an extraordinary one on her part, as an act that proves her greater worth as a person.
>
> Perhaps donation seems to the female to be a simple extension of her usual family obligations, while for the male it is an unusual type of gift. In our society the traditional female role is one in which altruism and sacrifice within the family is expected. . . .
>
> In fact, entering a hospital and suffering pain and body manipulation to give life to another is ordinarily a major part of her role and purpose in life. Giving birth to an infant is congruent psychologically with the act of giving a body-part so a loved one can be reborn. . . .
>
> From a male's point of view, there is no life experience or expectation like childbirth that prepares him for this act of donation. Thus he may have stronger ambivalences and doubts even after the transplant. In any case, whether his feelings are positive or negative, he is more likely to feel he has performed an exceptional act. If his feelings are positive, as the majority of men's are, he is more likely to reap self-image benefits from this extraordinary gift. (188–89)

Fertile wives of infertile men exhibit altruistic behavior whether or not they undergo treatment—they often protectively display a "courtesy stigma" by calling themselves infertile as well (Miall 1986). Given the findings on the way mothers, sisters, and daughters volunteer to donate a kidney, is there any doubt that fertile wives of infertile men, who have already taken the burden of the social stigma and the search for treatment on their shoulders, would undergo IVF, too? But are these acts true acts of altruism? An examination of the gender differences in reaction to childlessness and in use of the medical system indicates a marked lack of choice for women.

Manipulation by the Medical System

A study (Greil, Leitko and Porter 1988) in which twenty-two infertile couples were interviewed intensively found that no matter who had the physiological impairment, the women felt *they* were *physiologically* infertile. In their behavior, they are. Women tend to take the initiative in seeking treatment for failure to conceive—they are the ones who know with each menstrual period that they have not gotten pregnant, and they usually have been to gynecologists at some time during their adult lives (Greil, Leitko and Porter 1988; Miall 1986; Snarey, Son and Kuehne 1986). The male partner's procreative capacity may not be assessed until after a woman has gone though an infertility workup (Spark 1988, 126). The Norfolk program requires, as part of this workup, "cervical factor investigation, local and systemic immunologic factors, hysterosalpingogram, endometrial biopsy, laparoscopy, and basal body temperature chart" (Oehninger et al. 1988, 181). Such an extensive workup of the woman who is ostensibly fertile is likely to turn up some problem or anomaly which could justify the recommendation of IVF use.

More than a century ago, James Marion Sims, whose research on sterility had attributed barrenness in marriage to the woman and subjected her to numerous painful therapies, such as the surgical incision of the neck of the uterus, changed his views when he found that the newly developed microscope showed defects in male semen that could also account for infertility (Reiser 1978, 80–81). He then declared, in a paper published in the New York Journal of Medicine in 1869, that physicians could not, in good conscience, initiate therapy for sterility without first ascertaining the viability of sperm (cited in Reiser 1978, 264). If today the woman is not held automatically responsible for the couple's childlessness, she still ends up subject to traumatic and invasive procedures because physicians talk of a possible cure for " . . . a substantial population of infertile couples for whom before there was no effective treatment" (Yates and de Kretser 1987, 145). Such language ignores the fact that the treatment, IVF, does nothing about correcting low sperm count, misshapen sperm, or sperm that have little motility.

The recommendation of high-technology treatment of the woman to counteract the effects of the male's condition emerges from health care professionals taking it for granted that patients want the most sophisticated medical techniques. They rarely question patients on their motivations to undergo discomforting, expensive, and possibly dangerous treatments. This medical perspective so imbues interactions between patients and health professionals that patients' "lifeworld" concerns and hesitations are frequently ignored or discounted (Mishler 1984).

While many IVF programs have a psychologist or a social worker on their staff, most routinely see couples as part of the initial workup, for screening and for educational talks. They are available for counseling throughout the treatment process, but as part of the IVF team (Appleton 1986).

Most IVF psychologists, social workers, and counselors are women, and most of the physicians are men. Sympathetic male physicians could provide significant leverage if an infertile man must persuade his fertile female partner to undergo extensive invasive procedures in order for him to be a biological father. The enthusiasm with which male clinical researchers greeted the first reports of a way infertile men could become biological fathers, and the emphasis on the couple as the infertile unit lead very easily to physicians' recommendation of IVF as a favored alternative to donor insemination or adoption.

In kidney donation, some hospitals have established psychiatric review boards to protect the rights of ambivalent or anxious prospective donors who seem to be undergoing unbearable family pressure. Since the kidney patient's doctor may be placed in an ethical role conflict between his or her obligation to the donor and his or her commitment to save the life of the kidney patient, the kidney patient's physician often stays out of the appeal for donors. Care of the recipient is separated from care of the donor, each having his or her own physician. The prospective donor's personal physician can also act as an advocate in medical and family conflicts (Simmons, Klein Marine and Simmons 1987, 39–41, 217–218).

In order to similarly give a fertile woman the chance to withhold her consent to undergo IVF, both partners would have to have their own physicians, and there would have to be counseling entirely separated from the IVF program. This counseling would have to explore with each partner separately the advantages and disadvantages of all the alternative solutions to their childlessness. At the very least, if a woman indicated reluctance, ambivalence, or hesitation, she should be protected from undue coercion with a false medical excuse, which is a standard procedure in kidney donation.

Without such protective mechanisms, it is very likely that manipulation by the medical system is a significant factor in the use of IVF in male infertility, contaminating voluntary free choice. However, even if a woman consulted physicians and counselors separately, carefully weighed the advantages and disadvantages of IVF, donor insemination, and adoption, and opted for IVF because she wanted to try to have this particular man's child or she wanted to give her partner and his kin the chance to have biological kin, would it be a freely chosen act? In either case, only if she was an equal or dominant in the situation. Otherwise, I would argue, she is making a patriarchal bargain—resolving a situation in which she has limited options in the best way she can.

The Norms of Gift Giving

The norms of reciprocity in gift giving are that gifts should be given freely without thought of payment, but that until they are paid back with a gift of approximately equal value, the debtor is in a subordinate status. It is assumed that before the gift giving, the donor and recipient are of equal status, or the giver is of superior status and stays that way. Because the gift puts the giver in a superior position, it would be a presumption for an inferior to give a valuable gift to a superior. Reciprocal gift-giving is a way of building a relationship; the gifts keep relationships going, because as long as there is an outstanding debt, the relationship cannot be severed (Blau 1964; Mauss 1954).

Donation of a kidney is such an enormous gift that it seems as if it could not be reciprocated and that the giver would assume such a superior status that the relationship would be severely disturbed. However, only 7 percent of the 111 donors studied by Simmons, Klein Marine, and Simmons indicated a year later that the donation had disrupted their relationship with the recipient. Recipients felt betrayed when the donor requested a material return or a display of gratitude, or when there was evidence that the donor had been reluctant. In these cases, the value of the gift was diminished. Donors, in turn, felt betrayed when they did not get explicit gratitude (452).

But in most cases, the gift was freely given, and, while not "repaid," made for greater closeness between the donor and recipient. The authors suggest that the relationship itself—and its perpetuation because of the gift—is the donor's reward. Since the donor gave the great gift to maintain the relationship, the donor tries not to make the recipient feel enormously indebted. They may say they are paying back what the recipient has done for them already, or only extending what they already give, or doing what the other would do for them.

Rather than the gift being one which has to be repaid, the act is seen as an expression of love—"If you love me, you will do this unhesitatingly. If you do not do this unhesitatingly, then you do not truly love me." That is, the deeper the relationship, the more one can ask of the other:

> Family relationships and the professions of love that accompany them carry with them an assumption that one has earned great credit. . . . The credit . . . is normatively defined as almost unlimited—whatever the small child needs, whatever the spouse needs, will be forthcoming if at all within the realm of possibility. Only the life of the potential giver is excepted, and even then considerable risk to one's life is expected in a crisis. (Simmons, Klein Marine and Simmons 1987, 455)

In this sense, fertile women undergoing IVF could be seen as giving or paying back gifts of love, expressing their love, or doing what they would expect the other to do for them. However, given the unequal status of women and men in most heterosexual relationships, one can argue that undergoing IVF is not a true choice or a true act of altruism, but a patriarchal bargain.

BARGAINING WITH PATRIARCHY

Deniz Kandiyoti has argued that " . . . women strategize within a set of concrete constraints that reveal and define the blueprint of . . . the *patriarchal bargain* of any given society . . . " (1988, 275, emphasis in original). The impact of the hegemonic moral imperative that women must be mothers and that children should be biological, and the manipulation of women by the Western medical system make the use of IVF in female, male, or couple infertility a patriarchal bargain for women. Women and men are not equals in the situation because the burden of childlessness is greater for women. Greil, Leitko, and Porter's study (1988) found that whether the reproductive impairment was the wife's, the husband's, or the couple's together, not being able to conceive dominated the women's lives and became an everyday, pervasive concern. The husbands' attitudes were to distance themselves from the problem, or to deal with it in instrumental ways and if treatment did not work, "get on with their lives."

In order to become a mother, an infertile woman has to persuade her husband to join her in IVF treatment or adopt. A fertile woman has an additional choice— donor insemination—but if she wants to maintain her relationship with her male partner, she would need his consent, which is often difficult to obtain because the situation stigmatizes men (Lasker and Borg 1987; Novaes 1985; Pfeffer 1987). Sexual dysfunction seems to be a common reason why couples present themselves for infertility treatment and may be why there are so many "waiting list" pregnancies (Jarrell et al. 1986; Roh et al. 1987). It may also be the reason why the husband's inability to masturbate to ejaculation on demand is a perennial problem in IVF clinics the world over (Edwards and Purdy 1982, 199).

In sum, the sexual and emotional relationship of a childless couple who want children is often extremely fragile (Jones 1986). However, the marriages of couples undergoing IVF are reported to be strong, and the couples display a high degree of consensus (Lorber and Greenfeld 1990; Seibel and Levin 1987), suggesting that the woman who wants a baby with her current partner may have opted for IVF as the most likely way to obtain her mate's cooperation. If the treatment fails, as it will in the majority of cases, she is in a better position to bargain for donor insemination or adoption.

Despite our culture's emphasis on motherhood, men are often the dominant partner in childbearing decisions. A study of voluntarily childless couples found that it was the husband's wishes that prevailed (Marciano 1978). When the wife wanted a child and the husband did not, they stayed childless; when the husband wanted a child and the wife did not, they often divorced. In actuality, it is not that men per se control reproductive decisions, but that the dominant partner does, and in our society, the dominant partner is likely to be the man. Even if the woman is the dominant partner, if she wants a chance to have a child with her mate, she must persuade him to participate in infertility treatment with her, so he holds the power of the negative veto.

Male infertility exacerbates what Tangri (1976), a feminist population expert, has called men's "disability"—that they don't bear babies:

> . . . women's ability to bear babies in contrast to men's inability to do so, is a potential source of power unmatched in modern times by any physical advantages men have. Oddly enough, this advantage has been turned into a net disadvantage by a curious anomaly. Usually, in civilized societies, varying degrees of compensations have been created for the deprived. . . . In the case of fertility, however, instead of repairing the disabled—that is, men—they have received compensation in the form of social customs that give them power over the able—that is, over women's bodies—and fertility. (896)

In sum, while a fertile woman undergoing IVF to try to have a baby with an infertile man may be exchanging a gift of love or expressing love, it is more likely that she is making a patriarchal bargain—trying to maintain a relationship and have a child within the constraints of monogamy, the nuclear family structure, and the valorization of biological parenthood, especially for men. Even the gloss of love and altruism may be part of the bargain.

NOTES

Prepared with financial support from PSC-CUNY Grant #666–206 and 668–518. An earlier version was presented at the Eastern Sociological Society Annual Meeting, Philadelphia, March 1988. I would like to thank Barbara Katz Rothman and Patricia Mann for their helpful comments.

1. IVF treatment world-wide generally follows a protocol in which the woman is given fertility drugs to produce many ripe ova; sonograms and blood tests are used to determine readiness for ovulation; the ripe ova are removed surgically or vaginally, and are fertilized in a petri dish by semen produced by masturbation; after cell cleavage, the embryos are transferred directly into the uterus, usually via the vagina (Fredericks, Paulson and De-Cherney 1987; Holmes 1988). In a related procedure, gamete intrafallopian transfer (GIFT), the ova are layered in a tube with sperm and transferred immediately, without waiting for fertilization, into the fallopian tubes, not into the uterus. The woman must therefore have at least one intact tube. Both techniques have been used in female, male, and idiopathic infertility (Asch et al. 1988). After the first cycle of IVF or GIFT, some of the protocol can be bypassed by the use of frozen embryos (Testart et al. 1988).

Surgical treatment and aspiration of semen is used to correct or bypass male anatomical problems (Silber 1989; Spark 1988).

2. For recent feminist critiques of the emotional, financial, and societal costs of IVF for women for generally low rates of live births, see Baruch, D'Adamo and Seager 1988; Corea et al. 1987; Overall 1987; Rothman 1989; Spallone and Steinberg 1988; Stanworth 1987.

3. For research on procreatively impaired women's motivations to undergo IVF, see Bainbridge 1982; Callan et al. 1988; Crowe 1985; Williams 1988.

REFERENCES

Appleton, T. 1986. Caring for the IVF patient—counselling care. In In vitro fertilization: Past, present, future. S. Fishel and E. M. Symonds, eds. Oxford: IRL Press.

Asch, R. H., J. P. Balmaceda, E. Cittadini, P. Figueroa Casa, V. Gomel, M. K. Hohl, I. Johnston, J. Leeton, F. J. Rodriguez Escudero, U. Noss, and P. C. Wong. 1988. Gamete intrafallopian transfer: International cooperative study of the first 800 cases. Annals of the New York Academy of Sciences 541: 722–27.

Ashkenazi, J., D. Feldberg, M. B. David, M. Shelef, D. Dicker, and J. A. Goldman. 1987. Ovum pickup for in vitro fertilization: A cause of mechanical infertility? Journal of in Vitro Fertilization and Embryo Transfer 4: 242–45.

Bainbridge, I. 1982. With child in mind: The experiences of a potential IVF mother. In Test-tube babies. W. A. W. Walters and P. Singer, eds. Melbourne: Oxford.

Baruch, E. H., A. F. D'Adamo, Jr., and J. Seager, eds. 1988. Embryos, ethics and women's rights: Exploring the new reproductive technologies. New York: Harrington Park Press.

Blau, P. 1964. Exchange and power in social life. New York: Wiley.

Bourrit, B., R. Martin-Du, D. Benchouk, M. Biondo, and E. Stiksa. 1988. Psychotic reaction after in vitro fertilization (IVF). Journal of in Vitro Fertilization and Embryo Transfer 5: 114.

Callan, V. J., B. Kloske, Y. Kashima, and J. F. Hennessey. 1988. Toward understanding women's decisions to continue or to stop in vitro fertilization: The role of social, psychological, and background factors. Journal of in Vitro Fertilization and Embryo Transfer 5: 363–69.

Cixous, H. 1976. The laugh of the Medusa. Keith Cohen and Paula Cohen, trans. Signs: Journal of Women in Culture and Society 1: 875–893.

Cohen, J., C. B. Fehilly, S. B. Fishel, R. G. Edwards, J. Hewitt, G. F. Rowland, P. C. Steptoe, and J. Webster. 1984. Male infertility successfully treated by in vitro fertilization. Lancet 1 (June 2): 1238–39.

Cohen, J., R. Edwards, C. B. Fehilly, S. B. Fishel, J. Hewitt, J. Purdy, G. F. Rowland, P. C. Steptoe, and J. Webster. 1985. *In vitro* fertilization: a treatment for male infertility. *Fertility and Sterility* 43: 422–32.

Corea, G., J. Hanmer, B. Hoskins, J. Raymond, R. Duelli Klein, H. B. Holmes, M. Kishwar, R. Rowland, and R. Steinbacher. 1987. *Man-made women: How new reproductive technologies affect women.* Bloomington, IN: Indiana University Press.

Crowe, C. 1985. "Women want it": *In vitro* fertilization and women's motivations for participation. *Women's Studies International Forum* 8: 57–62.

Edwards, R. G., and J. M. Purdy, eds. 1982. *Human conception in vitro: Proceedings of the first Bourn Hall meeting.* New York: Academic Press.

Fredericks, C. M., J. D. Paulson and A. H. DeCherney, eds. 1987. *Foundations of in vitro fertilization.* Washington, DC: Hemisphere.

Gordon, J. W., and N. Laufer. 1988. Applications of micromanipulation to human *in vitro* fertilization. *Journal of in Vitro Fertilization and Embryo Transfer* 5: 57–60.

Greil, A. L., T. A. Leitko, and K. L. Porter. 1988. Infertility: His and hers. *Gender & Society* 2: 172–199.

Holmes, H. B. 1988. *In vitro* fertilization: Reflections on the state of the art. *Birth* 15: 134–145.

Holmes, H. B., and T. Tymstra. 1987. *In vitro* fertilization in the Netherlands: Experiences and opinions of Dutch women. *Journal of in Vitro Fertilization and Embryo Transfer* 4: 116–123.

Hull, M. G. R., and C. M. A. Glazener. 1984. Male infertility and *in vitro* fertilization. *Lancet* 2 (July 28): 231.

Jarrell, J., R. Gwatkin, R. N. Lumsden, K. G. Lamont, G. Boulter, S. Daya, and J. Collins. 1986. An *in vitro* fertilization and embryo transfer pilot study: Treatment-dependent and treatment-independent pregnancies. *American Journal of Obstetrics and Gynecology* 154: 231–35.

Johnston, W. I. H. 1987. The evolution of *in vitro* fertilization technology. In *Future aspects of in vitro fertilization.* W. Feichtinger and P. Kemeter, eds. Berlin: Springer Verlag.

Jones, H. W. 1986. The infertile couple. In *In vitro fertilization: Past, present, future.* S. Fishel and E. M. Symonds, eds. Oxford: IRL Press.

Kandiyoti, D. 1988. Bargaining with patriarchy. *Gender & Society* 2: 274–290.

Kruger, T. F., A. A. Acosta, K. F. Simmons, J. R. Swanson, J. F. Matta, and S. Oehninger. 1988. Predictive value of abnormal sperm morphology in *in vitro* fertilization. *Fertility and Sterility* 49: 112–117.

Lasker, J. N., and S. Borg. 1987. *In search of parenthood.* Boston: Beacon Press.

Leeton, J., C. King, and J. Harmon. 1988. Sister-sister *in vitro* fertilization surrogate pregnancy with donor sperm: The case for surrogate gestational pregnancy. *Journal of in Vitro Fertilization and Embryo Transfer* 5: 245–248.

Lorber, J. 1987. *In vitro* fertilization and gender politics. *Women & Health* 13: 117–33.

Lorber, J., and D. Greenfeld. 1990. Couples' experiences with *in vitro* fertilization: A phenomenological approach. In *Proceedings of the Sixth World Congress on In Vitro Fertilization and Alternate Assisted Reproduction.* Z. Ben-Rafael, ed. New York: Plenum.

Marciano, T. D. 1978. Male pressure in the decision to remain childfree. *Alternative Lifestyles* 1: 95–111.

Mauss, M. 1954. *The gift.* Glencoe, IL: Free Press.

Miall, C. E. 1986. The stigma of involuntary childlessness. *Social Problems* 33: 268–82.

Michelow, M. C., J. Bernstein, M. J. Jacobson, J. L. McLoughlin, D. Rubenstein, A. I. Hacking, S. Preddy, and J. Van Der Wat. 1988. Mother-daughter *in vitro* fertilization triplet surrogate pregnancy. *Journal of in Vitro Fertilization and Embryo Transfer* 5: 31–34.

Mishler, E. G. 1984. *The discourse of medicine: Dialectics of medical interviews.* Norwood, NJ: Ablex.

Novaes, S. B. 1985. Social integration of technical innovation: Sperm banking and AID in France and the United States. *Social Science Information* 24: 569–84.

Oehninger, S., A. A. Acosta, T. Kruger, L. L. Veeck, J. Flood, and H. W. Jones. 1988. Failure of fertilization in IVF: The 'occult' male factor. *Journal of in Vitro Fertilization and Embryo Transfer* 5: 181–187.

Overall, C. 1987. *Ethics and human reproduction: A feminist analysis.* Boston: Allen and Unwin.

Pfeffer, N. 1987. Artificial insemination, in vitro fertilization and the stigma of infertility. In *Reproductive technologies: Gender, motherhood and medicine.* M. Stanworth, ed. Minneapolis, MN: University of Minnesota Press.

Reiser, S. J. 1978. *Medicine and the reign of technology.* Cambridge: Cambridge University Press.

Roach, S. 1988. Surrogacy: For love or money? Unpublished paper, Department of Sociology, The Flinders University of South Australia.

Roh, S. I., S. G. Awadalla, J. M. Park, W. G. Dodds, C. I. Friedman, and M. H. Kim. 1987. In vitro fertilization and embryo transfer: Treatment-dependent versus treatment-independent pregnancies. *Fertility and Sterility* 48: 982–986.

Rothman, B. Katz. 1989. *Recreating motherhood: Ideology and technology in a patriarchal society.* New York: Norton.

Seibel, M. M., and S. Levin. 1987. A new era in reproductive technologies: The emotional stages of in vitro fertilization. *Journal of in Vitro Fertilization and Embryo Transfer* 4: 135–140.

Silber, S. L. 1989. New techniques in non-operable cases of male obstruction. Paper presented at Sixth World Conference on In Vitro Fertilization and Assisted Reproduction, Jerusalem.

Simmons, R. G., S. Klein Marine, and R. L. Simmons. 1987. *Gift of life: The effect of organ transplantation on individual, family, and societal dynamics.* New Brunswick, NJ: Transaction Books.

Simmons, R. G., and L. Abress. 1988. Ethics in organ transplantation. In *Organ transplantation and replacement.* J. Cerilli, ed. Philadelphia: Lippincott.

Spallone, P., and D. L. Steinberg. eds. 1988. *Made to order: The myth of reproductive and genetic progress.* New York: Pergamon Press.

Spark, R. F. 1988. *The infertile male: The clinician's guide to diagnosis and treatment.* New York: Plenum.

Stanworth, M., ed. 1987. *Reproductive technologies: Gender, motherhood and medicine.* Minneapolis, MN: University of Minnesota Press.

Tangri, Sandra Schwartz. 1976. A feminist perspective on some ethical issues in population programs. *Signs* 1:895–904.

Testart, J., B. Lasalle, J. Belaisch-Allart, R. Forman, A. Hazout, N. Fries, and R. Frydman. 1988. Human embryo freezing. *Annals of the New York Academy of Sciences* 541: 532–540.

Williams, L. S. 1988. "It's going to work for me." Responses to failures of IVF. *Birth* 15: 153–156.

Yates, C. A., and D. M. de Kretser. 1987. Male-factor infertility and in vitro fertilization. *Journal of In Vitro Fertilization and Embryo Transfer* 4: 141–147.

Yovich, J. L., J. D. Stanger, J. M. Yovich, S. R. Turner, and B. D. Newman. 1984. Treatment of male infertility by in vitro fertilization. *Lancet* 1 (July 21): 169–170.

Yovich, J. L., and J. D. Stanger. 1984. The limitations of in vitro fertilization from males with severe oligospermia and abnormal sperm morphology. *Journal of in Vitro Fertilization and Embryo Transfer* 1: 172–179.

Is Pregnancy Necessary?
Feminist Concerns about Ectogenesis

JULIEN S. MURPHY   ❖ ❖ ❖

To what extent are women obliged to be child-bearers? If reproductive technology could offer some form of ectogenesis, would feminists regard it as a liberating reproductive option? Three lines of reproductive rights arguments currently used by feminists are applied to ectogenesis. Each fails to provide strong grounds for prohibiting it. Yet, there are several ways in which ectogenesis could contribute to women's oppression, in particular, if it were used to undermine abortion rights, reinforce traditional views of fertility, increase fetal rights in pregnancy, and perpetuate the unequal 'distribution of scarce medical resources. A rethinking of women's relationship to pregnancy is needed in order to challenge ectogenetic research.

In the past few decades, great gains have been made in women's reproductive freedoms. Abortion, contraception, and sterilization techniques allow women greater control over fertility. Feminists are united in support of these techniques. The feminist issue is not whether there ought to be pregnancy preventatives for women, but that the techniques available ought to be more accessible to women, and researchers ought to develop more effective and safer methods including male contraceptives and an abortifacient.[1] While feminists have been unified in support of methods that enable women to control their own fertility, there is disagreement among feminists about new reproductive techniques designed to treat infertility and induce pregnancy, such as in vitro fertilization, embryo transfer, and research for ectogenesis. If one believes that reproductive freedoms ought to include both fertility and infertility control, it is puzzling that feminists are united in support of the former but divided about the latter.

The feminist debates over the new reproductive technologies which are aimed at treating infertility are very recent. Reproductive rights arguments that feminists have found effective in establishing rights to fertility control seem to have little effect in countering infertility techniques. Yet, given the rapid pace of infertility research and the large number of women involved, feminists need to develop coherent positions that either give valid grounds for making political distinctions between fertility and infertility research, or support both kinds of technology. Central to this task is an evaluation of women's relationship to pregnancy, since the last reproductive technique mentioned, ectogenesis, would replace pregnancy with alternative means of reproduction for some if not all women. Hence, a discussion of ectogenesis is central to the debates about infertility research. Must women be pregnant? Do fetuses belong in women's bodies? Would other alternatives undermine the role of women in society and impede our struggles for liberation?

The topic of ectogenesis is no longer confined to science fiction. Techniques that enable the short-term growth of embryos in vitro suggest the eventual possibility of total growth of embryos outside of women's bodies. Discussions of ectogenesis are commonplace in scientific research and in reports from ethics committees for new reproductive technologies. For instance, ectogenesis is mentioned in the the *Warnock Report* (1984). This report claims that it should be a criminal offense to develop a human embryo in vitro beyond fourteen days. This view has been stated even more strongly at a recent bioethics conference where Sir David Napley claimed, "It should be a serious criminal offense to develop a human embryo to full maturity outside the body of a woman."[2] An ectogenetic scenario has been vividly, albeit ironically, described by an editor of a leading journal in reproductive research. Referring to experiments for sustaining human uteri in vitro, he writes:

> Transvaginal oocyte recovery, fertilization in vitro, and embryo transfer to an artificially perfused uterus will render motherhood, as we recognize it, obsolete. Women may elect to avoid the disfigurement of pregnancy, pain of childbirth, postpartum blues, and the occasional ineptitudes of obstetricians. It seems like the perfect solution to the diminishing number of practicing obstetricians. Maternal-Fetal medicine specialists would ply their trade on this artificial womb, which would be referred to them by the specialist in techniques of assisted reproduction. The extracorporeal womb could be tossed aside after development was complete. The need for a continuing supply of temporary uteri would keep former obstetricians in work doing the necessary hysterectomies, unless someone should be resourceful enough to develop a method to recycle these used specimens. (McDonough 1988, 1001)

Feminists are concerned with how ectogenesis might increase the oppression of women. Clearly, there are other philosophical issues inherent in discussions of ectogenesis. One might question ectogenesis from the point of view of the embryo and ask whether there is any moral violation in sustaining embryos in vitro for either a portion of development (beyond fourteen days) or until full maturity. One might challenge the value scheme in a society that would utilize technological resources for out-of-the-body reproduction. This discussion, while recognizing these issues, takes for its focus the effects of ectogenesis on feminist assumptions about what it means to be a woman.

Would current feminist reproductive rights arguments provide protection from potential abuses of ectogenesis? Some assumptions must be made about the kind of techniques required and the political context in which they would be developed. In order to analyze ectogenesis, let us assume that ectogenetic techniques will not only exist in the future, but will be methodologically similar to and consistent with the current lines of ectogenetic research, and that the sociopolitical climate of the future society in which ectogenesis might occur will not vary greatly from the present.

Would there be good reasons for feminists to object to ectogenesis? A question central to any ectogenetic research and one that has received very little attention to date is: Must women reproduce? While this question is continually raised by individual women about their situations, it is rarely raised of women as a group. Should women, as a group, be liberated from the responsibility of childbearing? Or, despite our liberation in many areas, does our ability to reproduce dictate a responsibility to ourselves and to future generations to be childbearers? (Allen, 1984).

Do fetuses "belong" in women's bodies, as the *Warnock Report* and political conservatives claim? Abortion arguments currently do not address this issue. While feminist arguments for freedom to choose abortion affirm women's right to terminate a pregnancy, that affirmation does not imply that women as such ought not be childbearers, but merely that women should not be pregnant against their will. Hence, the reproductive freedom of women acknowledged by the abortion right claims that pregnancy ought to be a woman's choice. But what if very few women chose it? In order to explore the relationship between fetuses and women's bodies, the nature and scope of ectogenetic research must be established.

ECTOGENETIC RESEARCH

If ectogenesis is to be accomplished, replacements must be found for the series of biochemical processes performed by women's bodies in pregnancy: egg maturation; fertilization, implantation, and embryo maintenance; temperature control; waste removal and transport of blood, nourishment, and oxygen to the embryo. Such a procedure, if successful, would accomplish in vitro gestation (IVG) for human reproduction. I will be using the terms ectogenesis and in vitro gestation as equivalent throughout this discussion. Both refer to the creation of an artificial womb.

The initial steps to develop IVG include the following techniques. Ovulation induction techniques and superovulation techniques enable the control of egg maturation though the actual process remains in vivo. Techniques for in vitro fertilization (IVF) are already in use. IVF and embryo transfer (ET) techniques have resulted in over two thousand live births worldwide, and are a common treatment for some forms of female infertility.[3] Techniques for freezing and thawing sperm and embryos have also met with some success. The criterion for success in these procedures is live birth. None of these techniques is completely safe for women and some might be quite dangerous (Holmes 1988; Laborie 1987, 1988; Rowland 1987a).

Already existing reproductive techniques are pointing the way toward better research strategies for an artificial womb. For instance, it seems clear that a fetus does not need to be implanted in the uterus of its genetic mother in order to thrive, as a recipient uterus has been used in embryo transfer. Also, research techniques for sustaining pregnancies in brain-dead women have resulted in a few live births showing that fetuses can thrive in the bodies of brain-dead pregnant women if there is proper temperature regulation, intubation, and ventilation, and all vital organs remain unharmed (Murphy 1989).

Neonatal technology has advanced to enable the maintenance of fetuses—some as early as sixteen weeks or as small as two hundred grams—in incubators, though it is quite costly. The longer a fetus can be sustained in utero, the greater its chances of surviving after cesarean section. In one case, a fetus was sustained in a brain-dead pregnant patient for sixty-three days. One researcher, who was prepared to obtain a court order if any relatives of the brain-dead woman objected to the procedure, remarked that brain-dead women have no rights because they are considered legally dead, and besides, their bodies are "the cheapest incubators we have."[4]

Other research for artificial wombs uses an artificial medium or even removed human uteri. Gena Corea (1985) notes that techniques for artificial wombs, which have been under investigation since the late 1950s, include several perfusion experiments on aborted fetuses. One experimenter (Goodlin 1963) submerged several fetuses in a high pressure oxygen chamber and used tubes to transport oxygen and nourishment. The fetuses survived this crude form of IVG for less than two days. A research group in Italy has kept human uteri removed from women undergoing hysterectomies alive by perfusing them in an oxygenated medium. A human blastocyst injected into such a uterus survived for fifty-two hours, and implanted itself (Bulletti 1988). Research to determine the chemical environment necessary for IVG is under way in animal experiments with rat embryos removed from uteri on the tenth day of gestation and cultured with various teratogens (Daston 1987).

ECTOGENESIS: WHO WANTS IT?

The research indicates that ectogenesis is of interest to scientists. It is a major component if not the culmination of reproductive technology, for it would provide nearly complete control of the developing embryo throughout gestation. The scientific gains from ectogenesis would be substantial, and it could be used to provide a supply of organs and tissue for transplants (Singer and Wells 1984). Let us focus on the implications of IVG if it were chosen by women or men as an alternative to pregnancy.

Women might draw upon several medical, social, or professional reasons in their desire for IVG. Whether or not these reasons are sufficient to justify ectogenesis, and what assumptions stand behind these reasons need further discussion. A woman may desire ectogenesis because she is unable to maintain a pregnancy or may have had a hysterectomy. Her medical history might indicate that she would have a high risk pregnancy, or that her health might be impaired because of having endured pregnancy. Other reasons involve the effects that pregnancy can have on women's social and professional lives. A woman may find ectogenesis desirable because she is a smoker, drug user, or casual drinker and does not wish to alter her behavior or place her fetus at risk. Pregnancy might make a woman ineligible for certain career opportunities (for example, athletics, dancing, modeling, acting).

Her job may be hazardous for pregnant women, yet the temporary transfer to safer working conditions may be impossible or undesirable. A woman may be in good health and fertile but may not want the emotional and physical stress of pregnancy.

Women might desire ectogenesis in order to be freed from the burden of child-bearing within a spousal relationship. Childbearing has been a blessing and a curse to women. Sometimes, women have reveled in the delights of pregnancy, even finding the female body superior to that of the male for its complicated reproductive possibilities. Other times, childbearing has fallen to women as a burden. Even in the best of situations, in both heterosexual and lesbian relationships, pregnancy is a woman's job.[5] Finally, some men might find ectogenesis a desirable alternative for it would enable them to have a child on their own provided there were ova banks.

There are three assumptions that are fundamental to support for ectogenesis: i) that IVG would not harm fetal development; ii) IVG privileges a genetically related child over an adopted child, either for ego-centered reasons or because of the shortage of children for adoption; iii) IVG would not contribute to the further oppression of women. While all supporters of IVG might share the first assumption, along with one of the two positions in the second assumption, it would be feminists who would also be concerned with the third assumption. A discussion of each assumption will follow.

i) IVG and Fetal Harm

The desirability of ectogenesis is predicated on the assumption that IVG would not produce fetal harm. Feminist concern about fetal damage with respect to IVG need not collapse into a fetus-centered perspective on reproductive issues. Usually, in reproductive debates, one must choose one of two perspectives—either a primary focus on respect for women or on the fetus. Janice Raymond (1987) terms the latter a fetalist position and contrasts fetalists with feminists in their reasons for opposition to reproductive technologies. As long as alternative gestation practices require women's bodies, there can be a conflict between women's rights and concern for the fetus. This conflict is illustrated by Annette Burfoot, who writes that reproductive medicine "regards women servomechanically as parts of a biological machine whose sole purpose is to nurture embryos" (1988). However, since IVG would not involve women's bodies (assuming egg removal was safe and required consent), concern for fetal harm need not eclipse respect for women's rights. It would seem appropriate to object to a reproductive procedure that might bring harm to a fetus, just as one might object to procedures that harm animals, neonates, or other higher life forms. The goal of IVG must surely be to produce an infant indistinguishable in health and vigor from an infant born of a human pregnancy. Clearly IVG would lose supporters if it harmed fetuses.

It is not known whether techniques for IVG would be safe for the fetus. Even if IVG proved safe in animals, no one would be sure that IVG would be safe in humans until it was actually tried. But who would be the first to risk it? Certainly the fear of irreparable damage to the embryo would be enough to prevent anyone from pursuing the fantasy of ectogenesis. A similar concern marked the precursory stages of IVF. Yet IVF was tried, and dangers to fetal development seemed to be only slightly increased (Lancaster 1987; St. Clair and Wagner 1989).[6] One can suspect that when feasible, IVG will also be tried.

One potential horror would be if IVG damaged the fetus in ways only detectable long after birth. This might give the illusion that techniques were safe and IVG might be used on many embryos before its dangers were discovered. If active euthanasia and infanticide remained prohibited, the infants would be left to a life of suffering. What if severe fetal damage were detected in the later stages of development? Would it be morally permissible to "abort" a third trimester fetus damaged by IVG techniques?

If the fetus were harmed as a result of IVG techniques, one might feel a heavy sense of moral blame. For without IVG techniques, the suffering fetus would not have existed. The use of fetuses in experimental procedures would be questioned. Of course, it would be incumbent on researchers to prove that the fetal damage was caused by IVG techniques and not by defective sperm or eggs. If fetal damage did result from IVG, the ensuing philosophical debate would need to determine the point at which fetal damage was severe enough to make IVG ethically prohibitive.

ii) IVG AND THE PRIVILEGING OF GENETICALLY RELATED CHILDREN

Does a desire for ectogenesis privilege genetic resemblance? If so, is there anything wrong with preferring to parent a child produced by one's own genetic material rather than a child with a different genetic heritage who might be available for adoption? It could be argued that IVG should not be favored over adoption since adoption provides parents for children who already exist. This assumes that there are children available for adoption, and that the rules and procedures of adoption facilities do not discriminate against competent applicants on grounds of sexual preference, race, class, age, or marital status.

Even if adoption were possible for most people wanting children, some would still prefer to have a genetic offspring (James 1987). Is the desire for a genetic offspring merely the result of egocentric prejudice? And if so, is there anything wrong with this? Clearly the desire may be hard to fulfill since human reproduction does not guarantee that one's offspring will share many physical characteristics, or likeness in character or personality. Even if genetic offspring do not greatly resemble the parent, it is still possible to see resemblances to oneself in the body of one's genetically related child. This may be enough to satisfy the desire for a genetic offspring. To delight in these resemblances need not be to collapse into narcissism but rather to revel in the mysteries of reproduction.

At what price does IVG offer this? First, this view romanticizes physical resemblances and genetic material. Secondly, there is no valid ground for favoring a child that looks like oneself over another. After all, one's genetic material is so diverse that it does not guarantee that a genetically related child will bear any resemblance to oneself. But more importantly, this sort of genetic privileging may lead to discrimination against several groups of people: gay and lesbian couples who are unable to "make" a child "in their own likeness"; non-monogamous heterosexual couples whose children will not look like a matched set; and infertile couples, who might expend great economic and personal resources trying to have a "natural child" (rather than all of us spending our efforts on undoing the superiority of the "natural child").

The preference for the natural child reinforces the link between genetic parent and offspring, a link which is often dysfunctional. Such a preference can perpetuate dysfunctional families by social policies that keep the family together because the genetic ties are seen as binding. Also, preference for a genetically similar child reinforces race, class, and cultural prejudices in adoption practices. Families that continue to represent "matched sets" to some extent perpetuate these prejudices in the society at large. In short, the desire for a genetic offspring is loaded with political and social values. Even if our society did not discriminate on any of these grounds, one would need to decide at what point concerns for an overpopulated world ought to override an individual's right to procreate.

If adoption supplied an adequate number of children for people desiring parenthood, and if adoption could be restructured to eliminate long waiting periods, tedious bureaucratic procedures, and discrimination, then IVG would seem unnecessary. But what if there were not enough adoptive children available to meet the demand by prospective IVG clients? Should surrogacy arrangements or international adoptions be encouraged? If the latter, it would be important to guarantee that no coercive strategies were used to take children away from their mothers, and that governments were not deliberately negligent about methods of fertility control for women for the sake of profits from their children.

iii) WOULD IVG BE A TECHNIQUE OF LIBERATION?

This question is at the center of the feminist debate over the new reproductive technologies. Much of the discussion has presupposed strong feminist arguments about reproductive rights relevant to fertility control. I believe that an examination of these arguments shows that the oppressive nature of IVG requires challenging the entire context of reproduction. It also raises the question: Why are alternatives to pregnancy desirable?

Three lines of argument have been used by feminists to justify reproductive rights for women. The first two are grounded in the notion of individual freedoms implied by having rights over our bodies. They are 1) the protection-from-bodily-violation argument and 2) the right-to-bodily-control argument. I will show that neither can be used to reject appeals for ectogenesis. The protection from bodily violation argument, while primarily applicable to arguing against assault and rape, has been used extensively in debates about contraceptive methods. The argument states that achieving reproductive ends does not justify subjecting women to unsafe drugs or procedures. Women's health should not be jeopardized just to enable contraception.

Feminists have appealed to the first argument to protest experimentation with and use of oral contraceptives and unsafe illegal abortions, as well as unnecessary hysterectomies, cesarean sections, and other abuses (for example, thalidomide, DES, and the Dalkon Shield). It has also been used recently by feminists to protest embryo transfer techniques. The claim is that ovulation induction, superovulation, and embryo transfer techniques are unsafe, and medical researchers often fail to inform women about the low probability IVF-ET offers for pregnancy (Soules, 1985; Laborie, 1987, 1988; Corea and Ince, 1987).

The right to bodily control is the second line of argument used by feminists to object to reproductive technology. It is commonly used in defense of a woman's right to abortion, but it could be extended to include the freedom to choose or refrain from medical procedures in general, as well as against assault and rape, and in support of safe contraception. When applied to pregnancy, this argument claims that women have a right to control our bodies in pregnancy, specifically, to choose to not be pregnant. Hence, women ought to have access to safe abortions. Admittedly, for some feminists this right holds only during early stages of fetal development; others extend it throughout pregnancy.

Both lines of argument could be applied to IVG. Feminists could use the argument for protection from bodily violation to object to IVG if the techniques for obtaining eggs for fertilization were unsafe. For even though IVG eliminates the need for women to bear children, it still requires women to supply the eggs.[7] If the methods for egg removal were painful or dangerous, then feminists would object to IVG by appealing to the first argument—bodily violation. Originally laparoscopy, requiring general anesthesia, was used for egg removal, and some deaths occured (Holmes 1988; Gomez dos Reis 1987). Although local anesthetic and "ultrasonically directed" methods are now more commonly used, some morbidity has been reported (Holmes 1988). The techniques to control ovulation that almost always precede egg removal may pose risks to women's health. While no careful study has been made regarding these risks, some feminists believe they may be substantial (Klein and Rowland 1988; Laborie 1988). If these techniques are found to endanger women's health, IVG would be a suspect procedure until better techniques were found.

Even if egg removal techniques presented danger to women, some women might still defend IVG as their best option for obtaining a genetic offspring. They might claim that many women in the past chose pregnancy knowing it might very well be life-endangering. Women who survived high risk pregnancies might have found that their choice greatly enhanced their lives. Why then should choosing a high risk egg removal procedure for IVG not be equally justifiable? Of course IVG would not be the only option for these women. One could obtain a genetic offspring by being an egg donor and using a surrogate embryo recipient for IVF-ET. Yet this procedure still involves egg removal and if egg removal techniques are unsafe, women would be enduring health risks in order to pursue this goal. Feminists might argue that reproductive technology should not be used to offer women new ways to risk their lives in reproduction. While each infertile woman would need to weigh her desire for a genetic offspring with risks to her health, feminists might insist that such a wager is not a mark of a liberating technology. The right-to-bodily-control argument could also be applied to IVG and egg removal techniques. Both egg removal and egg disposition ought to require informed consent.

An expanded right-to-bodily-control argument is being used by some feminists who assume that "bodily control" means the right to have full charge of reproduction. IVF-ET and presumably IVG mediate women's access to our reproductive bodies. Several feminists claim that women who choose IVF-ET are reduced to experimental victims of scientific research. Janice Raymond writes that "as women become the penultimate research 'subjects' (read objects), the way is paved for women's wider and more drastic use in reproductive research and experimentation. Women become the scheduled raw material in the factory of legalized reproductive experimentation" (1987, 64). IVG might be seen as a case in which women lose all control over reproduction by losing the experience of pregnancy and depending on technicians for the maintenance of their IVG fetuses. Nonetheless, IVG might not be a violation of the expanded right to bodily control if one understood bodily control to include the expansion of options which may or may not be connected to women's direct control. IVG would enable some infertile women to do something they otherwise would not be able to do: reproduce. And IVG could enable fertile women to have genetic offspring without the risk of pregnancy. In short, IVG would expand our reproductive options. However the creation of additional options need not be a sign of liberation (Dworkin 1982; Rowland 1987a). New options could be exploitative. Imagine a new drug that enabled workers to work for eighteen hour shifts without feeling tired. This discovery, if used to lengthen the work week, would be enslaving, not liberating.

Can we envision a scenario where the availability of IVG did not involve exploitation? IVG certainly would not exploit women in a traditional way, by keeping them pregnant. And, as long as women's consent were required for IVG, and pregnancy remained an option for fertile women, IVG would not necessarily be exploitive at all. Whether or not one affirms an expanded sense of bodily control is contingent on how one sees modern medicine, as benefiting or harming health. Women who value the experience of pregnancy and see it as offering a deeply satisfying and unique connection to new life would still choose pregnancy. Women who see pregnancy as either life-threatening or simply undesirable might feel bodily control expanded by the option of IVG. Guidelines for informed consent might ensure that women's eggs would not be used for exploitative ends.

The most extreme objection to IVG might be termed the elimination-of-women argument; it could be derived from the two previous arguments. This argument claims that the aim of certain reproductive techniques is to do away with women altogether. Clearly women researchers are underrepresented in the field of repro-ductive technology. What is to prevent men from making women extinct once our unique contribution to society—reproduction—can be supplied another way?[8] IVG, accompanied by sex selection techniques and methods for producing synthetic eggs, could risk the reproduction of an all male population, the ultimate patriarchal culture.[9] The link between artificial wombs and the possibility of femicide is sug-gested by Steinbacher and Holmes (1987, 57): "There is no atrocity too terrible for human nature to contemplate and often carry out. This has, in fact, been the case numerous times throughout history, and has been justified as necessary to fulfil the needs and 'rights' of 'superior' individuals or races." They suggest that the fate of women might be similar to that of some other oppressed groups (for example, "witches," American Indians, European Jews). A similarly apocalyptic tone is sounded by Robyn Rowland:

Much as we turn from consideration of a nuclear aftermath, we turn from seeing
a future where children are neither borne or born or where women are forced to
bear only sons and to slaughter their foetal daughters. Chinese and Indian women
are already trudging this path. The future of women as a group is at stake and
we need to ensure that we have thoroughly considered all possibilities before
endorsing technology which could mean the death of the female. (1987b, 75)

Despite the ever-present threat of violence against the oppressed, the elimination-of-women argument is implausible. It assumes that women are allowed to
exist in patriarchy simply because of their childbearing function. Despite feminist
attacks on female socialization, women's roles in society remain steadfast. Women
continue to provide patriarchy with at least four other functions: nurturing, a
diligent work force, the maintenance of male egoism, and objects of sexual desire.
Almost as important as reproduction are the many nurturing roles delegated to
women in family life, the community, and the labor force (for example, nursing,
childcare, elementary education, social service, secretarial jobs). It is hard to imagine a sexist government eliminating women only to delegate these undesired nurturing roles to men. Women also provide patriarchy with cheap labor for tedious
jobs (in electronics, textiles, data processing, and so forth). Women's reputations
for small hands and docility make it all the easier to assign such work to them.
Men might think it worth while to keep women around to spare themselves these
forms of labor. Further, sexism has been part of society for so long that men have
grown accustomed to a position of superiority vis-à-vis women that would be hard
to give up. Male egoism is maintained by a sexist culture. Then of course there is
a heterosexual structure in patriarchy that is thousands of years old. Male heter-
osexuality would have to undergo radical transformation. In short, it would be hard
to eliminate women if women remained the objects of sexual desire for many men.
In addition to these four functions, women might wage a successful resistance
movement. All in all, it is hard to see how IVG could lead to such massive social
transformations as would be required for a transition to an all male society. The
existence of women is built into the sexist socialization patterns of society which
requires that women exist.[10]

None of the above three arguments defeat ectogenetic research. Furthermore,
feminists who see liberating potential in IVG might appeal to Shulamith Firestone,
a feminist who has argued that reproduction should not be seen as "women's work"
and has advocated ectogenesis. She claims that "pregnancy is barbaric," "a temporary deformation of the body of the individual for the sake of the species,"
physically dangerous and painful. Writing in 1970, Firestone envisioned a cultural,
economic, and sexual revolution which would use technology to expand human
freedoms. Ectogenesis would play a key role: "I submit, then, that the first demand
for any alternative system must be: *The freeing of women from the tyranny of their
reproductive biology by every means available, and the diffusion of the childbearing and
child rearing role to the society as a whole, men as well as women*" (1970, 206). Her
revolutionary plan requires abolition of capitalism, racism, sexism, the family,
marriage, sexual repression (in all of its forms), and all institutions that keep women

and children out of the larger society (such as female labor and elementary schools). But we should heed her warning: "in the hands of our current society and under the direction of current scientists (few of whom are female) any attempted use of technology to 'free' anybody is suspect" (1970, 206).

We are far from achieving the sort of revolution required in order for ectogenesis to be liberating. Capitalism, for instance, continues to be the dominant economic system. Marriages and families, although less prevalent than when Firestone wrote, are still the norm; schooling is still compulsory. Yet, advocates of ectogenesis Peter Singer and Deane Wells rely in part on Firestone's writings to claim that ectogenesis ought to be a feminist goal now. They argue that despite widespread sexism, ectogenesis can only enhance the status of women:

> Can it seriously be claimed that in our present society the status of women rests entirely on their role as nurturers of embryos from conception to birth? If we argue that to break the link between women and childbearing would be to undermine the status of women in our society what are we saying about the ability of women to obtain true equality in other spheres of life? We, at least, are not nearly so pessimistic about the abilities of women to achieve equality with men across the broad range of human endeavor. For that reason, we think women will be helped rather than harmed by the development of a technology that makes it possible for them to have children without being pregnant. (Singer and Wells 1984, 129)

This position ignores the theory of revolution implicit in Firestone's support for ectogenesis. In fact, it would be consistent with Firestone's vision to assume that technology itself would be thoroughly transformed by the transformation of society. Ectogenesis, for instance, could not be advocated as a cure for "infertility," since there would no emphasis on having a biological child. If ectogenesis were to exist at all it would be to create more desired children.

It would be hard to imagine a post-revolutionary society finding a place for IVG. IVG would definitely not replace pregnancy. For if it were to do so, that would suggest that women's bodies had been judged unfit for pregnancy. Is the best way to abolish sexism a method that downgrades a female capacity—pregnancy? This suggests that the way to deal with difference is to annihilate it.

The sexism of our current society makes evident that we are far from the goals Firestone envisioned. Debates about fertility and infertility as well as research protocols must be seen within this context. As long as egg removal does not produce severe and immediate harm to women, no doubt many will pursue ectogenesis as an alternative to pregnancy. However, while there may be valid reasons for women to seek alternatives to pregnancy, we need to consider possible detrimental effects of the availability of ectogenesis on abortion and pregnancy rights.

IVG presents some benefits for women, for instance, fetal surgery would not involve surgery on the mother. Yet even this benefit could be detrimental for women, since it could be used to undermine a woman's right to refuse treatment on her in utero fetus. Furthermore, since the IVG fetus is detached from the mother, and is able to be a patient in its own right, it could be harder to claim that any fetus is not (yet) a human being. If IVG fetuses are not dependent on women's bodies, they may seem to differ only slightly from neonates. Hence, if neonates are persons, why not IVG fetuses too? And what is the moral difference between an IVG fetus and an in utero one?

IVG could thus make it more difficult to justify elective abortions for pregnant women. With IVG, the thorny problem of fetal viability appears. If the definition from *Roe v. Wade* remains unchanged, then every IVG fetus is a viable fetus, for viability means the ability to survive outside the mother's womb, possibly aided by life-support technology. An IVG fetus would be viable in all stages of gestation provided it were able to thrive. Hence viability would no longer be a useful indicator of fetal development. Some other criteria would be needed if the fetus were to increase in status as birth approached. The tendency might be to discredit the notion of viability altogether, and prohibit abortion. For if IVG parents went to great expense to reproduce in this manner, they might be less sensitive to pregnant women who wanted to abort healthy fetuses. Should prospective parents of an IVG fetus have the right to terminate the fetus if they wish? This act, similar to an abortion, might be difficult to justify since IVG procedures do not conflict with a woman's right to control her body. The right over genetic material might be included in the overriding right to control one's body. It would be a right for both women and men, and so a way of resolving conflicting desires between the two gamete donors would be needed. While this right might justify termination of IVG fetuses, it could also be used by men to demand abortion on the part of their female partners.

IVG could also be implicated in efforts to place greater controls on pregnant women. First, pregnancy might come to be viewed as an inferior act. Women choosing pregnancy over IVG, especially if the latter were believed to provide ideal conditions for fetal development, might be seen as taking unnecessary risks with fetal life in order to have an experience of childbirth. Or pregnant women might feel the need to monitor their pregnancies and limit their lives in an attempt to duplicate as much as possible IVG conditions. We might come to see pregnancy as a mere biological function, repeatable in IVG, and not also as a human bond in formation of new life that can be had in no other way. We would need to decide, as a society, whether pregnancy per se had any intrinsic value. If not, we might judge the ideal conditions for fetal development and freedom from risk for women to outweigh *any* value for pregnancy. Hence, IVG could lead to the creation of a class system in reproduction with the rich reproducing in ectogenic labs while the poor continue to rely on women's bodies for pregnancy.

IVG might also contribute to excessive concern for "quality control" in fetal development. Sex-identification techniques are already in use on some embryos prior to implantation. Genetic research is under way for screening techniques to identify gene-linked traits. If IVG were advocated because it offered ideal conditions for fetal development, it would be hard to imagine researchers resisting the opportunity to ensure ideal fetal quality, despite the fact that such product-control endeavors might undermine respect for life's diversity. In fact, it is the opportunity for genetic engineering that has been seen as one of the greatest dangers of this research (Bradish 1987; Minden 1987; Bullard 1987). Linda Bullard claims that genetic engineering is "*inherently* eugenic in that it always requires someone to decide what is a good and a bad gene" (1987, 117). We might be able to develop a feminist criterion for genetic engineering, however, such as restricting choices to the prevention of genetic disease (for example, Down syndrome, muscular dystrophy, thalassemia, Tay-Sachs disease, cystic fibrosis).

Is Infertility a Feminist Issue?

Any feminist protest of IVG is likely to be seen as undermining the rights of infertile women to have appropriate medical treatment. What is not obvious is the sexist paradigm assumed by IVG.

This is the most important criticism of IVG for feminists. While those who desire IVG might attempt to justify the procedure on an individual basis, one must also examine the male paradigm of reproduction that any IVG research must assume. The feminist movement ought not to choose sides over which women's rights to support: those of fertile or infertile women. Nor is it appropriate to denigrate those women who choose IVG by assuming they desperately seek motherhood because they are "unenlightened" about their socialization to be mothers. This approach might be plausible if feminists, in large numbers, refuse pregnancy and motherhood as a mark of enlightenment. However, this is not the case. Given this context, it is unfair for a feminist who has chosen pregnancy or who merely admits to valuing pregnancy, to find an infertile woman's desire to reproduce indicative of patriarchal socialization. This does not mean that other reasons do not exist for condemning IVG. Before going any further, we must consider whether infertility is a disability at all.

Some advocates of reproductive technology argue that infertility is a disability and ought to be treated. Deane Wells claims "*prima facie* the inability to bring into the world one's own genetic children is a disability in the same way as is shortsightedness" (1987, 374). Wells argues that the same objections to the cost and research for infertility treatments could have been made about treatment for shortsightedness in times before the manufacturing of spectacles. Just as it would seem foolish to object to treating shortsightedness, it would similarly be foolish to object to treating infertility. Yet, one should not lose sight of an obvious difference between a reproductive impairment and a visual impairment. The major difference is that while everyone surely desires to have greater visual abilities, not everyone desires to reproduce. Hence, a reproductive impairment need not require treatment. Reproductive abilities, unlike visual abilities, are used seldom in our lives, particularly in the United States, where the birth rate continues to decrease.

There is another difficulty feminists might have in casting infertility as a "disability." Infertility is a social and political phenomenon. Pregnancy is linked to the essence of being female. Infertility ought not to mark women for the whole of our lives in any primary way. Nonetheless, women who are unable to reproduce have the right to pursue medical options. Feminist concerns about infertility options ought to center on whether or not infertility treatments restore or replace women's reproductive capacities.

It is imperative to consider the broader implications for women's status of any medical treatment for infertility beyond the actual restoration of women's reproductive functions. IVF-ET for example, could be seen as a new way of legitimating pregnancy as women's social "duty" (Crowe 1987; Soloman 1988). IVG breaks the necessary connection between women and reproduction, but could imply that pregnancy is merely a collection of bodily processes undermining the reproductive work women do in society. This is not to say that infertility should not be treated. It is merely to say that one should not be shortsighted about the broader social effects of new reproductive methods.

It is not that feminists should not support infertility research. Rather, we should demand a share in controlling its direction. If feminists are going to protest IVG and its precursory techniques (IVF-ET), then we ought also to support research into the causes of infertility. After all, approximately 10 percent of heterosexual couples in the United States are infertile, and most likely that number will increase with the growing number of environmental and reproductive hazards we are exposed to.

The issue then for society and for feminists ought not to be replacing the functions of women's bodies by technological alternatives, but rather developing non-exploitative ways to treat infertility that enable women to experience pregnancy and childbirth. Technology that is restorative, that enables women to experience our reproductive bodies without endangering our health is the sort of technology that feminists can support in a unified way.

Of all the reproductive techniques, ectogenesis, because it could eliminate pregnancy, poses the greatest challenge to women's reproductive rights. There appears to be nothing a priori that requires human gestation to occur in vivo anymore than there is an unwritten law requiring sex be the only means for egg fertilization. But in a patriarchal society we can expect the methods of infertility treatment to reflect sexist biases. IVG does this by suggesting that the way to treat infertility is to remove reproduction from women's bodies completely. Not only does IVG displace our bodily abilities, but it also suggests that gestation in a laboratory is equivalent to human pregnancy. Hence, what women contribute to their pregnancies is not essential to reproduction. Sexism proclaims pregnancy to be "inferior" and men recoil in fear of women's reproductive potential; such are the consequences when those in power do not themselves have such powers.

Clearly, many feminists would favor pregnancy over IVG in most cases, not because women are the most cost-effective uteri (what sort of artificial uterus could also hold down a job and run a family while maintaining a fetus?) but because IVG represents a misguided approach to infertility. That some women might prefer gestation of their fertilized eggs in a laboratory rather than in their own bodies is more of a mark of the oppressive ways in which women's bodies and pregnancy are seen in this culture rather than a sign of progressive social attitudes. The oppression that leads to such negative attitudes can only be changed by redirecting our priorities. We must ensure that everyone be provided with appropriate health care, as well as other prerequisites for health such as education and decent housing. The effects of poverty on women (not to mention children) are far more devastating than the effects of either infertility or reproductive technology.

We need a woman-centered reproductive agenda that makes visible the needs of all women, particularly poor women and women of color. We are only beginning to realize what this might mean. Without such an agenda, women will continue to be exploited by the sexist research system that is a product of our sexist society. More and more resources, including women's bodies, eggs, and uteri, will be wasted on experiments that undermine women, while social programs that would provide a better life will continue to be neglected. These considerations suggest that feminists must protest sexist research methods such as IVG and politicize not only those women most likely to use IVG, but also those most likely not to need it.

NOTES

1. RU486 is the abortifacient currently used in France and is at the center of controversy in the United States. See Suh (1989) and Navasky (1988).

2. A statement made by Sir David Napley, past president of the English Law Society, at the 1983 Mogul International Management Consultants Ltd. Conference on Bioethics and Law of Human Conception in Vitro. See Kirby (1984).

3. Cf. Spallone and Steinberg (1987) for a survey of IVF research in sixteen countries.

4. Conversations with medical researchers engaged in sustaining pregnancies in brain-dead pregnant women. See Murphy (1989).

5. Of course, in lesbian relationships both women can decide together which would "prefer" to have a child, provided both are fertile. While a lesbian relationship model removes some of the automatic "burden" (it is not assumed that one person instead of the other must be the one to be pregnant), still lesbians along with heterosexual women may wish that women could be spared pregnancy.

6. The National Perinatal Statistics Unit in Australia found that in 1985, IVF infants were four times more likely (than the general population) to die at birth due to prematurity (Australian 1985), and they found a larger than expected number of IVF babies with spina bifida and transposition of blood vessels to the heart (Lancaster 1987). See also Holmes (1988).

7. See my article (1984) for a discussion of the sexist language of egg removal in medical research.

8. IVG would be the second to the last technique in the series. The final technique might be the manufacture of synthetic eggs, which would enable a perpetual supply of eggs.

9. Cf. Holmes and Hoskins (1987) for a feminist critique of sex selection techniques.

10. It might be possible to have an "all male" society while still allowing those of us with female bodies to exist. This would be possible if the category "woman" could be destroyed without requiring the destruction of the category "man." This would assume that masculinity could survive without femininity. The society would be thoroughly masculine in its values. Everyone would be regarded as "men," though some would donate eggs to IVG procedures while others provided sperm. For this to come about women would have to be coerced to take on all the traits of masculinity and would come to be regarded not as a different gender, but rather as inferior men (undesirable mutations of men).

REFERENCES

Allen, Jeffner. 1984. Motherhood: The annihilation of women. In *Mothering: Essays in feminist theory.* Joyce Trebilcot, ed. New Jersey: Rowman and Allanheld, 315–330.

Arditti, Rita, Renate Duelli Klein, and Shelley Minden, eds. 1984. *Test-tube women.* London: Pandora Press.

Australian *In Vitro* Fertilisation. Collaborative Group. 1985. High incidence of preterm births and early losses in pregnancy after *in vitro* fertilisation. *British Medical Journal* 291:1160–1163.

Bradish, Paula. 1987. From genetic counseling and genetic analysis, to genetic ideal and genetic fate? In Spallone and Steinberg (1987).

Bullard, Linda. 1987. Killing us softly: Toward a feminist analysis of genetic engineering. In Spallone and Steinberg (1987).

Bulletti, C., V. M. Jasonni, S. Tabanelli, et al. 1988. Early human pregnancy in vitro utilizing an artificially perfused uterus. *Fertility and Sterility* 49 (6):1–6.

Burfoot, Annette. 1988. A review of the third annual meeting of the European Society of Human Reproduction and Embryology. *Reproductive and Genetic Engineering: Journal of International Feminist Analysis.* 1 (1):107–111.

Corea, Gena. 1985. *The mother machine: Reproductive technologies from artificial insemination to artificial wombs.* New York: Harper and Row.

Corea, Gena, Renate Duelli Klein, Jalna Hanmer, et al. 1987. *Man-Made women.* Bloomington: Indiana University Press.

Corea, Gena, and Susan Ince. 1987. Report of a survey of IVF clinics in the US. In Spallone and Steinberg (1987).

Crowe, Christine. 1987. Women want it: In vitro fertilization and women's motivations for participation. In Spallone and Steinberg (1987).

Daston, G. P., M. T. Ebron, B. Carver, et al. 1987. *In vitro* teratogenicity of ethylene-thiourea in the rat. *Teratology* 35 (2):239–245.

Dworkin, Gerald. 1982. Is more choice better than less? *Midwest Studies in Philosophy* 7:47–61.

Firestone, Shulamith. 1970. *The dialectic of sex.* New York: Bantam.

Gomes dos Reis, Ana Regina. 1987. IVF in Brazil: The story told by the newspapers. In Spallone and Steinberg (1987).

Goodlin, Robert C. 1963. An improved fetal incubator. *Transactions–American Society for Artificial Internal Organs* 9:348–350.

Holmes, Helen B., and Betty B. Hoskins. 1987. Prenatal and preconception sex choice technologies: A path to femicide. In Corea, et al. (1987).

Holmes, Helen B., 1988. In vitro fertilization: Reflections on the state of the art. *Birth: Issues in Perinatal Care and Education* 15 (3): 134–145.

James, David N. 1987. Ectogenesis: A reply to Singer and Wells. *Bioethics* 1 (1):80–99.

Kirby, M. D. 1984. Bioethics of IVF—The state of the debate. *Journal of Medical Ethics* 1:45–48.

Klein, Renate, and Robyn Rowland. 1988. Women as test-sites for fertility drugs: Clomiphene citrate and hormonal cocktails. *Reproductive and Genetic Engineering: Journal of International Feminist Analysis* 1 (3):251–273.

Laborie, Françoise. 1987. Looking for mothers you only find fetuses. In Spallone and Steinberg (1987).

Laborie, Françoise. 1988. New reproductive technologies: News from France and elsewhere. *Reproductive and Genetic Engineering* 1 (1):77–85.

McDonough, Paul G. 1988. Comment. *Fertility and Sterility* 50 (6):1001–1002.

Minden, Shelley. 1987. Patriarchal designs: The genetic engineering of human embryos. In Spallone and Steinberg (1987).

Murphy, Julien S. 1984. Egg farming and women's future. In *Test-Tube women*. Rita Arditti, Renate Duelli Klein, and Shelley Minden (1984).

Murphy, Julien S. 1986. Abortion rights and fetal termination. *Journal of Social Philosophy* 17:11–16.

Murphy, Julien S. 1989. Should pregnancy be sustained in brain-dead women? A philosophical discussion of postmortem pregnancy. In *Healing Technologies*. Kathryn Strother Ratcliff, Myra Marx Ferree, Gail Mellow, et al., eds. Ann Arbor: University of Michigan Press.

Navasky, Victor. 1988. Bitter pill. *The Nation* 247 (15):515–516.

Raymond, Janice G. 1987. Fetalists and feminists: They are not the same. In Spallone and Steinberg (1987).

Rowland, Robyn. 1987a. Of women born, but for how long? The relationship of women to the new reproductive technologies and the issue of choice. In Spallone and Steinberg (1987).

Rowland, Robyn. 1987b. Motherhood, patriarchal power, alienation and the issue of 'choice' in sex preselection. In Spallone and Steinberg (1987).

St. Clair, Patricia A., and Marsden G. Wagner. 1989. Are *in-vitro* fertilisation and embryo transfer of benefit to all? *The Lancet* ii:1027–1030.

Singer, Peter, and Deane Wells. 1984. *Making babies: The new science and ethics of conception.* New York: Charles Scribner's Sons.

Solomon, Alison. 1988. Integrating infertility crisis counseling into feminist practice. *Reproductive and Genetic Engineering* 1 (1):41–49.

Soules, Michael. 1985. The in vitro fertilization pregnancy rate—Let's be honest with one another. *Fertility and Sterility* 43 (4):511–513.

Spallone, Patricia, and Deborah Lynn Steinberg. 1987. *Made to order: The myth of reproductive and genetic progress.* Oxford: Pergamon Press.

Steinbacher, Roberta, and Helen B. Holmes. 1987. Sex choice: survival and sisterhood. In Corea et al. (1987).

Suh, Mary. 1989. RU Detour. *Ms* (January–February):135–136.

Warnock, Mary. 1984. *A question of life: The Warnock report on human fertilisation & embryology.* Oxford: Basil Blackwell.

Wells, Deane. 1987. Ectogenesis, justice and utility: A reply to James. *Bioethics* 1 (4): 372–379.

The Moral Significance of Birth

MARY ANNE WARREN ❖ ❖ ❖

Does birth make a difference to the moral rights of the fetus/infant? Should it make a difference to its legal rights? Most contemporary philosophers believe that birth cannot make a difference to moral rights. If this is true, then it becomes difficult to justify either a moral or a legal distinction between late abortion and infanticide. I argue that the view that birth is irrelevant to moral rights rests upon two highly questionable assumptions about the theoretical foundations of moral rights. If we reject these assumptions, then we are free to take account of the contrasting biological and social relationships that make even relatively late abortion morally different from infanticide.

English common law treats the moment of live birth as the point at which a legal person comes into existence. Although abortion has often been prohibited, it has almost never been classified as homicide. In contrast, infanticide generally is classified as a form of homicide, even where (as in England) there are statutes designed to mitigate the severity of the crime in certain cases. But many people—including some feminists—now favor the extension of equal legal rights to some or all fetuses (S. Callahan 1984, 1986). The extension of legal personhood to fetuses would not only threaten women's right to choose abortion, but also undermine other fundamental rights. I will argue that because of these dangers, birth remains the most appropriate place to mark the existence of a new legal person.

SPEAKING OF RIGHTS

In making this case, I find it useful to speak of moral as well as legal rights. Although not all legal rights can be grounded in moral rights, the right to life can plausibly be so construed. This approach is controversial. Some feminist philosophers have been critical of moral analyses based upon rights. Carol Gilligan (1982), Nel Noddings (1984), and others have argued that women tend to take a different approach to morality, one that emphasizes care and responsibility in interpersonal relationships rather than abstract rules, principles, or conflicts of rights. I would argue, however, that moral rights are complementary to a feminist ethics of care and responsibility, not inconsistent or competitive with it. Whereas caring relationships can provide a moral ideal, respect for rights provides a moral floor—a

Hypatia vol.4, no. 3 (Fall 1989).© Mary Anne Warren

minimum protection for individuals which remains morally binding even where appropriate caring relationships are absent or have broken down (Manning 1988). Furthermore, as I shall argue, social relationships are part of the foundation of moral rights.

Some feminist philosophers have suggested that the very concept of a moral right may be inconsistent with the social nature of persons. Elizabeth Wolgast (1987, 41–42) argues convincingly that this concept has developed within an atomistic model of the social world, in which persons are depicted as self-sufficient and exclusively self-interested individuals whose relationships with one another are essentially competitive. As Wolgast notes, such an atomistic model is particularly inappropriate in the context of pregnancy, birth, and parental responsibility. More-over, recent feminist research has greatly expanded our awareness of the historical, religious, sociological, and political forces that shape contemporary struggles over reproductive rights, further underscoring the need for approaches to moral theory that can take account of such social realities (Harrison 1983; Luker 1984; Petchesky 1984).

But is the concept of a moral right necessarily incompatible with the social nature of human beings? Rights are indeed individualistic, in that they can be ascribed to individuals, as well as to groups. But respect for moral rights need not be based upon an excessively individualistic view of human nature. A more socially perceptive account of moral rights is possible, provided that we reject two common assumptions about the theoretical foundations of moral rights. These assumptions are widely accepted by mainstream philosophers, but rarely stated and still more rarely defended.

The first is what I shall call the intrinsic-properties assumption. This is the view that the only facts that can justify the ascription of basic moral rights[1] or moral standing[2] to individuals are facts about *the intrinsic properties of those individuals*. Philosophers who accept this view disagree about which of the intrinsic properties of individuals are relevant to the ascription of rights. They agree, how-ever, that relational properties—such as being loved, or being part of a social community or biological ecosystem—cannot be relevant.

The second is what I shall call the single-criterion assumption. This is the view that there is some single property, the presence or absence of which divides the world into those things which have moral rights or moral standing, and those things which do not. Christopher Stone (1987) locates this assumption within a more general theoretical approach, which he calls "moral monism." Moral monists be-lieve that the goal of moral philosophy is the production of a coherent set of principles, sufficient to provide definitive answers to all possible moral dilemmas. Among these principles, the monist typically assumes, will be one that identifies some key property which is such that, "Those beings that possess the key property count morally . . . [while those] things that lack it are all utterly irrelevant, except as resources for the benefit of those things that do count" (1987, 13).

Together, the intrinsic-properties and single-criterion assumptions preclude any adequate account of the social foundations of moral rights. The intrinsic-properties assumption requires us to regard all personal or other relationships among indi-viduals or groups as wholly irrelevant to basic moral rights. The single-criterion assumption requires us to deny that there can be a variety of sound reasons for ascribing moral rights, and a variety of things and beings to which some rights may appropriately be ascribed. Both assumptions are inimical to a feminist approach to moral theory, as well as to approaches that are less anthropocentric and more environmentally adequate. The prevalence of these assumptions helps to explain why few mainstream philosophers believe that birth can in any way alter the infant's moral rights.

THE DENIAL OF THE MORAL SIGNIFICANCE OF BIRTH

The view that birth is irrelevant to moral rights is shared by philosophers on all points of the spectrum of moral views about abortion. For the most conservative, birth adds nothing to the infant's moral rights, since all of those rights have been present since conception. Moderates hold that the fetus acquires an equal right to life at some point after conception but before birth. The most popular candidates for this point of moral demarcation are (1) the stage at which the fetus becomes viable (i.e., capable of surviving outside the womb, with or without medical assistance), and (2) the stage at which it becomes sentient (i.e., capable of having experiences, including that of pain). For those who hold a view of this sort, both infanticide and abortion at any time past the critical stage are forms of homicide, and there is little reason to distinguish between them either morally or legally.

Finally, liberals hold that even relatively late abortion is sometimes morally acceptable, and that at no time is abortion the moral equivalent of homicide. However, few liberals wish to hold that infanticide is not—at least sometimes—morally comparable to homicide. Consequently, the presumption that being born makes no difference to one's moral rights creates problems for the liberal view of abortion. Unless the liberal can establish some grounds for a general moral distinction between late abortion and early infanticide, she must either retreat to a moderate position on abortion, or else conclude that infanticide is not so bad after all.

To those who accept the intrinsic-properties assumption, birth can make little difference to the moral standing of the fetus/infant. For birth does not seem to alter any intrinsic property that could reasonably be linked to the possession of a strong right to life. Newborn infants have very nearly the same intrinsic properties as do fetuses shortly before birth. They have, as L. W. Sumner (1983, 53) says, "the same size, shape, internal constitution, species membership, capacities, level of consciousness, and so forth."[3] Consequently, Sumner says, infanticide cannot be morally very different from late abortion. In his words, "Birth is a shallow and arbitrary criterion of moral standing, and there appears to be no way of connecting it to a deeper account" (52).

Sumner holds that the only valid criterion of moral standing is the capacity for sentience (136). Prenatal neurophysiology and behavior suggest that human fetuses begin to have rudimentary sensory experiences at some time during the second trimester of pregnancy. Thus, Sumner concludes that abortion should be permitted during the first trimester but not thereafter, except in special circumstances (152).[4]

Michael Tooley (1983) agrees that birth can make no difference to moral standing. However, rather than rejecting the liberal view of abortion, Tooley boldly claims that neither late abortion nor early infanticide is seriously wrong. He argues that an entity cannot have a strong right to life unless it is capable of desiring its own continued existence. To be capable of such a desire, he argues, a being must have a concept of itself as a continuing subject of conscious experience. Having such a concept is a central part of what it is to be a person, and thus the kind of being that has strong moral rights (41). Fetuses certainly lack such a concept, as do infants during the first few months of their lives. Thus, Tooley concludes, neither fetuses nor newborn infants have a strong right to life, and neither abortion nor infanticide is an intrinsic moral wrong.

These two theories are worth examining, not only because they illustrate the difficulties generated by the intrinsic-properties and single-criterion assumptions, but also because each includes valid insights that need to be integrated into a more comprehensive account. Both Sumner and Tooley are partially right. Unlike "genetic humanity"—a property possessed by fertilized human ova—sentience and self-awareness are properties that have some general relevance to what we may owe another being in the way of respect and protection. However, neither the sentience criterion nor the self-awareness criterion can explain the moral significance of birth.

THE SENTIENCE CRITERION

Both newborn infants and late-term fetuses show clear signs of sentience. For instance, they are apparently capable of having visual experiences. Infants will often turn away from bright lights, and those who have done intrauterine photography have sometimes observed a similar reaction in the late-term fetus when bright lights are introduced in its vicinity. Both may respond to loud noises, voices, or other sounds, so both can probably have auditory experiences. They are evidently also responsive to touch, taste, motion, and other kinds of sensory stimulation.

The sentience of infants and late-term fetuses makes a difference to how they should be treated, by contrast with fertilized ova or first-trimester fetuses. Sentient beings are usually capable of experiencing painful as well as pleasurable or affectively neutral sensations.[5] While the capacity to experience pain is valuable to an organism, pain is by definition an intrinsically unpleasant experience. Thus, sentient beings may plausibly be said to have a moral right not to be deliberately subjected to pain in the absence of any compelling reason. For those who prefer not to speak of rights, it is still plausible that a capacity for sentience gives an entity some moral standing. It may, for instance, require that its interests be given some consideration in utilitarian calculations, or that it be treated as an end and never merely as a means.

But it is not clear that sentience is a sufficient condition for moral equality, since there are many clearly-sentient creatures (e.g., mice) to which most of us would not be prepared to ascribe equal moral standing. Sumner examines the implications of the sentience criterion primarily in the context of abortion. Given his belief that some compromise is essential between the conservative and liberal viewpoints on abortion, the sentience criterion recommends itself as a means of drawing a moral distinction between early abortion and late abortion. It is, in some ways, a more defensible criterion than fetal viability.

The 1973 *Roe v. Wade* decision treats the presumed viability of third-trimester fetuses as a basis for permitting states to restrict abortion rights in order to protect fetal life in the third trimester, but not earlier. Yet viability is relative, among other things, to the medical care available to the pregnant woman and her infant. Increasingly sophisticated neonatal intensive care has made it possible to save many more premature infants than before, thus altering the average age of viability. Someday it may be possible to keep even first-trimester fetuses alive and developing normally outside the womb. The viability criterion seems to imply that the advent of total ectogenesis (artificial gestation from conception to birth) would automatically eliminate women's right to abortion, even in the earliest stages of pregnancy. At the very least, it must imply that as many aborted fetuses as possible should be kept alive through artificial gestation. But the mere technological possibility of providing artificial wombs for huge numbers of human fetuses could not establish such a moral obligation. A massive commitment to ectogenesis would probably be ruinously expensive, and might prove contrary to the interests of parents and children. The viability criterion forces us to make a hazardous leap from the technologically possible to the morally mandatory.

The sentience criterion at first appears more promising as a means of defending a moderate view of abortion. It provides an intuitively plausible distinction between early and late abortion. Unlike the viability criterion, it is unlikely to be undermined by new biomedical technologies. Further investigation of fetal neurophysiology and behavior might refute the presumption that fetuses begin to be capable of sentience *at some point in the second trimester*. Perhaps this development occurs slightly earlier or slightly later than present evidence suggests. (It is unlikely to be much earlier or much later.) However, that is a consequence that those who hold a moderate position on abortion could live with; so long as the line could still be drawn with some degree of confidence, they need not insist that it be drawn exactly where Sumner suggests.

But closer inspection reveals that the sentience criterion will not yield the result that Sumner wants. His position vacillates between two versions of the sentience criterion, neither of which can adequately support his moderate view of abortion. The strong version of the sentience criterion treats sentience as a sufficient condition for having full and equal moral standing. The weak version treats sentience as sufficient for having some moral standing, but not necessarily full and equal moral standing.

Sumner's claim that sentient fetuses have the same moral standing as older human beings clearly requires the strong version of the sentience criterion. On this theory, any being which has even minimal capacities for sensory experience is the moral equal of any person. If we accept this theory, then we must conclude that not only is late abortion the moral equivalent of homicide, but so is the killing of such sentient nonhuman beings as mice. Sumner evidently does not wish to accept this further conclusion, for he also says that "sentience admits of degrees . . . [a fact that] enables us to employ it both as an inclusion criterion and as a comparison criterion of moral standing" (144). In other words, all sentient beings have some moral standing, but beings that are more highly sentient have greater moral standing than do less highly sentient beings. This weaker version of the sentience criterion leaves room for a distinction between the moral standing of mice and that of sentient humans—provided, that is, that mice can be shown to be less highly sentient. However, it will not support the moral equality of late-term fetuses, since the relatively undeveloped condition of fetal brains almost certainly means that fetuses are less highly sentient than older human beings.

A similar dilemma haunts those who use the sentience criterion to argue for the moral equality of nonhuman animals. Some animal liberationists hold that all sentient beings are morally equal, regardless of species. For instance, Peter Singer (1981, 111) maintains that all sentient beings are entitled to equal consideration for their comparably important interests. Animal liberationists are primarily concerned to argue for the moral equality of vertebrate animals, such as mammals, birds, reptiles and fish. In this project, the sentience criterion serves them less well than they may suppose. On the one hand, if they use the weak version of the sentience criterion then they cannot sustain the claim that all nonhuman vertebrates are our moral equals—unless they can demonstrate that they are all sentient *to the same degree* that we are. It is unclear how such a demonstration would proceed, or what would count as success. On the other hand, if they use the strong version of the sentience criterion, then they are committed to the conclusion that if flies and mosquitos are even minimally sentient then they too are our moral equals. Not even the most radical animal liberationists have endorsed the moral equality of such invertebrate animals,[6] yet it is quite likely that these creatures enjoy some form of sentience.

We do not really know whether complex invertebrate animals such as spiders and insects have sensory experiences, but the evidence suggests that they may. They have both sense organs and central nervous systems, and they often act as if they could see, hear, and feel very well. Sumner says that all invertebrates are probably nonsentient, because they lack certain brain structures—notably fore-brains—that appear to be essential to the processing of pain in vertebrate animals (143). But might not some invertebrate animals have neurological devices for the processing of pain that are different from those of vertebrates, just as some have very different organs for the detection of light, sound, or odor? The capacity to feel pain is important to highly mobile organisms which guide their behavior through perceptual data, since it often enables them to avoid damage or destruction. Without that capacity, such organisms would be less likely to survive long enough to reproduce. Thus, if insects, spiders, crayfish, or octopi can see, hear, or smell, then it is quite likely that they can also feel pain. If sentience is the sole criterion for moral equality, then such probably-sentient entities deserve the benefit of the doubt.

But it is difficult to believe that killing invertebrate animals is as morally objectionable as homicide. That an entity is probably sentient provides a reason for avoiding actions that may cause it pain. It may also provide a reason for respecting its life, a life which it may enjoy. But it is not a sufficient reason for regarding it as a moral equal. Perhaps an ideally moral person would try to avoid killing any sentient being, even a fly. Yet it is impossible in practice to treat the killing of persons and the killing of sentient invertebrates with the same severity. Even the simplest activities essential to human survival (such as agriculture, or gathering wild foods) generally entail some loss of invertebrate lives. If the strong version of the sentience criterion is correct, then all such activities are morally problematic. And if it is not, then the probable sentience of late-term fetuses and newborn infants is not enough to demonstrate that either late abortion or infanticide is the moral equivalent of homicide. Some additional argument is needed to show that either late abortion or early infanticide is seriously immoral.

THE SELF-AWARENESS CRITERION

Although newborn infants are regarded as persons in both law and common moral conviction, they lack certain mental capacities that are typical of persons. They have sensory experiences, but, as Tooley points out, they probably do not yet think, or have a sense of who they are, or a desire to continue to exist. It is not unreasonable to suppose that these facts make some difference to their moral standing. Other things being equal, it is surely worse to kill a self-aware being that wants to go on living than one that has never been self-aware and that has no such preference. If this is true, then it is hard to avoid the conclusion that neither abortion nor infanticide is quite as bad as the killing of older human beings. And indeed many human societies seem to have accepted that conclusion.

Tooley notes that the abhorrence of infanticide which is characteristic of cultures influenced by Christianity has not been shared by most cultures outside that influence (315–322). Prior to the present century, most societies—from the gatherer-hunter societies of Australia, Africa, North and South America, and elsewhere, to the high civilizations of China, India, Greece, Rome, and Egypt—have not only tolerated occasional instances of infanticide but have regarded it as sometimes the wisest course of action. Even in Christian Europe there was often a de facto toleration of infanticide—so long as the mother was married and the killing discreet. Throughout much of the second millennium in Europe, single women whose infants failed to survive were often executed in sadistic ways, yet married women whose infants died under equally suspicious circumstances generally escaped legal penalty (Piers 1978, 45–46). Evidently, the sanctions against infanticide had more to do with the desire to punish female sexual transgressions than with a consistently held belief that infanticide is morally comparable to homicide.

If infanticide has been less universally regarded as wrong than most people today believe, then the self-awareness criterion is more consistent with common moral convictions than it at first appears. Nevertheless, it conflicts with some convictions that are almost universal, even in cultures that tolerate infanticide. Tooley argues that infants probably begin to think and to become self-aware at about three months of age, and that this is therefore the stage at which they begin to have a strong right to life (405–406). Perhaps this is true. However the customs of most cultures seem to have required that a decision about the life of an infant be made within, at most, a few days of birth. Often, there was some special gesture or ceremony— such as washing the infant, feeding it, or giving it a name—to mark the fact that it would thenceforth be regarded as a member of the community. From that point on, infanticide would not be considered, except perhaps under unusual circumstances. For instance, Margaret Mead gives this account of birth and infanticide among the Arapesh people of Papua New Guinea:

> While the child is being delivered, the father waits within ear-shot until its sex is determined, when the midwives call it out to him. To this information he answers laconically, "Wash it," or "Do not wash it." If the command is "Wash it," the child is to be brought up. In a few cases when the child is a girl and there are already several girl-children in the family, the child will not be saved, but left, unwashed, with the cord uncut, in the bark basin on which the delivery takes place. (Mead [1935] 1963, 32–33)

Mead's account shows that among the Arapesh infanticide is at least to some degree a function of patriarchal power. In this, they are not unusual. In almost every society in which infanticide has been tolerated, female infants have been the most frequent victims. In patriarchal, patrilineal and patrilocal societies, daughters are usually valued less than sons, e.g., because they will leave the family at marriage, and will probably be unable to contribute as much as sons to the parents' economic support later. Female infanticide probably reinforces male domination by reducing the relative number of women and dramatically reinforcing the social devaluation of females.[7] Often it is the father who decides which infants will be reared. Dianne Romaine has pointed out to me that this practice may be due to a reluctance to force women, the primary caregivers, to decide when care should not be given. However, it also suggests that infanticide often served the interests of individual men more than those of women, the family, or the community as a whole.

Nevertheless, infanticide must sometimes have been the most humane resolution of a tragic dilemma. In the absence of effective contraception or abortion, abandoning a newborn can sometimes be the only alternative to the infant's later death from starvation. Women of nomadic gatherer-hunter societies, for instance, are sometimes unable to raise an infant born too soon after the last one, because they can neither nurse nor carry two small children.

But if infanticide is to be considered, it is better that it be done immediately after birth, before the bonds of love and care between the infant and the mother (and other persons) have grown any stronger than they may already be. Postponing the question of the infant's acceptance for weeks or months would be cruel to all concerned. Although an infant may be little more sentient or self-aware at two weeks of age than at birth, its death is apt to be a greater tragedy—not for it, but for those who have come to love it. I suspect that this is why, where infanticide is tolerated, the decision to kill or abandon an infant must usually be made rather quickly. If this consideration is morally relevant—and I think it is—then the self-awareness criterion fails to illuminate some of the morally salient aspects of infanticide.

PROTECTING NONPERSONS

If we are to justify a general moral distinction between abortion and infanticide, we must answer two questions. First, why should infanticide be discouraged, rather than treated as a matter for individual decision? And second, why should sentient fetuses not be given the same protections that law and common sense morality accord to infants? But before turning to these two questions, it is necessary to make a more general point.

Persons have sound reasons for treating one another as moral equals. These reasons derive from both self-interest and altruistic concern for others—which, because of our social nature, are often very difficult to distinguish. Human persons—and perhaps all persons—normally come into existence only in and through social relationships. Sentience may begin to emerge without much direct social interaction, but it is doubtful that a child reared in total isolation from human or other sentient (or apparently sentient) beings could develop the capacities for self-awareness and social interaction that are essential to personhood. The recognition of the fundamentally social nature of persons can only strengthen the case for moral equality, since social relationships are undermined and distorted by inequalities that are perceived as unjust. There may be many nonhuman animals who have enough capacity for self-awareness and social interaction to be regarded as persons, with equal basic moral rights. But, whether or not this is true, it is certainly true that if any things have full and equal basic moral rights then persons do.

However we cannot conclude that, because all persons have equal basic moral rights, it is always wrong to extend strong moral protections to beings that are not persons. Those who accept the single-criterion assumption may find that a plausible inference. By now, however, most thoughtful people recognize the need to protect vulnerable elements of the natural world—such as endangered plant and animal species, rainforests, and rivers—from further destruction at human hands. Some argue that it is appropriate, as a way of protecting these things, to ascribe to them legal if not moral rights (Stone 1974). These things should be protected not because they are sentient or self-aware, but for other good reasons. They are irreplaceable parts of the terrestrial biosphere, and as such they have incalculable value to human beings. Their long-term instrumental value is often a fully sufficient reason for protecting them. However, they may also be held to have inherent value, i.e., value that is independent of the uses we might wish to make of them (Taylor 1986). Although destroying them is not murder, it is an act of vandalism which later generations will mourn.

It is probably not crucial whether or not we say that endangered species and natural habitats have a moral right to our protection. What is crucial is that we recognize and act upon the need to protect them. Yet certain contemporary realities argue for an increased willingness to ascribe rights to impersonal elements of the natural world. Americans, at least, are likely to be more sensitive to appeals and demands couched in terms of rights than those that appeal to less familiar concepts, such as inherent value. So central are rights to our common moral idiom, that to deny that trees have rights is risk being thought to condone the reckless destruction of rainforests and redwood groves. If we want to communicate effectively about the need to protect the natural world—and to protect it for its own sake as well as our own—then we may be wise to develop theories that permit us to ascribe at least some moral rights to some things that are clearly not persons.

Parallel issues arise with respect to the moral status of the newborn infant. As Wolgast (1987, 38) argues, it is much more important to understand our responsibilities to protect and care for infants than to insist that they have exactly the same moral rights as older human beings. Yet to deny that infants have equal basic moral rights is to risk being thought to condone infanticide and the neglect and abuse of infants. Here too, effective communication about human moral responsibilities seems to demand the ascription of rights to beings that lack certain properties that are typical of persons. But, of course, that does not explain why we have these responsibilities towards infants in the first place.

WHY PROTECT INFANTS?

I have already mentioned some of the reasons for protecting human infants more carefully than we protect most comparably-sentient nonhuman beings. Most people care deeply about infants, particularly—but not exclusively—their own. Normal human adults (and children) are probably "programmed" by their biological nature to respond to human infants with care and concern. For the mother, in particular, that response is apt to begin well before the infant is born. But even for her it is likely to become more intense after the infant's birth. The infant at birth enters the human social world, where, if it lives, it becomes involved in social relationships with others, of kinds that can only be dimly foreshadowed before birth. It begins to be known and cared for, not just as a potential member of the family or community, but as a socially present and responsive individual. In the words of Loren Lomasky (1984, 172), "birth constitutes a quantum leap forward in the process of establishing . . . social bonds." The newborn is not yet self-aware, but it is already (rapidly becoming) a social being.

Thus, although the human newborn may have no intrinsic properties that can ground a moral right to life stronger than that of a fetus just before birth, its emergence into the social world makes it appropriate to treat it as if it had such a stronger right. This, in effect, is what the law has done, through the doctrine that a person begins to exist at birth. Those who accept the intrinsic-properties assumption can only regard this doctrine as a legal fiction. However, it is a fiction that we would have difficulty doing without. If the line were not drawn at birth, then I think we would have to draw it at some point rather soon thereafter, as many other societies have done.

Another reason for condemning infanticide is that, at least in relatively priv-ileged nations like our own, infants whose parents cannot raise them can usually be placed with people who will love them and take good care of them. This means that infanticide is rarely in the infant's own best interests, and would often deprive some potential adoptive individual or family of a great benefit. It also means that the prohibition of infanticide need not impose intolerable burdens upon parents (especially women). A rare parent might think it best to kill a healthy[8] infant rather than permitting it to be reared by others, but a persuasive defense of that claim would require special circumstances. For instance, when abortion is un-available and women face savage abuses for supposed sexual transgressions, those who resort to infanticide to conceal an "illegitimate" birth may be doing only what they must. But where enforcement of the sexual double standard is less brutal, abortion and adoption can provide alternatives that most women would prefer to infanticide.

Some might wonder whether adoption is really preferable to infanticide, at least from the parent's point of view. Judith Thomson (1971, 66) notes that "a woman may be utterly devastated by the thought of a child, a bit of herself, put out for adoption and never seen or heard of again." From the standpoint of narrow self-interest, it might not be irrational to prefer the death of the child to such a future. Yet few would wish to resolve this problem by legalizing infanticide. The evolution of more open adoption procedures which permit more contact between the adopted child and the biological parent(s) might lessen the psychological pain often as-sociated with adoption. But that would be at best a partial solution. More basic is the provision of better social support for child-rearers, so that parents are not forced by economic necessity to surrender their children for adoption.

These are just some of the arguments for treating infants as legal persons, with an equal right to life. A more complete account might deal with the effects of the toleration of infanticide upon other moral norms. But the existence of such effects is unclear. Despite a tradition of occasional infanticide, the Arapesh appear in Mead's descriptions as gentle people who treat their children with great kindness and affection. The case against infanticide need not rest upon the questionable claim that the toleration of infanticide inevitably leads to the erosion of other moral norms. It is enough that most people today strongly desire that the lives of infants be protected, and that this can now be done without imposing intolerable burdens upon individuals or communities.

But have I not left the door open to the claim that infanticide may still be justified in some places, e.g., where there is severe poverty and a lack of accessible adoption agencies or where women face exceptionally harsh penalties for "illegit-imate" births? I have, and deliberately. The moral case against the toleration of infanticide is contingent upon the existence of morally preferable options. Where economic hardship, the lack of contraception and abortion, and other forms of sexual and political oppression have eliminated all such options, there will be instances in which infanticide is the least tragic of a tragic set of choices. In such circumstances, the enforcement of extreme sanctions against infanticide can constitute an additional injustice.

WHY BIRTH MATTERS

I have defended what most regard as needing no defense, i.e., the ascription of an equal right to life to human infants. Under reasonably favorable conditions that policy can protect the rights and interests of all concerned, including infants, biological parents, and potential adoptive parents.

But if protecting infants is such a good idea, then why is it not a good idea to extend the same strong protections to sentient fetuses? The question is not whether sentient fetuses ought to be protected: of course they should. Most women readily accept the responsibility for doing whatever they can to ensure that their (voluntarily continued) pregnancies are successful, and that no avoidable harm comes to the fetus. Negligent or malevolent actions by third parties which result in death or injury to pregnant women or their potential children should be subject to moral censure and legal prosecution. A just and caring society would do much more than ours does to protect the health of all its members, including pregnant women. The question is whether the law should accord to late-term fetuses *exactly the same* protections as are accorded to infants and older human beings.

The case for doing so might seem quite strong. We normally regard not only infants, but all other postnatal human beings as entitled to strong legal protections *so long as they are either sentient or capable of an eventual return to sentience.* We do not also require that they demonstrate a capacity for thought, self-awareness, or social relationships before we conclude that they have an equal right to life. Such restrictive criteria would leave too much room for invidious discrimination. The eternal propensity of powerful groups to rationalize sexual, racial, and class oppression by claiming that members of the oppressed group are mentally or otherwise "inferior" leaves little hope that such restrictive criteria could be applied without bias. Thus, for human beings past the prenatal stage, the capacity for sentience—or for a return to sentience—may be the only pragmatically defensible criterion for the ascription of full and equal basic rights. If so, then both theoretical simplicity and moral consistency may seem to require that we extend the same protections to sentient human beings that have not yet been born as to those that have.

But there is one crucial consideration which this argument leaves out. It is impossible to treat fetuses *in utero* as if they were persons without treating women as if they were something less than persons. The extension of equal rights to sentient fetuses would inevitably license severe violations of women's basic rights to personal autonomy and physical security. In the first place, it would rule out most second-trimester abortions performed to protect the woman's life or health. Such abortions might sometimes be construed as a form of self-defense. But the right to self-defense is not usually taken to mean that one may kill innocent persons just because their continued existence poses some threat to one's own life or health. If abortion must be justified as self-defense, then it will rarely be performed until the woman is already in extreme danger, and perhaps not even then. Such a policy would cost some women their lives, while others would be subjected to needless suffering and permanent physical harm.

Other alarming consequences of the drive to extend more equal rights to fetuses are already apparent in the United States. In the past decade it has become increasingly common for hospitals or physicians to obtain court orders requiring women in labor to undergo cesarean sections, against their will, for what is thought to be the good of the fetus. Such an extreme infringement of the woman's right to security against physical assault would be almost unthinkable once the infant has been born. No parent or relative can legally be forced to undergo any surgical procedure, even possibly to save the life of a child, once it is born. But pregnant women can sometimes be forced to undergo major surgery, for the supposed benefit of the fetus. As George Annas (1982, 16) points out, forced cesareans threaten to reduce women to the status of inanimate objects—containers which may be opened at the will of others in order to get at their contents.

Perhaps the most troubling illustration of this trend is the case of Angela Carder, who died at George Washington University Medical Center in June 1987, two days after a court-ordered cesarean section. Ms. Carder had suffered a recurrence of an earlier cancer, and was not expected to live much longer. Her physicians agreed that the fetus was too undeveloped to be viable, and that Carder herself was probably too weak to survive the surgery. Although she, her family, and the physicians were all opposed to a cesarean delivery, the hospital administration—evidently believing it had a legal obligation to try to save the fetus—sought and obtained a court order to have it done. As predicted, both Carder and her infant died soon after the operation.[9] This woman's rights to autonomy, physical integrity, and life itself were forfeit—not just because of her illness, but because of her pregnancy.

Such precedents are doubly alarming in the light of the development of new techniques of fetal therapy. As fetuses come to be regarded as patients, with rights that may be in direct conflict with those of their mothers, and as the *in utero* treatment of fetuses becomes more feasible, more and more pregnant women may be subjected against their will to dangerous and invasive medical interventions. If so, then we may be sure that there will be other Angela Carders.

Another danger in extending equal legal protections to sentient fetuses is that women will increasingly be blamed, and sometimes legally prosecuted, when they miscarry or give birth to premature, sick, or abnormal infants. It is reasonable to hold the caretakers of infants legally responsible if their charges are harmed because of their avoidable negligence. But when a woman miscarries or gives birth to an abnormal infant, the cause of the harm might be traced to any of an enormous number of actions or circumstances which would not normally constitute any legal offense. She might have gotten too much exercise or too little, eaten the wrong foods or the wrong quantity of the right ones, or taken or failed to take certain drugs. She might have smoked, consumed alcohol, or gotten too little sleep. She might have "permitted" her health to be damaged by hard work, by unsafe employment conditions, by the lack of affordable medical care, by living near a source of industrial pollution, by a physically or mentally abusive partner, or in any number of other ways.

Are such supposed failures on the part of pregnant women potentially to be construed as child abuse or negligent homicide? If sentient fetuses are entitled to the same legal protections as infants, then it would seem so. The danger is not a merely theoretical one. Two years ago in San Diego, a woman whose son was born with brain damage and died several weeks later was charged with felony child neglect. It was said that she had been advised by her physician to avoid sex and illicit drugs, and to go to the hospital immediately if she noticed any bleeding. Instead, she had allegedly had sex with her husband, taken some inappropriate drug, and delayed getting to the hospital for what might have been several hours after the onset of bleeding.

In this case, the charges were eventually dismissed on the grounds that the child protection law invoked had not been intended to apply to cases of this kind. But the multiplication of such cases is inevitable if the strong legal protections accorded to infants are extended to sentient fetuses. A bill recently introduced in the Australian state of New South Wales would make women liable to criminal prosecution if they are found to have smoked during pregnancy, eaten unhealthful foods, or taken any other action which can be shown to have adversely affected the development of the fetus (*The Australian*, July 5, 1988, 5). Such an approach to the protection of fetuses authorizes the legal regulation of virtually every aspect of women's public and private lives, and thus is incompatible with even the most minimal right to autonomy. Moreover, such laws are apt to prove counterproductive, since the fear of prosecution may deter poor or otherwise vulnerable women from seeking needed medical care during pregnancy. I am not suggesting that women whose apparent negligence causes prenatal harm to their infants should always be immune from criticism. However, if we want to improve the health of infants we would do better to provide the services women need to protect their health, rather than seeking to use the law to punish those whose prenatal care has been less than ideal.

There is yet another problem, which may prove temporary but which remains significant at this time. The extension of legal personhood to sentient fetuses would rule out most abortions performed because of severe fetal abnormalities, such as Down syndrome or spina bifida. Abortions performed following amniocentesis are usually done in the latter part of the second trimester, since it is usually not possible to obtain test results earlier. Methods of detecting fetal abnormalities at earlier stages, such as chorion biopsy, may eventually make late abortion for reasons of fetal abnormality unnecessary; but these methods are not yet widely available.

The elimination of most such abortions might be a consequence that could be accepted, were the society willing to provide adequate support for the handicapped children and adults who would come into being as a result of this policy. However, our society is not prepared to do this. In the absence of adequate communally-funded care for the handicapped, the prohibition of such abortions is exploitative of women. Of course, the male relatives of severely handicapped persons may also bear heavy burdens. Yet the heaviest portion of the daily responsibility generally falls upon mothers and other female relatives. If fetuses are not yet persons (and women are), then a respect for the equality of persons should lead to support for the availability of abortion in cases of severe fetal abnormality.[10]

Such arguments will not persuade those who deeply believe that fetuses are already persons, with equal moral rights. How, they will ask, is denying legal equality to sentient fetuses different from denying it to any other powerless group of human beings? If some human beings are more equal than others, then how can any of us feel safe? The answer is twofold.

First, pregnancy is a relationship different from any other, including that between parents and already-born children. It is not just one of innumerable situations in which the rights of one individual may come into conflict with those of another; it is probably the *only* case in which the legal personhood of one human being is necessarily incompatible with that of another. Only in pregnancy is the organic functioning of one human individual biologically inseparable from that of another. This organic unity makes it impossible for others to provide the fetus with medical care or any other presumed benefit, except by doing something to or for the woman. To try to "protect" the fetus other than through her cooperation and consent is effectively to nullify her right to autonomy, and potentially to expose her to violent physical assaults such as would not be legally condoned in any other type of case. The uniqueness of pregnancy helps to explain why the toleration of abortion does not lead to the disenfranchisement of other groups of human beings, as opponents of abortion often claim. For biological as well as psychological reasons, "It is all but impossible to extrapolate from attitudes towards fetal life attitudes toward [other] existing human life" (D. Callahan 1970, 474).

But, granting the uniqueness of pregnancy, why is it *women's* rights that should be privileged? If women and fetuses cannot both be legal persons then why not favor fetuses, e.g., on the grounds that they are more helpless, or more innocent, or have a longer life expectancy? It is difficult to justify this apparent bias towards women without appealing to the empirical fact that women are already persons in the usual, nonlegal sense—already thinking, self-aware, fully social beings—and fetuses are not. Regardless of whether we stress the intrinsic properties of persons, or the social and relational dimensions of personhood, this distinction remains. Even sentient fetuses do not yet have either the cognitive capacities or the richly interactive social involvements typical of persons.

This "not yet" is morally decisive. It is wrong to treat persons as if they do not have equal basic rights. Other things being equal, it is worse to deprive persons of their most basic moral and legal rights than to refrain from extending such rights to beings that are not persons. This is one important element of truth in the self-awareness criterion. If fetuses were already thinking, self-aware, socially responsive members of communities, then nothing could justify refusing them the equal protection of the law. In that case, we would sometimes be forced to balance the rights of the fetus against those of the woman, and sometimes the scales might be almost equally weighted. However, if women are persons and fetuses are not, then the balance must swing towards women's rights.

CONCLUSION

Birth is morally significant because it marks the end of one relationship and the beginning of others. It marks the end of pregnancy, a relationship so intimate that it is impossible to extend the equal protection of the law to fetuses without severely infringing women's most basic rights. Birth also marks the beginning of the infant's existence as a socially responsive member of a human community. Although the infant is not instantly transformed into a person at the moment of birth, it does become a biologically separate human being. As such, it can be known and cared for as a particular individual. It can also be vigorously protected without negating the basic rights of women. There are circumstances in which infanticide may be the best of a bad set of options. But our own society has both the ability and the desire to protect infants, and there is no reason why we should not do so.

We should not, however, seek to extend the same degree of protection to fetuses. Both late-term fetuses and newborn infants are probably capable of sentience. Both are precious to those who want children; and both need to be protected from a variety of possible harms. All of these factors contribute to the moral standing of the late-term fetus, which is substantial. However, to extend equal legal rights to fetuses is necessarily to deprive pregnant women of the rights to personal autonomy, physical integrity, and sometimes life itself. *There is room for only one person with full and equal rights inside a single human skin.* That is why it is birth, rather than sentience, viability, or some other prenatal milestone that must mark the beginning of legal personhood.

NOTES

My thanks to Helen Heise, Dianne Romaine, Peter Singer, and Michael Scriven for their helpful comments on earlier versions of this paper.

1. Basic moral rights are those that are possessed equally by all persons, and that are essential to the moral equality of persons. The intended contrast is to those rights which arise from certain special circumstances—for instance, the right of a person to whom a promise has been made that that promise be kept. (Whether there are beings that are not persons but that have similar basic moral rights is one of the questions to be addressed here.)

2. "Moral standing," like "moral status," is a term that can be used to refer to the moral considerability of individuals, without being committed to the existence of moral rights. For instance, Sumner (1983) and Singer (1981) prefer these terms because, as utilitarians, they are unconvinced of the need for moral rights.

3. It is not obvious that a newborn infant's "level of consciousness" is similar to that of a fetus shortly before birth. Perhaps birth is analogous to an awakening, in that the infant has many experiences that were previously precluded by its prenatal brain chemistry or by its relative insulation within the womb. This speculation is plausible in evolutionary terms,

since a rich subjective mental life might have little survival value for the fetus, but might be highly valuable for the newborn, e.g., in enabling it to recognize its mother and signal its hunger, discomfort, etc. However, for the sake of the argument I will assume that the newborn's capacity for sentience is generally not very different from that of the fetus shortly before birth.

4. It is interesting that Sumner regards fetal abnormality and the protection of the woman's health as sufficient justifications for late abortion. In this, he evidently departs from his own theory by effectively differentiating between the moral status of sentient fetuses and that of older humans—who presumably may not be killed just because they are abnormal or because their existence (through no fault of their own) poses a threat to someone else's health.

5. There are evidently some people who, though otherwise sentient, cannot experience physical pain. However, the survival value of the capacity to experience pain makes it probable that such individuals are the exception rather than the rule among mature members of sentient species.

6. There is at least one religion, that of the Jains, in which the killing of any living thing—even an insect—is regarded as morally wrong. But even the Jains do not regard the killing of insects as morally equivalent to the killing of persons. Laypersons (unlike mendicants) are permitted some unintentional killing of insects—though not of vertebrate animals or persons—when this is unavoidable to the pursuit of their profession (See Jaini 1979, 171–3).

7. Marcia Guttentag and Paul Secord (1983) argue that a shortage of women benefits at least some women, by increasing their "value" in the marriage market. However, they also argue that this increased value does not lead to greater freedom for women; on the contrary, it tends to coincide with an exceptionally severe sexual double standard, the exclusion of women from public life, and their confinement to domestic roles.

8. The extension of equal basic rights to infants need not imply the absolute rejection of euthanasia for infant patients. There are instances in which artificially extending the life of a severely compromised infant is contrary to the infant's own best interests. Competent adults or older children who are terminally ill sometimes rightly judge that further prolongation of their lives would not be a benefit to them. While infants cannot make that judgment for themselves, it is sometimes the right judgment for others to make on their behalf.

9. See Civil Liberties 363 (Winter 1988), 12, and Lawrence Lader, "Regulating Birth: Is the State Going Too Far?" Conscience IX: 5 (September/October, 1988), 5–6.

10. It is sometimes argued that using abortion to prevent the birth of severely handicapped infants will inevitably lead to a loss of concern for handicapped persons. I doubt that this is true. There is no need to confuse the question of whether it is good that persons be born handicapped with the very different question of whether handicapped persons are entitled to respect, support, and care.

REFERENCES

Annas, George. 1982. Forced cesareans: The most unkindest cut of all. Hastings Center Report 12(3):16–17;45.

The Australian, Tuesday, July 5, 1988, 5.

Callahan, Daniel. 1970. Abortion: Law, choice and morality. New York: Macmillan.

Callahan, Sydney. 1984. Value choices in abortion. In Abortion: Understanding differences. Sydney Callahan and Daniel Callahan, eds. New York and London: Plenum Press.

Callahan, Sydney. 1986. Abortion and the sexual agenda. Commonweal, April 25, 232–238.

Gilligan, Carol. 1982. *In a different voice: Psychological theory and women's development.* Cambridge, Massachusetts: Harvard University Press.

Guttentag, Marcia, and Paul Secord. 1983. *Too many women: The sex ratio question.* Beverly Hills: Sage Publications.

Harrison, Beverly Wildung. 1983. *Our right to choose: Toward a new ethic of abortion.* Boston: Beacon Press.

Jaini, Padmanab S. 1979. *The jaina path of purification.* Berkeley, Los Angeles, London: University of California Press.

Lomasky, Loren. 1984. Being a person—does it matter? In *The problem of abortion.* Joel Feinberg, ed. Belmont, California.

Luker, Kristen. 1984. *Abortion and the politics of motherhood.* Berkeley, Los Angeles and London: University of California Press.

Manning, Rita. 1988. Caring for and caring about. Paper presented at conference entitled *Explorations in Feminist Ethics,* Duluth, Minnesota. October 8.

Mead, Margaret. [1935] 1963. *Sex and temperament in three primitive societies.* New York: Morrow Quill Paperbacks.

Noddings, Nel 1984. *Caring: A feminine approach to ethics and moral education.* Berkeley, Los Angeles and London: University of California Press.

Petchesky, Rosalind Pollack. 1984. *Abortion and women's choice.* New York, London: Longman.

Piers, Maria W. 1978. *Infanticide.* New York: W. W. Norton and Company.

Singer, Peter. 1981. *The expanding circle: Ethics and sociobiology.* New York: Farrar, Straus and Giroux.

Stone, Christopher. 1974. *Should trees have standing: Towards legal rights for natural objects.* Los Altos: William Kaufman.

Stone, Christopher. 1987. *Earth and other ethics.* New York: Harper & Row.

Sumner, L. W. 1983. *Abortion and moral theory.* Princeton, New Jersey: Princeton University Press.

Taylor, Paul W. 1986. *Respect for nature: A theory of environmental ethics.* Princeton, New Jersey: Princeton University Press.

Thomson, Judith Jarvis. 1971. A defense of abortion. *Philosophy and Public Affairs* 1 (1): 47–66.

Tooley, Michael. 1983. *Abortion and infanticide.* Oxford: Oxford University Press.

Wolgast, Elizabeth. 1987. *The grammar of justice.* Ithaca and London: Cornell University Press.

Women in Labor: Some Issues about Informed Consent

ROSALIND EKMAN LADD   ❖ ❖ ❖

Women wishing hospital admission for childbirth are asked to sign very general pre-admission consent forms. The use of such forms suggests that women in labor are considered incompetent to give informed consent. This paper explores some of the problems with advance directives and general consent, and argues that since women in labor are not generally incompetent, it is not appropriate to require this kind of consent of them.

Women who plan to give birth in hospitals, like other persons agreeing to medical care, are asked to give written informed consent. An example of a consent form, typical of those used as a condition of admission to maternity hospitals or obstetrics services in general hospitals, is reproduced here.

Consent for Obstetrical Care, Delivery and Anesthesia

Date: _____   Time: _____
1. I _____ (or _____
for _____) am pregnant and plant to deliver my baby
at _____ Hospital, do hereby consent to
hospital care, including such diagnostic procedures and medical treatment, by
Dr. _____ his/her assistants or designees as is judged
necessary. I also consent to the provision of needed treatment to my newborn(s).

2. I authorize the performance of either a vaginal or cesarean delivery, by the above named physician or his/her designees. The various methods of delivery have been discussed with me.

3. My physician has discussed, and I understand that unforeseeable problems or complications sometimes occur. These risks include:

[Here follows a list of six specific risks.]

I understand that this list is not complete, that other unforeseen risks do exist and these have been discussed with me. Additional procedures which may be required have been discussed with me and I consent to those which my physician deems necessary.

Hypatia vol. 4, no. 3 (Fall 1989). © by Rosalind Ekman Ladd

4. I consent to the administration of anesthesia to be administered by or under the supervision of an anesthesiologist.

5. I consent to and authorize the transfusion or administration of blood or blood components whenever deemed necessary by physicians attending to my care.

6. **[A paragraph giving consent for use of specimens for research.]**

7. I acknowledge that no guarantee or promise has been given to me by anyone as to the results of the treatment for me or my baby hereby consented to.

8. This form has been explained to me and I understand it.

[Spaces for signature, witness, and physician's acknowledgment.]

Consent forms such as this are generally signed at a pre-natal appointment well before the ninth month of pregnancy, and thus function as advance directives, giving permission ahead for procedures, and as a general consent, covering a wide range of contingencies.

It will be argued here that the use of this kind of consent form raises philosophical issues. Specifically, requiring such consent seems to imply that later the signer will be incompetent to make informed, voluntary decisions. It will be argued further that while in other cases this implication may be justified, it is not justified generally in the case of women in labor, and that a different process of decision-making would be more appropriate.

INFORMED CONSENT

Informed consent is both a moral and a legal requirement for non-emergency, non-mandatory medical treatment. It assumes the patient's capacity to understand and evaluate information offered and the ability freely and without coercion to accept, refuse, or choose between alternative treatments. Incompetence, strictly speaking, is a legal concept, to be applied by the courts; the standards vary from state to state and in different contexts, ranging from the bare ability to say yes or no to a very high level of understanding of alternatives and consequences. Often, however, an informal, non-legal determination of incompetency is made for unconscious patients or controversial cases involving medication or severe stress, pain, or fear.

The use of consent forms is intended to protect the signer, by guaranteeing disclosure of information—procedures, risks, and alternatives—and allowing the exercise of autonomy, in this case, voluntary admission to the hospital under the stated conditions. It is also intended to protect the institution and staff against various forms of assault and battery charges.

In general, it is agreed that any person has the right to refuse medical treatment; that is, treatment cannot be given without informed consent. Exceptions to the informed consent requirement include care in life-threatening, emergency situations, court-ordered mandatory treatment (e.g. AIDS testing, court-ordered psychiatric examination or treatment when a person is thought to be a threat to self or others), therapeutic privilege, where giving information poses serious harm to the patient, and treatment of minors and incompetents, in which case proxy consent is required. Controversial possible exceptions include requiring treatment of the pregnant woman for the benefit of her fetus (Kolder, Gallagher, and Parsons 1987). The discussion here will concern only decision-making in situations which are not life-threatening to either woman or fetus.

ADVANCE DIRECTIVES

Compare, as an example of giving permission ahead for anticipated procedures, informed consent for surgery. When general or total anesthetic is to be used, then the anticipation of temporary patient incompetency is justified: decisions must be made ahead.

According to 1980 figures, however, only 41% of women in labor receive general anesthetic, and that is not administered throughout the whole period of labor. The increase in childbirth preparation has led to a decrease in the overall use of anesthesia (Cogan 1980). Thus, women in labor do not have the same need as surgery patients to consent ahead.

There are further differences. Up until the time of the administration of general anesthetic or the actual beginning of a procedure under local anesthetic, the surgery patient can always change her mind and retract consent. Non-emergency surgery is postponable and patients are allowed to leave the hospital, if they insist, signing out "AMA," that is, against medical advice (Jonsen, Siegler, and Winslade 1982, 99).

There is good precedent for the principle that a person should be able to withdraw from a medical commitment. According to the principles of both the Helsinki Declaration and the Nuremberg Code, consent for participation in research must always explicitly give the signer the right to withdraw from the project at any time. The recipient of the first artificial heart, for example, had a "key" with which he could turn off the machine if he decided to withdraw from the experiment.

By contrast, the process of labor and birth is not postponable or reversible in the same way as elective surgery or participation in research. Although a woman could, theoretically, get up and leave the hospital, this is rarely a feasible alternative. Women in labor do not have the same "escape hatches" from pre-consent available to them that other signers have. Pre-consent is in a sense, then, more coercive for them than for others.

Obstetric pre-consent forms may also be compared to advance directives such as living wills or durable powers of attorney. A living will specifies what "extraordinary" life support measures one will or will not accept when one can no longer express one's own wishes, and a durable power of attorney designates a proxy decision-maker to make medical decisions, either according to written instructions or carte blanche, when one is unable to make one's own decisions.

A living will or durable power of attorney specifies that it will go into effect only when the signer is unable to decide for himself; at any point before that, the provisions of the document may be changed and in some cases the entire document must be reviewed and reaffirmed at stated intervals in order to retain its legal force.

By contrast, a general consent form for care during labor and delivery goes into effect as soon as the woman enters the hospital. Although many physicians may continue to consult the woman and defer to her decisions when choices arise, this may be seen as a courtesy and not a legal or ethical requirement or a right which the woman can claim. For those medical staff who do not continue to consult the woman in decision-making, it is as if they were treating her as incompetent, i.e. competent at the time of signing but incompetent at the time of labor and delivery. The justification for treating all women in labor as if they were incompetent needs further exploration.

GENERAL CONSENT FORMS

The fact that some consent forms, such as the one reproduced above, are general enough to give permission for alternative procedures and cover a wide range of contingencies suggests that the signer will not be considered competent to make decisions when the contingencies arise. There are three ways that the argument for the incompetency of women in labor can be made, and each must be examined critically.

1. Competency to give informed consent requires that two conditions be met: a) that the agent or patient be informed, i.e. be given information and understand it, and b) that the consent be given freely, i.e. not coerced. It is argued that fear, stress, and pain can negate at least the first of these conditions by impairing the person's cognitive, rational capacities. Doubts are also raised about voluntariness (van Liev 1986), but these will not be discussed here.

Generally, the argument is that the effect of the emotional stress of illness and pain impairs any person's cognitive, rational capacities, making it impossible for her to understand and appreciate the information offered (Ingelfinger 1972; Jonsen, Siegler, and Winslade 1982). Empirical studies (Robinson and Merav 1976; Meisel and Roth 1983) seem to confirm this, yet most studies are post-tests, measuring how much and how well someone has remembered information which was received under stress several days or weeks earlier. What the studies do not establish is that the person failed to understand at the time the decision was made (Applebaum, Lidz, and Meisel 1987, 139). Unless that can be shown, the presumption of incompetence under stress in medical decision-making is not justified.

Specifically, the argument about impaired judgment is made about women in labor. One version of the argument about cognitive, rational capacities appears in the book, *Medical Choices, Medical Chances*. That it appears in a book which argues for a new model of the doctor-patient relationship, one which rests on trust, caring, and shared decision-making, illustrates the pervasiveness of the presumption. In the model dialogue, the physician says,

> I think you have to decide about analgesics *before* labor. I say that because it's almost too hard a decision to make while you're in labor. . . . It's almost not fair

to expect someone whose feelings are so intense to think rationally. (Bursztajn, et al. 1981)

The main difficulty with presuming all women in labor are incompetent to give informed consent is that it seems to be a generalization made without sufficient evidence. There is good reason to think otherwise. First, cross-cultural comparisons suggest that in other cultures, the locus of decision-making is with the woman (Ekstrom 1980). Secondly, prepared childbirth, visualization, controlled breathing and other methods have been shown to decrease fear, stress, and perhaps even pain (Cogan 1980). And thirdly, there must be a difference in fear and stress between first deliveries and subsequent deliveries, between those expecting a normal delivery and those anticipating a difficult delivery.

Since incompetency in other cases of medical decision-making must be determined on an individual basis, and since there is evidence of individual differences among women in labor, it seems reasonable to question the generalization that all women in labor have their cognitive capacities impaired to the extent that they cannot comprehend information.

Moreover, there is medical precedent for giving full choice and opportunity for informed consent even in situations of extreme fear, anxiety, and stress. One often-cited case involved allowing severely burned patients, while still alert, to decide to refuse treatment (Beauchamp and Childress 1983, 297). Other examples abound: deciding for oneself or for loved ones after an automobile accident, after a serious heart attack, after the birth of an infant requiring immediate surgery.

2. A person who signs a pre-consent form may change her mind, and this raises questions about which decision to honor, the earlier or the later. Is one the same person one was when the document was signed? Can one make commitments for one's later self? What if one has changed one's values? What if one changes one's mind (Buchanan 1988)? It is generally assumed that the moment of greatest knowledge, judgment, and free choice is in the calm time before a decision must take effect, not when one is immersed in the situation and can feel its full emotional impact.

The case of the Odysseus contracts illustrates this. Anticipating that he will be irresistibly attracted by the voices of the Sirens but wanting to hear their beautiful song, Odysseus instructs his sailors to tie him to the mast before they sail within earshot of the Sirens and not to heed his later pleas for release.

The analogy can be made to the pregnant woman who resolves ahead of time to forego pain medication, instructs her physician to ignore her later pleas, and then at the time of pain, regrets her decision. Although Dworkin (1972) argues that Odysseus's sailors are right to keep their promise to him and that to do so does not constitute unjustified paternalism, in medical cases, there can be legitimate doubt whether consent can be truly informed before one experiences the situation.

Different physicians respond differently when faced with an Odysseus-like situation. I have heard one physician say he would ignore a prior promise not to try to resuscitate an elderly heart-attack victim, and I have heard another physician relate how she reminded a dying cystic fibrosis patient of the patient's own wish not to accept ventilator support when it would have to become a permanent dependency.

There seems to be no consensus about how to assess someone else's true wishes, but the use of general consent forms seems to rule out honoring a change of mind.

It could be argued, though, that the case of the woman in labor is not like that of Odysseus. Because many decisions regarding the conduct of labor and birth depend on circumstances which cannot be known in advance, the prior consent of the women in labor seems less informed than that of Odysseus. For example, a woman might be willing to consent to a cesarean operation after trying to deliver vaginally for a certain length of time, but how long depends on a complicated set of factors, such as position of fetus, degree of discomfort, whether or not labor commenced at the end of a good night's sleep, etc. It is not feasible to try to spell out all the possibilities in advance,[1] thus only general consent is possible ahead of time. But, when the woman learns how these factors play out in her case and how she feels, both physically and emotionally, then she is able to make an informed decision. Thus, contrary to the general assumption, she is perhaps in a better position to decide at the later time than in the calm but uninformed time before.

3. It might be argued that all steps that physicians take after the onset of labor are "medically indicated," i.e. determined by clear and widely accepted criteria. This would mean that they are medically necessary and thus only those people with medical knowledge are competent to decide about them. The woman in labor, as a non-professional, cannot understand.

Although this is undoubtedly true in many medical situations, and may be true of some obstetrical situations, there is good reason to think that it is not true of all. The wide variety of obstetrical practices and the history of abuse of the cesarean option, for example, suggest that there are "gray zones" with no precise medical guidelines. Whitbeck (1987) makes the stronger point that decisions to use fetal monitors involve assessment of risks and are thus value questions. The same may be true of deciding how much pain medication should be given and, within certain limits, how long one should wait before opting for a cesarean. Thus, these issues could and should be decided by the woman's preference, after appropriate informing and advising.

SUMMARY AND CONCLUSION

I have argued that the use of very general, pre-admission consent forms implies that the signer will not be competent at a later time to give informed consent for her own treatment. I have argued further that this is not always true of women in labor, and thus the use of such consent forms is not appropriate.

Using a general consent form results in giving physicians a great deal of discretion, in effect making them and other medical staff surrogate decision-makers. Such general consent forms amount to a waiver of the right to decide (Applebaum, Lidz, and Meisel 1987, 69ff.), rather than a consent to certain procedures. However, if we accept that women in labor are not usually incompetent, why should they be required to waive their right to decision-making?

One of the first challenges of the women's movement to American gynecologists and obstetricians was made in 1974 (Kaiser and Kaiser 1974). The challenge needs repeating even today. If medical practitioners could be persuaded to approach women in labor just as they approach other individuals under their care, questioning competency only when indicated by the standard tests, the issues raised here would be resolved. More generally, if physicians and patients reevaluate the traditional doctor-patient relationship, recognize and challenge unstated presumptions, and strive for a more cooperative model of mutual respect and shared decision-making in all areas of medicine, then the practice of obstetrics will present fewer problems.

A story told to me by a young physician suggests a better model of doctor-patient relationship. "One time I had a patient who did not want to sign the general consent form the hospital required. Knowing that the hospital might refuse admission without it, I urged the woman to sign it, saying, 'Look, I will be with you all the time. I promise I will not do anything or let others do anything that you don't want.' The woman signed and the labor and delivery was accomplished as promised." How significant is it that this young physician is female?

NOTE

1. One attempt to spell out "childbirth requests" results in a three-page document, copies to be delivered to nine different people (Herzfeld 1985). While a few women may have the education, leisure, and motivation to do this, most will not, nor should they be expected to.

REFERENCES

Applebaum, Paul S., Charles W. Lidz, and Alan Meisel. 1987. *Informed consent: Legal theory and clinical practice.* New York: Oxford Univ. Press.

Beauchamp, Tom L., and James F. Childress. 1983. *Principles of biomedical ethics.* (2nd ed.). New York: Oxford Univ. Press.

Buchanan, Allen. 1988. Advance directives and the personal identity problem. *Philosophy and Public Affairs* 17 (4): 277–303.

Bursztajn, Harold, Richard I. Feinbloom, Robert M. Hamm, and Archie Brodsky. 1981. *Medical choices, medical chances: How patients, families, and physicians can cope with uncertainty.* New York: Delta/Seymour Lawrence.

Cogan, Rosemary. 1980. Effects of childbirth preparation. *Clinical Obstetrics and Gynecology* 23 (1): 1–14.

Dworkin, Gerald. 1972. Paternalism. *Monist* 56 (1): 64–84. Reprinted in *Moral problems in medicine.* Samuel Gorovitz, Andrew L. Jameton, Ruth Macklin, John M. O'Connor, Eugene V. Perrin, Beverly Page St. Clair, and Susan Sherwin, eds. 1976. Englewood Cliffs, New Jersey: Prentice Hall.

Ekstrom, Susan Cope. 1980. A report on birth in three cultures. In *Birth control and controlling birth: Women-centered perspectives.* Helen B. Holmes, Betty B. Hoskins, and Michael Gross, eds. Clifton, NJ: Humana Press.

Herzfeld, Judith. 1985. *Sense and sensibility in childbirth.* New York: W. W. Norton.

Ingelfinger, Franz J. 1972. Informed (but uneducated) consent. *New England Journal of Medicine* 287 (9): 465–466. Reprinted in *Contemporary issues in bioethics*. Tom L. Beauchamp and LeRoy Walters, eds. 1978. Encino, CA: Dickenson.

Jonsen, Albert R., Mark Siegler, and William J. Winslade. 1982. *Clinical ethics*. New York: Macmillan.

Kaiser, Barbara L., and Irwin H. Kaiser. 1974. *American Journal of Obstetrics and Gynecology* 120 (5): 652–661.

Kolder, Veronica E. B., Janet Gallagher, and Michael T. Parsons. 1987. Court-ordered obstetrical interventions. *New England Journal of Medicine* 316 (19): 1192–1196.

Meisel, Alan, and L. H. Roth. 1983. Toward an informed discussion of informed consent: A review and critique of the empirical studies. *Arizona Law Review* 25: 265–346.

Robinson, George, and Avraham Merav. 1976. Informed consent: Recall by patients tested postoperatively. *The Annals of Thoracic Surgery* 22 (3): 209–212. Reprinted in *Moral problems in medicine*. (2nd ed.). Samuel Gorovitz, Ruth Macklin, Andrew L. Jameton, John M. O'Connor, and Susan Sherwin, eds. 1983. Englewood Cliffs, NJ: Prentice Hall.

van Liev, Donna, and Joyce E. Roberts. 1986. Promoting informed consent of women in labor. *Journal of Obstetrics, Gynecology, and Neonatal Nursing* 15 (5): 419–422.

Whitbeck, Caroline. 1987. Fetal imaging and fetal monitoring: Finding the ethical issues. *Women and Health* 13 (1/2): 45–57.

Women, Fetuses, Medicine, and the Law

JOAN C. CALLAHAN and JAMES W. KNIGHT ❖ ❖ ❖

In recent years, we've seen a growing interest in preventing prenatal harm to human beings. This interest has issued in concerns about certain behaviors of pregnant women (e.g., use of teratogenic drugs) and concerns about pregnant women's decisions to decline medical/surgical interventions thought to be fetal-helping. In turn, these concerns have issued in a number of court-ordered medical/surgical interventions on pregnant women, prosecutions of women for harming their fetuses, incarcerations of women to protect their fetuses, and proposals of various criminal and legal sanctions to be applied to women to protect their fetuses. In this essay, we argue against all these uses of the law as attempts to prevent prenatal harm.

INTRODUCTION

Although American law has traditionally treated prenatal human beings as part of the women bearing them, courts, legal commentators, and medical practitioners have suggested with increasing frequency that prenatal human beings are entities having moral rights of their own that should be legally recognized.[1] Motivating some court decisions and arguments for recognizing fetal rights is, doubtlessly, discontent with the U.S. Supreme Court's decision in *Roe v. Wade* (1973), which allows American women to seek an abortion for any reason whatever through the end of the second trimester of pregnancy. But some of the motivation springs from a concern to prevent harm to human beings consequent to events taking place before they are born. Insofar as such harm can result from a pregnant woman's behaviors (e.g., use of teratogenic drugs) or decisions (e.g., refusal of a medical or surgical intervention), it has been argued that some pregnant women should be interfered with to prevent prenatal harm or subject to criminal or civil sanctions for causing prenatal harm to their offspring. In what follows, we want to show why these suggestions should be rejected.

PRENATAL PERSONHOOD: A MATTER OF DECISION, NOT DISCOVERY

The questions of concern in this paper cannot be addressed without first touching on the abortion debate which, in much of the world, centers on the question of the moral status of the prenatal human being. Frequently, this question is debated in terms of the personhood of prenatal human beings, and those who hold that abortion is intrinsically morally wrong generally believe that the prenatal human being is a person and therefore is a being with the moral rights of any person. But if prenatal human beings are persons this is not obvious, since they lack the kinds of characteristics which compel the recognition of strong moral rights and are possessed by paradigm cases of persons. Among these are certain mental characteristics, for example, a concept of oneself as an ongoing being with at least some kinds of plans and stakes (cf. Warren 1975; Callahan 1986). Prenatal human beings simply do not have any of the characteristics which compel an immediate recognition of personhood. These characteristics are emergent, and this makes the matter of accepting human beings as persons prior to the full emergence of these characteristics (which is long after birth) a matter of decision rather than discovery. That is, we need to decide whether beings which do not yet have the characteristics of paradigm persons ought to be treated in custom and law as persons prior to the emergence of those characteristics and, if so, how early in their development. If we need to *decide* whether to treat developing human beings as persons before the full emergence of characteristics that morally compel a recognition of personhood, then we are confronted with setting a convention.

One possible convention is to set the recognition of personhood at birth. Another is to set it at conception. Other conventions might set recognition of personhood at various prenatal stages or at various points after birth. Those who oppose elective abortion generally insist that we must decide that personhood is to be recognized from the point of fertilization onward. The secular argument given for this conclusion rests on the assumption that unless beings are radically different, treating them in radically different ways cannot be morally justified. The argument begins by starting with human beings, whom everyone recognizes as having powerful moral rights. It then points out that a person at twenty-five, for example, is not radically different from one at twenty-four and a half, and that person is not radically different from one at twenty-four, and so on. The argument presses us back from twenty-four to twenty-three to twenty-two, through adolescence and childhood to infancy. From infancy, it is a short step to late-term fetuses, because (the argument goes) change in location does not constitute an essential change in a being itself. Thus, change of place from the womb to the wider world is not, it is argued, sufficient to justify treating late-term fetuses and infants in radically different ways. The argument then presses us back to embryos and finally to fertilization, which is the only point in human development where a clear line can be drawn between radically different kinds of beings. Logic and fairness, it is argued, force us to accept that even the human zygote has the same fundamental rights as the mature human being (see, for example, Wertheimer 1971).

One significant objection to this wedge argument for prenatal personhood is that it turns on the assumption that we can never treat beings that are not radically different from one another in radically different ways. But if we accept this assumption we shall be unable to justify all sorts of public policies that we believe are both necessary and fair. For example, this assumption entails that we cannot be justified in setting ages for the commencement of important privileges, since withholding these privileges until a certain age unfairly discriminates against those who are close to that age: We must give the four-year-old the right to vote, the five-year-old the right to drink, the six-year-old the right to drive. But these implications show that this kind of argument for adopting a convention of recognizing personhood at fertilization is unsound (cf. Glover 1977).

It might be objected to this criticism of the wedge argument that such reasoning cannot be correct, since it not only rules out our being committed to the personhood of prenatal human beings; it also entails that we are not compelled to accept that human infants are beings that must be recognized as having the rights of persons, since infants are, it can be argued, more like (say) very young kittens in regard to the characteristics in question than they are like paradigmatic persons.

But this objection is not devastating. For, again, the question is one of deciding what convention we shall adopt. Even if infants do not yet have the characteristics that compel us to accept them as persons, there are other considerations that provide excellent reasons for taking birth as the best place to set the conventional recognition of personhood with its full range of fundamental moral and legal rights, despite the fact that infants are far more like very young kittens than they are like beings whose characteristics compel us to accept them as full members of the moral community. Chief among these considerations are that persons other than an infant's biological mother are able to care for the infant and have an interest in doing so (cf. Warren 1975). Although there are intriguing physiological changes accompanying birth, there is no change in the morally relevant characteristics of a human being itself just before birth and just after birth; all else being equal, if the life of a late-term fetus is sustained, it will develop the characteristics of paradigmatic persons. But once a viable human being emerges from the womb and others are able and willing to care for it, there are radical changes in what is involved in preserving its life. And the crucial change is that sustaining its life does not violate its biological mother's rights to self-direction and bodily integrity. Thus, even though birth, unlike fertilization, is not a point at which we have a radically new kind of being, it is *not* a morally arbitrary point for commencing recognition of young human beings as persons in moral custom and public policy. Prenatal human beings, then, ought not to be treated as persons with the full range of fundamental rights attaching to persons. Rather, we should take birth as the place to set the convention of commencing treatment as persons human beings that do not yet possess the characteristics of paradigmatic persons. Recognizing personhood at birth has the moral advantage of taking the actual, unequivocal personhood of women far more seriously than setting conventional recognition of personhood at any prenatal stage.[2]

Our position on commencing treatment of human beings as persons at birth is consistent with the U.S. Supreme Court's abortion-liberalizing decision in Roe v. Wade (1973). For, as Glantz (1983) emphasizes, the court in Roe did not argue that a fetus is to be recognized as a person at viability (having the attendant moral and legal rights of other persons). On the other hand, the court also did not contend that the state has no interest in protecting even pre-viable human beings from injury. That is, although the Roe decision guarantees women the right to fully elective abortion through the end of the second trimester of pregnancy, a very different issue regarding protection of the prenatal human being arises when a woman elects not to abort a pregnancy, and her actions (or the actions of another) result in the birth of a damaged child. Indeed, the decision in *Roe* has increasingly been used in U.S. legal decisions and by legal commentators to shore up other arguments for expanding liability for prenatal harm, for restricting the behaviors of pregnant women, and for imposing medical and surgical interventions on women to protect prenatal human beings that are expected to be born as infants.[3] At least some of these commentators may be unhappy with the *Roe* decision's refusal to recognize prenatal human beings as persons in either the moral or legal sense, and therefore they want to do whatever they can to force a recognition of fetal rights. However, a moral position holding that prenatal human beings are not persons, that elective abortion is acceptable, yet that people may be held legally liable for or may be prevented by the law from contributing to nonfatal prenatal harm because such harms involve persons can be perfectly consistent. In order to see this, we need to distinguish between actual persons, potential persons, and future persons.

PERSONS, POTENTIAL PERSONS, AND FUTURE PERSONS

We have distinguished between (1) the time when a human being has developed the kinds of characteristics that compel us to recognize beings as persons (we shall call these 'metaphysical' or 'actual persons') and (2) the time set by convention when a human being that does not yet have these characteristics is to be accepted by convention into the community of persons (we shall call these 'conventional persons'). We have argued that the conventional recognition of personhood should be set at birth. We now need to distinguish between potential persons and future persons in order to address the questions at hand.

A prenatal human being is a potential person when it is the case that (1) *if* that being were supported, it would eventually develop into a being that has the kinds of characteristics that would compel us to recognize it as a person, and (2) *if* that being were supported, it would also be born, gaining conventional entry into the class of persons. Notice that not every prenatal human being is a potential person (in either the metaphysical or conventional sense), since many conceptions terminate in spontaneous abortion, and often this is because the being has an anomaly incompatible with life or that will prevent its ever developing the kinds of characteristics which would compel recognition of a being as a person.

A prenatal human being is a future person (1) *if* it has the capacity to develop the characteristics that are morally relevant to compelling a recognition of personhood and (2) it *will* gain conventional entry into the class of persons through birth. All future persons are potential persons, but since not all potential persons will endure to reach either actual or conventional personhood (they may die because of anomalies incompatible with life, intentional abortion, accidents, etc.), not all potential persons are future persons. The complex moral and legal issues that concern us involve prenatal human beings as both potential and future persons. Our focus, however, will be on harm to prenatal future persons.

Protecting Future Persons

In the United States, recovery for prenatal injury was first granted to persons if the injury was sustained after viability (*Bonbrest v. Kotz* 1946). But a number of legal decisions have gone further and allowed recovery for injuries sustained prior to viability.[4] What is more, over the last decade, we have begun to see cases in which a plaintiff has recovered for injuries resulting from the actions of others prior to the plaintiff's conception. *Renslow v. Mennonite Hospital* (1977), for example, involved a child who was born suffering from hyperbilirubinemia (an excess of bilirubin in the blood, which, when sufficiently high, produces visible jaundice and may cause severe neurological damage, often occurring in fetuses as a result of blood group incompatibility). The child recovered for permanent brain and nervous system damage alleged to have resulted from the hospital's twice negligently transfusing her mother with blood from the wrong blood group nine years prior to the child's birth. By allowing recovery for preconceptive harm, such decisions have helped to pave the way for controversial restrictions on allowing fertile women to work in environments that might have deleterious effects on their capacity to reproduce healthy children, a topic we take up elsewhere.[5] Today, most courts hold that the time of prenatal injury is irrelevant if a causal connection can be "shown" between the harm suffered and someone's actions or omissions (Glantz 1983).[6]

Central to the reasoning in decisions granting recovery for prenatal injuries is the state's interest in protecting the interests of liveborn persons (Glantz 1983), or using our distinction, future persons, an interest that is underpinned by our widely shared moral conviction that innocent persons should not be harmed.[7] This morally grounded state interest was articulated in a Canadian decision, quoted by the court in *Bonbrest* (1946):

> If a right action be denied to the child it will be compelled without any fault on its own part to go through life carrying the seal of another's fault and bearing a very heavy burden of infirmity and inconvenience without any compensation therefore. To my mind, it is but natural justice that a child, if born alive and viable, should be allowed to maintain an action in the courts for injuries wrongfully committed upon its person while in the womb of its mother. (*Montreal Tramways v. Leveille* 1933)

This same concern is captured more succinctly in *Smith v. Brennan* (1960), in the claim that a child has a legal right to begin life with a sound mind and body.[8]

Such reasoning can be used to argue for recovery for both nonfatal prenatal injury and wrongful life (recovery where the plaintiff's claim is that, given his or her predictable afflictions, having been born constitutes an injury). Wrongful life actions have enjoyed little success in the courts to date. But a California appellate court decision suggests that courts may be about to change that trend, not only in allowing more recoveries for wrongful life in general, but in allowing recovery from parents as well as third parties. The case involved the failure of a laboratory (which had previously been alerted to failures in its testing) to diagnose a couple as carriers of Tay-Sachs disease (a recessive disorder characterized by progressive retardation in development, paralysis, dementia, blindness, and death by age three or four). The child's claim was recognized, and the court added this comment:

> If a case arose where, despite due care by the medical profession in transmitting the necessary warnings, parents made a conscious choice to proceed with a pregnancy, with full knowledge that a seriously impaired infant would be born, that conscious choice would provide an intervening act of proximate cause to preclude liability insofar as defendants other than the parents were concerned. Under such circumstances, we see no sound public policy which would protect those parents from being answerable for the pain, suffering, and misery which they have wrought upon their offspring. (*Curlender v. Bio-Science Laboratories* 1980, *in dictum*)

In cases where potential for a severe genetic defect is discovered prior to conception, this kind of reasoning entails that unless potential parents practice contraception or seek abortion if they do conceive, they may well find themselves legally liable for producing a wrongful life. In cases where a severe genetic defect is discovered or a severe prenatal harm is suspected after conception, such reasoning clearly places parents in the position of choosing abortion or potentially facing legal liability for bringing a pregnancy to term. And since biological fathers (at least at present) have no legal right to interfere with a woman's right to abort or not abort a pregnancy,[9] any such liability for wrongful life must fall on women who do not abort.[10]

As regards prenatal injury more generally, there is also a rising trend toward holding women legally liable for causing prenatal harm and toward imposing medical and surgical procedures on women to prevent prenatal harm.[11] The reasoning in many of the relevant American post-*Roe* cases and commentaries turns on the position that (1) if a woman has decided to carry a pregnancy to term, *ceteris paribus*, she carries what we have suggested be understood as a future person, and (2) that future person has a compelling moral right not to begin its independent life disadvantaged by avoidable harms resulting from the actions or omissions of others, including its mother—a moral right, it is further assumed, which is appropriately captured in law, as is the right of any existing person not to be harmed. This reasoning has led to using child protection statutes to impose transfusions and cesarean sections on women to save their fetuses, and it has also given rise to arguments for holding women criminally liable for acting in ways thought to cause prenatal harm during pregnancies expected to be brought to full term.[12]

In one California action, a woman, Pamela Stewart, was criminally prosecuted when her failure to follow medical instructions (including instructions not to take amphetamines, to stay off her feet, to abstain from intercourse, and to seek immediate medical treatment if she began bleeding) was held to have caused severe brain damage to her fetus. The infant died five weeks after birth, and Stewart was arrested for causing the death of her son. Annas (1986) reports that police officials wanted Stewart charged with murder, but the district attorney decided instead to prosecute under a California child support statute.[13] Stewart was charged with a misdemeanor that carried a possible sentence of a year in prison or a fine of $2,000. The case was dismissed only because the defendant was able to convince the court that the 1872 law under which she was being prosecuted was intended to ensure that fathers provide child support, including (following a 1925 amendment) financial support for women pregnant by them (Annas 1986; Brown et al. 1987; Johnsen 1987; *People v. Stewart* 1987).[14]

PRENATAL HUMAN BEINGS AS PATIENTS

The situation becomes even more complex as prenatal therapies, including prenatal surgical techniques, are developed. As these procedures pass from experimental status to being recognized by practitioners as safe and effective treatments, we are likely to see increasing support for requiring women to submit to them for the sake of future persons. It is not uncommon for those supportive of intrusive prenatal protection policies to suggest that recent advances in medicine that make prenatal human beings potential patients somehow change their moral status, endowing them with the right to treatment we recognize other human beings as having (e.g., Bowes and Selgestad 1981).

But it should be obvious that nothing about the moral status of a being follows from the bare fact that it can be effectively treated medically or surgically. Veterinarians, after all, are able to provide remarkable treatments for a great variety of animals; and some treatment of nonhuman animal fetuses is also now possible. But we do not think that this fact endows these beings with personhood and an attendant right to treatment. On the contrary, the question of the moral status of a being is prior to the question of entitlements, and those who argue from the fact that a prenatal human being can now be treated as a patient to the moral claim that prenatal human beings (but not prenatal pigs, prenatal cattle, etc.) have a right to treatment fail to understand that they are simply begging the question in favor of prenatal personhood for human beings.

Again, however, arguments for requiring women to submit to therapies for the good of prenatal human beings need not be based on any claim or assumption that these beings are already persons. All that needs to be claimed is that insofar as a prenatal human being is a *future* person, it is morally (and must be legally) required that it not be injured in a way that will importantly set back the interests it will have as an actual person. A crucial question, then, is whether the fact that a woman intends to bring a pregnancy to term justifies imposing medical and surgical procedures on her or otherwise legally restricting her behavior for the sake of a prenatal future person.

DIRECT INTERFERENCE WITH PREGNANT WOMEN AND THE
ANALOGY TO PEDIATRIC CASES

Much of the case for such impositions rests on the argument that in deciding to bring a pregnancy to term, a woman thereby waives her legal right to abortion and thereby takes on a set of special, legally enforceable moral duties of care toward a prenatal human being as the current embodiment of a future person. But, in fact, a woman never waives her right to abortion (Smith 1983; Annas 1987). She may decide not to exercise that right, but this does not count as a waiver of the right itself any more than the decision not to buy a certain kind of car amounts to a waiver of the right to buy that kind of car. Given the decision in *Roe*, a woman in the United States retains a legal right to elect abortion for any reason at all through the end of the second trimester of pregnancy and even after the second trimester if the pregnancy is sufficiently threatening to her health.

Further, those who argue for the view in question commonly assume that in making the decision not to abort, a pregnant woman waives both her moral and legal rights to bodily integrity in favor of the welfare of the future person she carries (e.g., Mathieu 1985; Green and Brill 1987). But waiving a right involves voluntarily relinquishing it, and in just the kinds of cases that concern us (i.e., cases in which a woman refuses a surgical or medical procedure thought to prevent prenatal harm or in which a woman acts in a way that is thought to cause prenatal harm) we find women who clearly have *not* voluntarily relinquished their moral and legal rights to bodily integrity. As Smith (1983) has rightly pointed out, the concept working here is not one of waiver at all. It is, rather, the concept of forfeiture. Felons, for example, forfeit, but do not waive, their moral and legal rights to be at liberty in the community. The argument, then, is one from forfeiture of moral and legal rights; and once this is understood, the picture is substantially altered to a far less benign one than one in which a woman voluntarily relinquishes legal protection of her bodily integrity to protect the welfare of another, in this case future, person. The pregnant woman becomes analogous to the criminal who can no longer demand that he or she not be interfered with by the state. Indeed, in arguing for the position that impingements on a pregnant woman's bodily integrity to protect a future person are justified, legal commentators often point out that bodily seizures and bodily intrusions without a person's consent are not unknown to the law. The examples given include imposing prison sentences, execution, forced medical and surgical treatment, forced feeding for the sake of prison discipline, and imposing surgery to retrieve evidence of a crime (e.g., Robertson 1982, 1985, 1986; Robertson and Schulman 1987). The analogy is chilling. Pregnant women are not felons; nor are they, to use another example in the literature, incompetents who may be ordered by courts to submit to bodily invasions to aid others because they are not capable of making such judgments for themselves.[15]

The argument from presumed waiver of a woman's moral and legal rights generally includes (explicitly or implicitly) analogizing the prenatal cases to ordinary pediatric cases (e.g., Robertson and Schulman 1987). It is widely accepted that the state may interfere with parents to provide treatment for a child or to provide for other fundamental needs of a child. Although it is generally recognized that there is an important difference between the prenatal and pediatric cases (since preventing harm in prenatal cases necessarily involves providing treatment through the woman's body or otherwise directly interfering with a woman's behaviors and preventing harm in pediatric cases does not), recommendations for when women might be imposed upon tend to be discussed in terms of comparing the risks of harm to the woman attendant to the bodily invasion (or other interference or imposition) and the risks of prenatal harm to a future person if there is no intervention (e.g., Robertson 1982, 1985, 1986). But the move to the pediatric model is too quick, and the presumption of waiver of rights accompanying it is mistaken, as we have already seen, and too strong, as we shall see shortly.

The very serious problem with all the arguments for imposing prenatal treatment on a woman or forcibly interfering with a woman's behavior to prevent prenatal harm is the failure of proponents of these arguments to address the issue from the point of view of pregnant women. Using the pediatric model to resolve the prenatal cases fails precisely because preventing pediatric harm does not involve the violations of autonomy or bodily integrity involved in the prenatal cases. What is more, the obligation not to harm proposed for the prenatal cases involves much more than what is involved in ordinary cases of avoiding harming other persons, even one's own children. The duty to avoid harming others is generally dischargeable by simply refraining from running them over with cars, avoiding dropping things on them, and so on. But, as Bolton (1979) has observed, if pregnant women have a duty to avoid causing prenatal harm, this requires actually nurturing a future person. Although this makes the prenatal cases unlike most cases of not harming others, it does make them somewhat like the pediatric cases, because we do recognize that parents have special positive duties of nurturing and aiding their children. But to avoid speciousness, proponents of the analogy must be willing to hold that morality requires court-ordered invasions of the bodily integrity of parents for their children's welfare, as well as severe restrictions on parental behaviors when those behaviors are believed to be damaging to children. Once the move is made to comparing the potential harms to parents resulting from intervention with the potential harms to children resulting from nonintervention, it follows from the analogy that parents could be forcibly taken to medical centers to donate blood, bone marrow, or even transplantable paired organs, such as eyes or kidneys. And since it is well known that substance abuse in parents is severely psychologically harmful to children, the position requires that the state must attempt to ensure that no such abuse goes on in families.

Rather than so dramatically interfere with individual lives, however, we have not allowed such forcible interventions. Where parents grossly fail to nurture their children or where their behaviors otherwise seriously harm their children, the acceptable intervention is physical separation of the children from the family. In the prenatal cases, however, protecting pre-viable future persons requires taking custody of pregnant women, and separation involves forcible removal of viable fetuses, a draconian measure not even the most strident supporters of prenatal protection have explicitly endorsed, although the cases involving forced cesarean sections are *extremely* close to this.[16]

The implications of making the prenatal and pediatric cases analogous are, we submit, simply too morally costly. On the one hand, upholding the analogy would require applying to the pediatric cases the doctrine of forfeiture of rights to bodily integrity and giving to the state a right to extreme and constant interference with parental behavior. On the other hand, it would involve giving the state the right to take a pregnant woman into custody, disable her, and induce labor in her or cut her open against her will to rescue her viable fetus. We describe the implications of the analogical argument this way, not as an exercise in inflammatory rhetoric, but to make evident the very harsh implications for pregnant women and for parents of accepting the view in question. And we submit that confronting these realities lucidly should make it evident that the moral costs of giving such intrusive powers to the state are just too high.

Thus, overriding a woman's right to control what will be done to or through her body for the sake of a future person cannot be conceptually, legally, or morally justified on the basis of an argument from the analogy between prenatal and pediatric cases, since these kinds of cases are crucially different empirically and the moral costs of accepting the analogy are too high. Since an argument from this analogy is the only argument which holds out any real hope of justifying the kinds of impositions on pregnant women that are currently being proposed, these proposals must be rejected. As Rothman (1986) argues, then, pregnant women may not be treated as mere "maternal environments"; and as Annas (1986) argues, neither may they be treated as mere "fetal containers" that may be opened and shut or otherwise forcibly manipulated for the protection of future persons.

LEGAL SANCTIONS FOR WOMEN WHO CAUSE PRENATAL HARM?

(1) *Criminal sanctions.* One suggested alternative to allowing direct interference with pregnant women is to apply sanctions to them after they have caused prenatal harm, relying on the deterrent value of the criminal law (e.g., Parness 1985, 1986). We have argued that the analogy of prenatal to pediatric cases fails to justify direct interference with pregnant women, but it has been argued that child protection statutes might be interpreted in such a way that women causing prenatal harm could be charged with crimes. For example, Leiberman et al. (1979) argue this way, contending that since pregnant women are the natural guardians of prenatal offspring, it is logical to construe rejection of a potentially lifesaving prenatal intervention (which does not put the woman's life at comparable risk) as a felony, and they suggest that physicians should be able to warn refusing patients that they are committing a felony. Parness (1983) suggests that a woman who risks addicting to heroin a fetus she intends to bring to term could be deemed to have undertaken both tortious and criminal conduct. And we have seen that an attempt to interpret an existing statute as criminalizing a woman's causing prenatal harm was made in the Pamela Stewart case. We believe that the arguments against the justifiability of directly interfering with women tell as well against using criminal sanctions against women to attempt to prevent prenatal harm, since such sanctions would coerce women into "accepting" intrusive interventions. But there are also other problems with this use of the criminal law that need to be pointed out.

First, it needs to be realized that the move to criminality by interpreting existing statutes to include prenatal harm caused by pregnant women will bear neither moral nor legal scrutiny. If we are to make women who act (or refuse to act) in the ways at issue into criminals, this requires that we enact new statutes or revise existing statutes to expressly and unambiguously make criminal the behaviors and refusals of medical/surgical interventions in question. This is a widely accepted requirement of any morally acceptable system of law—people must be able to predict which of their behaviors may lead to a loss of their liberty. In the United States, this moral requirement is captured by disallowing crimes (unlike torts) to emerge through case law. Common law crimes were abolished many years ago (see, for example, *In re Greene* 1892), and it is now a well-established principle in U.S. law that crimes must clearly be identified as such so that people are provided with advance notice that engaging in certain behaviors will mark them as enemies of the community and may justify the state's removing them from the community. Thus, unless criminal codes are revised to amply warn pregnant women who intend to continue their pregnancies to term that behaviors thought to cause prenatal harm and refusals of prenatal medical or surgical interventions are now crimes, criminal prosecution of women under existing statutes (be they child protection statutes or more general criminal neglect or battery statutes) cannot be morally or legally justified in the United States.

Rewriting criminal codes to expressly protect prenatal future persons has been suggested (e.g., Parness 1985). And if we take Leiberman et al. (1979) seriously, at least some medical/surgical intervention refusals ought to be felonious. But felonies are crimes punishable by death or imprisonment. What would be a morally acceptable and legally appropriate punishment for felonious refusals of medical and surgical interventions believed to prevent prenatal harm? Laying the possibility of execution aside, imprisonment of nonconsenting pregnant women is neither morally nor legally justifiable, since such women cannot reasonably be construed as societal menaces.

In cases where a woman's behaviors or omissions lead to prenatal harm, criminal sanctions are equally unacceptable. Prenatal harm resulting from maternal behaviors or omissions nearly always involves low birthweight and/or fetal drug addiction. Low birthweight is a major cause of infant mortality and has been identified as the single greatest hazard for surviving infants, since it results in heightened vulnerability to various developmental problems and substantially increased risk of death from common childhood diseases (e.g., National Academy of Sciences 1985). Low birthweight is associated with poor prenatal nutrition, pregnancy in the very young, smoking tobacco and drinking alcohol during pregnancy, and other kinds of drug use, including use of crack, the extremely potent form of cocaine, which is thought to account for a 20 percent rise in infant deaths in at least one American community in 1986 (Monmaney et al. 1987). That community is the impoverished black community in Harlem, New York, which has a high rate of teenage pregnancy, and in which, like many similar communities, prenatal education and prenatal care have not been readily available.

The Harlem example is a telling one, and proponents of holding women criminally liable for prenatal harm need to realize that the harms they seek to prevent are neither justifiably nor effectively dealt with by bringing the massive powers of the state to bear against women to coerce medical or surgical intervention or by treating as criminals women (often teenaged women), who frequently know very little about proper prenatal care. The often-interrelated problems of pregnancy in the very young, chemical abuse, poor nutrition, ignorance, and poverty are social problems, appropriately and most effectively dealt with by positive measures which enhance the social, economic, and intellectual position of the least well-off members of society and of women generally. Treating women as mere uterine environments that can be invaded or punished involves the kind of blaming the victim that can only seem correct when one flatly ignores the complex social conditions that typically give rise to the evil that is to be avoided—in this case, the evil of prenatal harm to future persons. As Annas (1986) argues, the best chance the state has for protecting prenatal future persons is through positive actions that benefit pregnant women, rather than by cutting funds for maternal education, health care, and nutrition and then assailing often resourceless women for not doing the best that can be done for their future children.

(2) *Civil sanctions.* Designing civil sanctions for use against women who cause prenatal harm is equally unacceptable; although holding a woman financially responsible for the costs associated with caring for a child who is handicapped as a result of her actions or omissions seems, in principle at least, to involve no violation of a woman's moral or civil rights. But one problem here is that such sanctions seem pointless, since parents with the resources to support their children are already commonly required to support them; thus, adding specific sanctions for pregnant women who cause prenatal harm is redundant. And requiring full support of parents who haven't the necessary resources is as futile in these cases as it is in other cases where children of impoverished parents require special care.

Further, adding in punitive sanctions for women seems gratuitously hostile to women, since the arguments for such sanctions ignore the fact that prenatal human beings are begotten by fathers, and fathers often encourage precisely the kinds of behaviors—alcohol and other drug use, for example—that may cause prenatal harm. Part of the case against Pamela Stewart, for instance, was that she had intercourse with her husband after being advised to refrain from doing so. Yet her husband was not prosecuted (Annas 1986).

Other problems with legal sanctions applicable to pregnant women include worries about abuse by fathers and prosecutors, as well as the concern that fear of lawsuits will surely motivate unnecessary interventions, as has been the case with cesarean deliveries. What is more, many medical interventions are unproven and this should make us *very* reluctant to press women into accepting them out of a fear of legal reprisal. That physicians tend to overestimate the need for intrusive interventions to prevent prenatal harm is demonstrated by a number of cases involving attempts to force cesarean deliveries on women who subsequently successfully delivered vaginally (see, for example, Rhoden, 1986).

Finally, introducing any of these forms of interference with women will surely encourage precisely those pregnant women most likely cause prenatal harm (e.g., those using teratogenic drugs) to avoid the medical establishment as completely as possible, leading to hidden pregnancies, births away from needed medical assistance, and increased abandonment of damaged infants, making such policies patently counterproductive (cf. Gallagher 1989). One need not be a jurist to realize that laws which are likely to contribute to the harm that they are instituted to prevent are bad laws.

CONCLUSION

Our conclusion, then, is that the arguments for interfering with pregnant women to protect prenatal human beings and for holding women legally liable for prenatal harm cannot bear the weight of their conclusions. The proper course is to find the political will to take positive action to reduce both the ignorance that underpins some (but certainly not all) maternal refusals of prenatal medical and surgical interventions (Shriner 1979; cf. Leiberman et al. 1979), and the ignorance that so often leads to poor prenatal nutrition. The task is to introduce and sustain policies that will increase, rather than decrease, the welfare of pregnant women (Annas 1986, 1987), and to encourage through education the avoidance of pregnancy among those who are not prepared to be committed to the welfare of the future persons whose interests will be so closely tied to their behaviors and decisions during pregnancy.

NOTES

This paper has been adapted from Callahan (1986) and Knight and Callahan (1989), chapters 7 and 9. We are grateful to *Commonweal* and to the University of Utah Press for permission to use the material here, and to Carolyn Bratt, Patricia Smith, and Deborah Mathieu for helpful comments on an earlier draft.

1. We use the term "prenatal human being" to refer to human beings from fertilization through the fetal stage. We use the term in its biological sense. That is, we do not take prenatal human beings to be persons. We explain and argue for this distinction in the next section.

2. For an expanded discussion, see Knight and Callahan (1989), chapter 7.

3. See, for example, *Jefferson v. Griffin Spalding County Hospital Authority* (1981); Bowes and Selgestad (1981); Parness and Pritchard (1982); Robertson (1982, 1985, 1986); the discussion in Lenow (1983); Dougherty (1986); Mathieu (1985); Parness (1985, 1986, 1987); Green and Brill (1987).

4. See, for example, *Hornbuckle v. Plantation Pipe Line* (1956); *Bennett v. Hymers* (1958); *Smith v. Brennan* (1960).

5. Knight and Callahan (1989), chapter 9.

6. Whether omissions are properly understood as causes of harm is a question beyond the scope of this essay, and we shall ignore it here. For a discussion of this question see Callahan (1988).

7. Traditionally, the class of liveborn persons includes all infants, even those with an anomaly (e.g., anencephaly—an invariably fatal condition involving absence of the cerebral hemispheres of the brain) that precludes their ever developing the kinds of characteristics that are relevant to compelling recognition of a being as a person. Thus, as the class is traditionally understood, all liveborn persons will not qualify as members of the class of future persons, since the class of future persons does not include beings incapable of developing the kinds of characteristics that are relevant to compelling recognizing the moral rights attendant to personhood. We shall not pursue this distinction here, since the position we defend will not depend on it.

8. This judgment has been reiterated in other cases; see, for example, *Womack v. Buckhorn* (1976); *Berger v. Weber* (1978); *In re Baby* X (1980).

9. But see *Taft v. Taft* (1983), in which the husband of a woman in her fourth month of pregnancy sought a court order giving him authority to require that she submit to a surgery involving suturing her cervix (a cerclage or "purse string" operation) to minimize her risk of a miscarriage—a surgery the woman had refused on religious grounds. The lower court appointed a guardian *ad litem* for the fetus, and granted the husband authority to consent to the surgery. Although the Massachusetts Supreme Court reversed the decision, it did so only because no legal precedent ordering such a submission to protect a pre-viable fetus was cited by the husband or found by the court and because no facts had been presented to show that the surgery would be a genuinely lifesaving one as opposed to a merely precautionary one. The reasons for the reversal leave open the possibility that the original decision might have been upheld in another case. The court makes this explicit in saying, "We do not decide whether, in some circumstances there would be justification for ordering a wife to submit to medical treatment in order to assist in carrying a child to term."

10. Wrongful life cases and the growing emphasis on prenatal testing raise a number of concerns. Pregnant women are increasingly pressured to undergo such testing and increasingly face the expectation that they will abort a fetus with any potential of disability. Such pressures foster already worrisome societal attitudes that both pressure women to produce "perfect" babies and disenfranchise the disabled. See, for example, Blatt 1987; Henifin 1987; Henifin et al. 1987; Saxton 1987).

11. See, for instance, *Application of President and Directors of Georgetown College* (1964); *Raleigh Fitkin-Paul Morgan Memorial Hospital v. Anderson* (1964); *People V. Estergard* (1969); *Jefferson v. Griffin Spalding County Memorial Hospital Authority* (1981); *Taft v. Taft* (1983); Leiberman et al. (1979); Bowes and Selgestad (1981); Parness and Pritchard (1982); Robertson (1982, 1985, 1986); Shaw (1983); Mathieu (1985); Parness (1985, 1986, 1987); Mackenzie and Nagel (1986); Johnsen (1987).

12. See, for example, Leiberman et al. (1979); Bowes and Selgestad (1981); Annas (1982, 1986); Parness (1983, 1985); Johnsen (1987).

13. Cal. Penal Code, Sec. 270 (West Publishing Company, 1986).

14. Cases like this raise some additional puzzles. For example, if physicians in such cases fail to so advise women, should *they* be subject to prosecution? What medical advice must be explicitly stated and what may be left up to "common sense"? Must a woman be told about *all* the drugs and other potentially hazardous chemicals that could possibly harm her fetus and be advised to avoid them; must she be advised not to skydive, etc.?

15. See, for example, *Strunk v. Strunk* (1969) and *Hart v. Brown* (1972), where kidney transplants from incompetents were ordered to save the life of a sibling, and the argument from these examples in Bowes and Selgestad (1981). See also the discussion of court-ordered bodily invasions in Mathieu (1985).

16. See also Parness's (1983) discussion of taking custody of prospective parents, with examples of several attempts by states to take custody of fetuses by taking custody of pregnant women.

REFERENCES

Annas, George J. 1987. Letters. *Hastings Center Report* 17/3: 26.

Annas, George J. 1986. Pregnant women as fetal containers. *Hastings Center Report* 16/6: 13.

Annas, George J. 1982. Forced cesareans: The most unkindest cut of all. *Hastings Center Report* 12/3: 16.

Application of President and Directors of Georgetown College. 1964. 331 F 2d 1000 (DC Cir.). Cert. den. 337 U.S. 978.

Bennett v. Hymers. 1958. 101 NH 483, 147 A 2d 108.

Berger v. Weber. 1978. 82 MI App 199, 267 NW 2d 124.

Blatt, Robin J. R. 1987. To choose or refuse prenatal testing. *Genewatch* 4: 3.

Bolton, Martha Brandt. 1979. Responsible women and abortion decisions. In *Having children: Philosophical and legal reflections on parenthood*. Ed. Onora O'Neill and William Ruddick. New York: Oxford University Press, pp. 40–51.

Bonbrest v. Kotz. 1946. 65 F.Supp. 138.

Bondeson, William B., H. Tristram Engelhardt, Jr., Stuart F. Spicker, and Daniel H. Winship, eds. 1983. *Abortion and the status of the fetus*. Boston: D. Reidel.

Bowes, Watson A., Jr., and Brad Selgestad. 1981. Fetal versus maternal rights: Medical and legal perspectives. *Obstetrics and Gynecology* 58: 209.

Brown, Edward, Chris Hackler, Helga Kuhse, and Colin Thomson. 1987. The latest word. *Hastings Center Report* 17/2: 51.

Callahan, Joan C. 1988. Acts, omissions, and euthanasia. *Public Affairs Quarterly* 2/2: 21.

Callahan, Joan C. 1986. The fetus and fundamental rights. *Commonweal* 11 April: 203. Revised, expanded version in *Abortion and catholicism: The American debate*. Ed. Thomas A. Shannon and Patricia B. Jung. New York: Crossroads, 1988, pp. 217–30.

Curlender v. Bio-Science Laboratories and Automated Laboratory Sciences. 1980. 165 CA Rpt 477.

Dougherty, Charles. 1986. The right to begin life with sound body and mind: Fetal patients and conflicts with their mothers. *University of Detroit Law Review* 63/1–2: 89.

Gallagher, Janet. 1989. Fetus as patient. In *Reproductive laws for the 1990s*. Ed. Sherrill Cohen and Nadine Taub. Clifton, NJ: Humana Press, pp. 185–235.

Glantz, Leonard. 1983. Is the fetus a person? A lawyer's view. In Bondeson et al., eds., above. pp. 107–17.

Glover, Jonathon. 1977. *Causing death and saving lives*. New York: Penguin.

Green, Willard, and Charles Brill. 1987. Letters. *Hastings Center Report* 17/3: 25.

Hart v. Brown. 1972. 29 CT Supp. 368, 289 A 2d 386 (CT Sup.Ct.).

Henifin, Mary Sue. 1987. What's wrong with "wrongful life" court cases? *Genewatch* 4: 1.

Henifin, Mary Sue, Ruth Hubbard, and Judy Norsigian. 1989. Prenatal screening. In *Reproduction laws for the 1990s*. Ed. Sherrill Cohen and Nadine Taub. Clifton, NJ: Humana Press, pp. 155–83.

Hornbuckle v. Plantation Pipe Line. 1956. 212 GA 504, 93 SE 2d 727.

In re Baby X. 1980. 97 MI App 111, 293 NW 2d 736.

In re Greene. 1892. 52 F 104 (CCW OH).

Jefferson v. Griffin Spalding County Hospital Authority. 1981. 247 GA 86, 274 SE 2d 457.

Johnsen, Dawn. 1987. A new threat to pregnant women's autonomy. *Hastings Center Report* 17/4: 33.

Knight, James W., and Joan C. Callahan. 1989. *Preventing birth: Contemporary methods and related moral controversies*. Salt Lake City: University of Utah Press.

Leiberman, J. R., M. Mazor, W. Chaim, and A. Cohen. 1979. The fetal right to live. *Obstetrics and Gynecology* 53: 515.

Lenow, Jeffrey L. 1983. The fetus as patient: Emerging legal rights as a person? *American Journal of Law and Medicine* 9: 1.

Mackenzie, Thomas B., and Theodore C. Nagel. 1986. When a pregnant woman endangers her fetus: Commentary. *Hastings Center Report* 16/1: 24.

Mathieu, Deborah. 1985. Respecting liberty and preventing harm. *Harvard Journal of Law and Public Policy* 8: 19.

Monmaney, Terrence, Mary Hager, Karen Springen, and Lisa Drew. 1987. A black health crisis. *Newsweek* 13 July: 53.

Montreal Tramways v. Leveille. 1933. 4 Dom. LR 337.

National Academy of Sciences. 1985. *Preventing low birthweight.* (Prep. by the Committee to Study the Prevention of Low Birthweight, Institute of Medicine.) Washington: National Academy Press.

Parness, Jeffrey A. 1987. Letters. *Hastings Center Report* 17/3: 26.

Parness, Jeffrey A. 1986. The abuse and neglect of the human unborn. *Family Law Quarterly* 20: 197.

Parness, Jeffrey A. 1985. Crimes against the unborn: Protecting and respecting the poten-tiality of human life. *Harvard Journal on Legislation* 22: 97.

Parness, Jeffrey A. 1983. The duty to prevent handicaps: Laws promoting the prevention of handicaps to newborns. *Western New England Law Review* 5: 431.

Parness, Jeffrey A., and Susan K. Pritchard. 1982. To be or not to be: Protecting the unborn's potentiality of life. *University of Cincinnati Law Review* 51: 257.

People v. Estergard. 1969. 457 P 2d 698 (CO S.Ct.).

People v. Stewart. 1987. No. M508197, San Diego Mun Ct, 23 February.

Raleigh Fitkin-Paul Morgan Memorial Hospital v. Anderson. 1964. 42 NJ 421, 201 A 2d 337 (NJ S.Ct.).

Renslow v. Mennonite Hospital. 1977. 67 IL 2d 348, 369 NE 2d 1250.

Rhoden, Nancy K. 1986. The judge in the delivery room: The emergence of court-ordered cesareans. *California Law Review* 74: 1951.

Robertson, John A. 1986. Legal issues in prenatal therapy. *Clinical Obstetrics and Gynecology* 29: 603.

Robertson, John A. 1985. Legal issues in fetal therapy. *Seminars in Perinatology* 9: 136.

Robertson, John A. 1982. The right to procreate and in utero fetal therapy. *Journal of Legal Medicine* 3: 333.

Robertson, John A., and Joseph D. Schulman. 1987. Pregnancy and prenatal harm to offspring: The case of mothers with PKU. *Hastings Center Report* 17/4: 23.

Roe v. Wade. 1973. 410 U.S. 113.

Rothman, Barbara Katz. 1986. When a pregnant woman endangers her fetus: Commentary. *Hastings Center Report* 16/1: 25.

Saxton, Marsha. 1987. Prenatal screening and discriminatory attitudes about disability. *Genewatch* 4: 8.

Shaw, Margery W. 1983. The destiny of the fetus. In Bondeson et al., eds., above, pp. 273–79.

Shriner, Thomas L. 1979. Maternal versus fetal rights—A clinical dilemma. *Obstetrics and Gynecology* 53: 518.

Smith, Holly M. 1983. Intercourse and responsibility for the fetus. In Bondeson et al., eds., above, pp. 229–45.

Smith v. Brennan. 1960. 31 NJ 353, 157 A 2d 497.

Strunk v. Strunk. 1969. 445 SW 2d 145 (KY Ct.App.).

Taft v. Taft. 1983. 338 MA 331, 446 NE 2d 395.

Warren, Mary Anne. 1975. On the moral and legal status of abortion. In *Today's Moral Problems.* Ed. Richard A. Wasserstrom. New York: Macmillan, pp. 120–36.

Wertheimer, Roger. 1971. Understanding the abortion argument. *Philosophy and Public Affairs* 1:67.

Womack v. Buckhorn. 1976. 384 MI 718, 187 NW 2d 218.

Sex Selection Through Prenatal Diagnosis: A Feminist Critique

DOROTHY C. WERTZ and JOHN C. FLETCHER   ❖ ❖ ❖

New prenatal techniques make possible the detection and abortion of fetuses of undesired sex. Feminists should take a stand against sex selection, which would increase sexism and sex role stereotyping, undo advances of the women's movement, and lead to restrictive laws against abortion. There is no moral justification for sex selection, even in India. Legal prohibition of sex selection would threaten the gains women have made in reproductive rights. The practice is best discouraged by not routinely providing information on fetal sex.

Reliable methods of detecting sex in the fetus or embryo pose difficult moral questions for women. Feminists need to examine ethical arguments about sex selection because it provides a rationale for restrictions on abortion. In November 1989, Pennsylvania passed a law prohibiting abortions under a variety of circumstances, including sex choice. The new law was one response to popular beliefs that such abortions are occurring. Indeed, recent data suggest that many physicians in the United States and some other nations are receptive to parents' requests for prenatal diagnosis merely to determine sex (Wertz and Fletcher 1989a–c). No study has ever been done of what actually occurs in practice in the United States with respect to sex selection by prenatal diagnosis.

New methods of sex detection earlier in pregnancy have increased the urgency of these issues.[1] It is already possible to determine fetal sex from ultrasound, sometimes as early as nine to eleven weeks, and ultrasound is becoming routine in most pregnancies (Wertz and Wertz 1989, 246–52). Women having ultrasound are usually told the fetus's sex. Furthermore, in the near future, minimally invasive methods such as maternal blood tests may be applied to all pregnant women (Holtzman 1989, 108).

By revealing fetal sex, prenatal diagnosis and ultrasonography present prospective parents with a new and troubling possibility: choosing their children's sex through selective abortion. To a sizeable number of doctors today, sex choice may seem to be a logical extension of parents' rights to control the number, timing, spacing, and quality of their offspring.[2] As abortion is available on demand, they may believe that it should not be denied for specific purposes. Some doctors may think of themselves as technicians who provide services nonjudgmentally; what patients subsequently do with the information is not their business.

What explains a current moral tolerance of sex selection? In the background is a popular desire for the perfect, tailor-made child, a desire to which medicine has contributed by offering the possibility of control over more and more aspects of pregnancy and birth. For some, control over the child's sex seems a logical extension of other kinds of control and of respect for reproductive freedom.

Further, the consumer movement in the United States has forced doctors to reveal test results. Many doctors now regard injecting their moral beliefs into the doctor–patient relationship as paternalistic. To feminists, an attempt at persuasion or the giving of advice on the part of doctors represents a reassertion of patriarchal authority. Nevertheless, few women desire to remove all moral values from the doctor–patient relationship. There is something distinctly unnerving about the idea of a doctor as a pure technician or an amoral individual who will do anything requested. Most patients would prefer that the doctor have a personal moral stance and code of values, as long as this is not imposed upon the patient. Sometimes it is difficult to adhere to personal and professional standards without appearing paternalistic. Nevertheless, the alternative—the doctor as amoral technician—poses grave moral dangers both to women and society.

Geneticists[3] are in a peculiarly sensitive position, because giving advice or withholding services leaves them open to accusations of practicing eugenics or acting as the gatekeepers to life. The new fields of medical genetics and genetic counseling that developed after World War II stressed "nondirectiveness," support for patients' decisions, whatever these decisions were, and refusal to "tell patients what to do." Today the stance of nondirectiveness (ethical neutrality) in genetic counseling is ubiquitous (Wertz and Fletcher 1988). A stated practice of nondirectiveness (Fraser 1974) makes it difficult for some practitioners to refuse a service without appearing judgmental.

FEMINIST VIEWS ON THE ETHICS OF SEX SELECTION

Sex selection through prenatal diagnosis is an issue that tests limits to reproductive choice. Mary Anne Warren and other feminist authors have considered some central moral arguments on sex selection (Warren 1985; Overall 1987, 17–39; Holmes 1985, 1987). Warren (1985), after a thorough, book-length feminist analysis of ethical arguments for and against sex selection, concludes on a basically positive note. Other feminists are more negative (Holmes 1985, 1987; Overall, 1987).

Overall (1987, 23–27), however, observes that even in a nonsexist society there would remain a natural desire for a child of one's own sex. This desire is not necessarily sexist, but a desire for companionship with which most of us sympathize. In her discussion, Overall is careful to distinguish between gender stereotyping, which is inherently sexist, and sexual identification, which is not. Preference for companionship with a person with a particular sexual identification (e.g., for a male partner if a woman is heterosexual or a female partner if she is lesbian) is not sexist. Overall believes that preferences for sexual identification can be extended to one's offspring without gender stereotyping and that they represent perhaps the only nonsexist argument for sex selection. Bayles, however, argues that *all* sex preferences "mask an irrational sexism" because they are premised on a belief in sexual inequality (1984, 35).

Overall (1987, 21–23) also examines three claims put forward by Warren: that sex choice, first, would enhance quality of life more for a child of the "wanted" sex than a child of the "unwanted" sex; second, would provide better quality of life for the family that has the "balance" it desires; and third, would bring a better quality of life to the mother, because she will undergo fewer births to have the desired number of children of each sex. Overall then demonstrates that each of these arguments is premised upon the existence of a sexist society with defined gender roles, because the perception of "better quality of life" would not be comprehensible except against the background of preferential treatment of one sex (usually the male). To practice sex selection for these reasons, Overall (1987, 29–35) maintains, not only would serve to perpetuate a sexist society, but further would not, in the context of a sexist society, lead to improved quality of life for the child, the family, or the mother. Overall claims that sex selection would worsen the quality of family life in several ways. Sex selection could encourage favored treatment of a child whose sex was deliberately selected by parents and result in neglect of existing children whose sex was determined by nature. Sex selection could also occasion marital conflict about family composition, and, in societies where women possess little power, foreclose their only chance to have a girl.

In addition, improved quality of life for women in general by sex choice is an illusion. Overall argues on consequentialist grounds that (assuming persons would act on their preferences, if they could) in most societies, sex selection would tend to be used against females (1987, 34). Even in the United States, where most couples desire to have one child of each sex, there are preferences for boys (Pebley and Westhoff 1982; Westhoff and Rindfuss 1974; Steinbacher and Holmes 1987). Overall concludes that there appear to be no valid arguments for sex selection on the basis of "quality of life."

Could sex selection improve the position of wives and daughters in India? A wife who bears no sons may face a real threat to her life. "Bride-burning" has become common. Unwanted daughters frequently die through selective neglect in childhood.[4] Although sex selection might ameliorate the situation of some individuals, it lowers the status of women in general and only perpetuates the situation that gave rise to it. Indian feminists are aware of this and have lobbied for the new laws against sex selection.[5]

Another argument used to justify sex selection is that it would help to limit the population. Families would not have six girls to have their desired son, for example (Postgate 1976). If fewer girls were born, there would be fewer fertile women available to produce the next generation. But there is no evidence that population trends result from a desire to have sons. Rather, most families try to have the number of children that seems most economically advantageous. If they could select sex, and if one sex presented an economic advantage over the other, some families might actually have more children than they would have had in the absence of sex selection. Holmes concludes that

> sex selection as a means to cure overpopulation is likely to be pernicious. Proposing such a method is particularly ironic when existing evidence has already demonstrated that population growth slows with improvement in social welfare and extension of the roles of women beyond that of childbearing. Family planning programs are generally unsuccessful when there is no improvement in providing the necessities of life. Birth rates are lowered with increases in income levels, health care, employment opportunities, education, and the status of women. (1985, 58)

Can other reasons be offered for sex preferences that are defensible in terms of serious tests of rationality? According to Overall (1987, 34), the sex of one child does not make her or him any more "my" child than one of the other sex; genetically, parents contribute equally to each child. Women can carry on the family name. They do so increasingly in the United States by retaining their maiden names, hyphenating their last names, or using the husband's family name only in society's private sector. In almost all nations, males and females are now more equal in the capacity to inherit the estates of parents or others. Few jobs exist that women cannot perform as well as or better than men, when performance is the criterion for evaluation.

Gender roles and stereotypes, however, are still prevalent in our society and influence children's preferences at an early age. Because of peer pressure on the child, it would be difficult to pursue one's hobby, say, of dressmaking with a son, or football with a daughter. Yet the women's movement has influenced many schools to offer homemaking courses to boys and the full range of sports to girls. Widespread adoption of sex selection of children would, in our view, turn back the clock on such gains. For example, if parents were to select daughters in order to have someone to care for them in their old age, this would merely reinforce women's subservient gender role as caregivers for the elderly. The daughter would be used as a means to an end rather than as an autonomous person. If we believe that sexual equality is necessary for a just society, then we should oppose sex selection. Any normal pleasure that can be enjoyed with a child of one sex, such as sports, vacations, hobbies, games, art, and literature, can be enjoyed with a child of the other sex (Bayles 1984, 35). Sex selection would turn back the clock on all this.

Moreover, to force a child to participate in one's own hobbies or sports primarily for one's own pleasure is unethical, because it uses the child as a means to an end (Powledge 1981, 203; Ryan, 1990). According to Hoskins and Holmes, "Treating people according to the sex role we envision, instead of according to their individuality, is sexism. What is more sexist than to *create* a person to fit a sex role ideology?" (1984, 248).

Can there be an altruistic reason for sex selection? What if parents clearly want to reduce the harms of sexism and to do so by balancing the sexes in their family?

Suppose a future in which a proven, safe, and inexpensive method of sex detection exists. Further, suppose that like most Americans you would use natural sex determination with your first child. Whatever the sex of your first child, by prior agreement with your spouse, for subsequent births you want to use sex selection to balance your family.

Prima facie there is no reason to condemn the desire to balance sex in families, especially among parents who want their children to respect sex-based differences and to learn fairness to the opposite sex by practicing it at home. Yet the desire for a balanced family assumes sex role stereotyping. Why desire to balance a family unless you already hold stereotypes about sex?

Furthermore, one can never guarantee that the interactions between children in a family will reduce sexism. Suppose a girl remains angry at her brother because she feels she is deprived of a sister? Suppose one child is cruel, selfish, and narcissistic? Suppose one child makes sexual advances on a sibling of the opposite sex? From family interactions siblings may develop gender role prejudices far different from what their parents hoped.

A Misuse of Prenatal Diagnosis?

Abortions for sex, however few in number, contribute to the backlash against abortion rights. The 1989 Pennsylvania law prohibiting abortion for sex selection may be a first step toward prohibiting abortions for characteristics of the fetus, and ultimately prohibiting abortion for reasons of women's life situations. Feminists have long opposed sex-choice abortions because these acts "trivialize" the moral seriousness of abortion decisions (Asch 1989, 82). Reproductive choices should not be unlimited, especially when they threaten fairness to others (Ryan 1990).

Societal arguments against using prenatal diagnosis for sex selection include the possibility of unbalancing the sex ratio, diminishing the status of women (assuming that sex preference would be for males), and unbalancing the birth order if, for example, most families acted upon their preference for first-born boys. There is, of course, no real proof that any of these things would happen in Western societies. Although families in Western nations may state sex or birth order preferences when answering a survey, these preferences are slight. It is doubtful that many would go to the length of having trial pregnancies and abortions for the purpose of tailoring their families to fit their survey responses. Unbalancing sex ratios through prenatal diagnosis alone seems a very remote possibility. (Attempting to select the child's sex before conception, by separating X-bearing and Y-bearing sperm, although at present not a reliable option, may be a greater social danger.)

Yet this use of prenatal diagnosis may contravene distributive justice. In rural and remote sections of the United States, prenatal diagnosis is still a scarce resource; and the majority of women for whom prenatal diagnosis is medically indicated on the basis of age (over thirty-five) do not receive it (Mulvihill et al. 1989, 423). As long as there are women with medical/genetic indications who need this service and who cannot afford it, the provision of this service for sex selection is a misuse of medical resources.

Even if there were an abundance of prenatal diagnostic services—as now in a few United States communities—a stronger reason to oppose sex selection by prenatal diagnosis is that it undermines the major moral reason that justifies prenatal diagnosis and selective abortion—the prevention of suffering for parents and children.[6] Originally, prenatal diagnosis was developed to detect serious disorders in the fetus, such as Down syndrome and spina bifida. A host of other disorders, however, including some relatively mild and some that are treatable, can also be diagnosed. Medical definitions of "seriousness" are rightly giving way to patients' definitions. What one family considers an acceptable burden, another family may find unbearable. No one except the mother herself—who will raise the child— should have the right to say what burdens are bearable. Nevertheless, there is a qualitative difference between even a treatable disorder (such as cleft palate) and gender itself.[7] Being born female is not a departure from the human norm. Any suffering that is attached to sex is suffering created by the family or society, not suffering created by nature. This suffering caused by society is indeed serious and needs to be removed; however, aborting fetuses of the sex that suffers more would be a rationale to reinforce and abet the conditions causing suffering, not one that would alleviate them.

PERFECT CHILDREN?

Another argument against sex selection—one that anticipates completion of the human genome map—is that by selecting for sex we set precedents for attempts to select other characteristics that have nothing to do with disease, for instance, height, eye and hair color, thinness, skin color, and straight teeth. Many parents already include some of these characteristics in visualizing their perfect children. Sex selection may well be the beginning of a "slippery slope." If sex selection becomes commonplace, will it not set a precedent for other requests from anxious parents in the next century? What else will geneticists be asked to do if and when they can understand and determine the expression of several genes? Parents could argue that having a child with "undesirable" characteristics—shortness, nearsightedness, color-blindness, or just an average IQ—would make them miserable, make the child miserable, and lower the quality of their family life (especially if they already had several such children)—many of the same arguments given for sex selection. For some minority groups, this precedent could lead in another direction: the temptation to select lighter-skinned fetuses, knowing that skin color is historically related to upward mobility in the United States. Although these choices are still in the realm of science fiction, sex selection is not. Within the next twenty years, or sooner, however, some of the more exotic choices may be technically possible, especially those related to body size and height.

No matter how desirable a trait is—20/20 vision, let us say—creating a child with such a trait (positive eugenics) is making a product, reducing a person to a marketplace commodity that is wanted only if it meets certain specifications. How will that child fare in its sense of identity and personal relationships? Suppose the parents feel that he/she is not sufficiently grateful for the expense they underwent in prenatal testing and aborting less perfect siblings? Suppose the child loses its eyesight in a motorcycle accident or adopts a trade (etching microchips, for example) that eventually leads to blindness?

At the extreme, such prenatal tinkering with desired characteristics could lead to selective breeding, reinforcing racism and the gap between social classes. Unless there are radical changes in the United States system of medical care, the capacity to use genetic knowledge will reside with the upper and middle classes, who can pay for eugenic interventions, sex selection, and "cosmetic" selections. These same classes will set the fashion for socially desired characteristics. If geneticists and allied professionals were to adopt a code of ethics that opposed sex selection through prenatal diagnosis, this could help to prevent classist uses of genetic knowledge in the future (Fletcher et al. 1985).

In this case, respect for the individual woman threatens justice for all women. In the long run, eugenic programs may result from individual actions as well as from social and political movements. Individual choices must be tempered by what is required for a just society.

For a final reason it is important to take a stand on sex selection now. In the preceding arguments, we discussed fetuses. In the future, preconceptual sex selection (by separation of X- from Y-bearing sperm) may become available. Unlike sex selection through abortion, preconceptual selection could gain widespread popular acceptance (among both pro-choice and anti-abortion advocates) and could more easily affect sex ratios or birth order, with unknown social repercussions. This is more likely to happen if there has been previous cultural acceptance of or neutrality toward sex selection through prenatal diagnosis.

THE ETHICS OF CARING AND RELATIONSHIPS

Gilligan (1982) demonstrates that women's upbringing and experience can lead to a focus on care rather than autonomy and justice. According to Gilligan,

> A progressively more adequate understanding of the psychology of human relationships—an increasing differentiation of self and other and a growing comprehension of the dynamics of social interaction—informs the development of an ethic of care. This ethic, which reflects a cumulative knowledge of human relationships, evolves around a central insight, that self and other are interdependent. (74)

In summarizing, Gilligan (274) says that "while an ethic of justice proceeds on the premise of equality—that everyone should be treated the same—an ethic of care rests on the premise of nonviolence—that no one should be hurt." An ethic of care looks at a situation from the points of view of all parties concerned, including society, and from the viewpoint of the future as well as the present. An ethic of care does not argue on the basis of individuals' "rights," but on the basis of the avoidance of harm, including harm to human relationships. Those following an ethic of care would welcome and accept a child as a person, not as someone who exists to fill a gender role (Hoskins and Holmes 1985, 36). In the feminist vision of community, all are welcome (Ryan 1990).

KNOWLEDGE AS TEMPTATION

The moral and social arguments seem to weigh heavily against performing prenatal diagnosis *solely* for sex selection. However, in this area most moral dilemmas will evolve from the knowledge about sex that is incidental to prenatal diagnosis performed for other purposes. In an actual case known to one of us, a couple had three boys and the husband wanted no more children. When the wife unexpectedly became pregnant, he threatened to leave her. She wanted the child, whatever the sex, but also wanted to preserve the family. She was over thirty-five and therefore had medical indications for prenatal diagnosis, on account of the higher risk for Down syndrome among older women. She knew that a prenatal diagnosis for Down syndrome would also reveal the fetal sex. Finally she and her husband struck a bargain: if the fetus were female, she would carry it to term. Otherwise she would abort, and he would not abandon the family.

Some parents may welcome the possibility of making such decisions, but for many it is an unwanted, agonizing choice. They are faced with a decision that may cause moral agony, not so much because they make the "wrong" choice, but because the choice exists. In William Styron's novel *Sophie's Choice* (1980), Sophie is forced to decide which of her two children to send to the gas chamber. Her subsequent nightmare is not that she chose the wrong child, but that *she* had to make the *choice*. The possibility of sex selection presents parents with a similar moral nightmare. Most would not seek to have prenatal diagnosis solely for sex selection, but their eligibility for the procedure on other grounds presents a temptation.[8]

The problem will be exacerbated if prenatal diagnosis is used in borderline situations like "maternal anxiety." By providing the procedure to any woman who says she is anxious about the fetus's health, doctors also open the gate to the possibility of sex selection. "Anxiety" is already a medical indication in Denmark, Sweden, and Switzerland, and accounts for roughly 10 percent of prenatal diagnoses in these nations (Wertz and Fletcher 1989a, c). Doctors may argue that women who work in institutions for the mentally retarded or whose friends have given birth to children with Down syndrome have special anxieties. Others believe that every pregnant woman should have the opportunity to have her anxieties relieved. They see prenatal diagnosis as a beneficent procedure that promotes the mother's mental health and that may thereby lead to a healthier pregnancy.

Prenatal diagnosis could soon become routine in most pregnancies. Although the more invasive and riskier methods, such as amniocentesis and CVS, may in the future be restricted to those at genuinely high risk, ultrasound, a noninvasive method, has already become routine. Fetal chromosome analysis may one day be possible through an inexpensive maternal blood test that poses no risk to mother or fetus. If such tests become routine, the sex of the fetus will be detected in the first trimester as part of everyday routine prenatal care. Thus it is imperative to face the impending moral and social problems.

SOME POSSIBLE SOLUTIONS

Laws against using prenatal diagnosis for sex selection would probably be disadvantageous in most Western nations. Women have only recently won control over their reproductive lives, and legal measures prohibiting prenatal diagnosis or abortion for a specific purpose would be a step backward toward other restrictive controls. Furthermore, laws against sex selection would be impossible to enforce, for few people in Western nations would make direct requests. In the United States it would be possible, within the framework of *Roe v. Wade* and recent Supreme Court decisions, to prohibit abortions done for a specific reason, such as sex selection, using the analogy of laws that prohibit the sale of guns to those who say they will use them to murder people. This is not a particularly helpful analogy, for few would-be murderers tell gun-shop owners that they intend to shoot people, and few prospective parents tell doctors that their real reason for having prenatal diagnosis is to discover fetal sex. Even unenforceable laws against sex selection in Western societies, however, pose real dangers to civil liberties and abortion rights.

Appropriate hospital and laboratory policy might be a possible solution, especially in countries with a national health service. In nations such as the United States, professional codes of medical ethics, including those of national specialty boards and state medical societies, could be used to discourage private doctors from using prenatal diagnosis merely for sex selection. The codes of state medical societies are particularly important, because these societies ordinarily control licensure and can discipline or suspend physicians who flagrantly violate the code. Of course, only the most obvious violators would be disciplined. Nevertheless, a professional stand on the question could go a long way toward preventing widespread abuse.

Most prospective parents would probably agree with this approach, which helps to remove a "Sophie's choice." A few doctors would continue to practice sex selection, but it is better to permit this freedom to the few than to start hedging reproduction with restrictive laws. Discouraging the use of prenatal diagnosis for sex selection will not necessarily result in fewer abortions; it may actually result in more, because those who are undecided about continuing a pregnancy may be more willing to abort if they are unable to find out the fetus's sex.

Why not simply withhold information about sex, rather than withholding prenatal diagnosis? Prima facie, this seems logical. Sex is not a disease, and it would probably be legal for doctors to withhold the information about sex as clinically irrelevant.

Withholding information, however, is a feminist issue. Information is power, particularly in the hands of a male-dominated medical establishment. The women's health movement has campaigned to transfer control of information to women patients, thereby empowering them. Patients in the United States have become used to asking for full disclosure, and ethicists have tried to educate professionals to convey the "whole truth" to competent patients. Withholding information puts control into the hands of doctors, not patients, and sets a precedent for a resurgence of medical paternalism.

Yet doctors do withhold some types of nonmedical information routinely. For instance, they may discover that the husband is not the biological father of a child.[9] The decision to withhold information from the husband in the interests of maintaining relationships is analogous to withholding other types of "incidental" information learned from genetic testing. A similar practice of not revealing incidental information routinely could be applied to fetal sex.[10] Information would not be withheld if patients take the initiative to ask for it. The doctor would not know something that the patient does not know, because the information would be not provided in the laboratory report. The information would reside in the laboratory. Thus patient and doctor would be equals in ignorance, a situation that would tend to equalize power. Nevertheless, unless women take medicine into their own hands or create an alternative system, *some* imbalance of power will inevitably remain, because the medical establishment still has the information. This may be a lesser evil than providing patients with the temptation to select sex. Parents would also avoid gender stereotyping their fetuses as "strong, vigorous, active" males or "sweet, gentle" females, as many prospective parents do after learning fetal sex (Rothman 1986, 116–54).

CONCLUSION

In sum, then, women should take a stance now against sex selection. Sex selection would increase sexism and sex role stereotyping, and could undo the hard-won advances of the women's movement. There is no moral justification for sex selection even in India, where it will only exacerbate the low status of women. Use of prenatal diagnosis for sex selection will discredit its use to detect serious genetic disorders. Sex selection is likely ultimately to lead to an anti-abortion backlash and to restrictive laws limiting abortion choices.

Legislators are already hastening to pass laws prohibiting abortion for sex selection; because these laws are the beginning of other restrictions on abortion, they are not in women's best interests. Restrictive laws against sex selection may be worse than the abuses they are intended to prevent. Abortion for sex selection should remain legal, even if morally unjustified. Concerned feminists using moral suasion on geneticists and other appropriate health care workers is a better avenue of prevention than legal restraint.

NOTES

The International Survey of Ethics and Human Genetics was supported by the Medical Trust, one of the Pew Memorial Trusts administered by the Glenmede Trust Company,

Philadelphia, PA, by the Muriel and Maurice Miller Foundation, Washington, DC, and by the Norwegian Marshall Fund.

1. Women who do not wish to wait until sixteen weeks for amniocentesis can now have chorionic villus sampling (CVS) at eight or nine weeks, before the fetus "quickens" in the womb. In CVS, fetal cells are obtained from the lining of what will become the amniotic sac, by means of a plastic cannula inserted into the vagina (Holmes 1985). Soon it may be possible to test pre-embryos at the four-cell stage that have been fertilized in vitro, and to select only healthy embryos of the desired sex for implantation. This procedure avoids abortion; embryos of the sex not desired can be frozen for future use. Sex detection at the four-cell stage has already occurred in research laboratories (Coutelle et al. 1989). This procedure will be costly, and, because it involves in vitro fertilization, will ultimately produce few babies.

2. When presented with a hypothetical case vignette describing a couple with four healthy daughters who desire a son, 62 percent in a 1985 survey of 295 United States geneticists said that they would either perform prenatal diagnosis for this couple (34 percent) or would refer them to someone who would perform it (28 percent). When asked why, most phrased their answers in terms of respect for patients' autonomy and rights of choice. Women doctors, who comprised 35 percent of the respondents, were twice as likely as men to say that they would actually perform prenatal diagnosis for sex (Wertz and Fletcher 1989a, 1989b, 57; Wertz et al. 1990).

In 1975, Fraser and Pressor learned that among 149 clinically oriented genetic counselors, 15 percent would recommend amniocentesis for sex selection or refer, while 28 percent indicated that they would do so in response to a case where a well-informed couple with one girl wanted to be sure that their second and final child was a son (Fraser and Pressor 1977). Apparently, attitudes of clinical geneticists about sex selection are more tolerant now than in 1975.

3. Geneticists are specialists who do counseling, diagnosis, and research (few treatments are available). About four-fifths are M.D.'s, usually pediatricians; the rest are Ph.D.'s or master's-level specialists in counseling. About one-third of doctoral-level geneticists, in the United States and elsewhere, are women. Almost all master's-level genetic counselors (a specialty that exists only in the United States and Canada) are women. Geneticists perform prenatal diagnosis through amniocentesis or CVS, but do not ordinarily perform abortions. If a woman chooses abortion on genetic grounds, the geneticist refers her to an obstetrician or other physician for the procedure.

4. In parts of northern India, preference for sons is so strong that the sex ratio reached a low of 935 women to 1,000 men in 1981 (India, Ministry of Welfare 1985). The imbalance, which has increased steadily since 1910, results from the preferential medical treatment and nutrition given male children from birth to age ten, coupled with occasional female infanticide. Prenatal diagnosis has offered a new method of obtaining sons. Government reports estimate that 8,000 to 10,000 female feticides occurred between 1978 and 1982 in the Bombay area (Joseph 1986; Verma and Singh 1989, 258–59; 267–68).

5. Banning sex selection in India will not remove the underlying economic causes of sexual inequality and the selective neglect of female children, but would be an important symbolic step in affirming the value of women. In 1988, the state of Maharashtra, which includes Bombay, passed a law prohibiting use of prenatal diagnosis for sex selection. The new law made it a crime to reveal the fetus's sex when procedures are done for legitimate medical indications, and provided a minimum penalty of Rs. 1,000 ($67.00) and one year in jail and suspension of license for two years for doctors who perform prenatal diagnosis for sex selection or reveal fetal sex (Maharashtra Legislature Secretariat, L.C. Bill No. VIII of 1988). The law assumed that a woman who seeks such procedures "has been compelled to do so by her husband or members of his family," and provided the same punishment for them as for the doctor. On account of the decentralization of private medical care in India into thousands of small clinics, it has been extremely difficult to enforce this law, though there have been several prosecutions. One effect of the new law has been to raise the price

of sex selection to about $750.00, still within the range of the well-to-do. Other states are considering similar laws, and the central government in New Delhi has forbidden the procedure in government-supported clinics.

6. The U.S. public's view of the indications for genetic testing relies on the principles of relief or prevention of suffering. The best study, among a national probability sample of 1,273 American adults by the Harris organization, shows overwhelming support (89 percent) for making genetic testing available for *serious and fatal genetic diseases*. Eighty-three percent would take such a test themselves for that reason, including 81 percent who describe themselves as very religious (U.S. Congress Office of Technology Assessment 1987, 74–75).

7. In our view, prenatal diagnosis for "X-linked disorders" is morally acceptable because it is for the detection of serious defects, not for the detection of sex per se. X-linked disorders are caused by genes on the "X" chromosome and affect mostly males, who carry only one X chromosome.

8. In a Swedish study, 16 percent of women having prenatal diagnosis on the basis of advanced age said that the fetus's sex would affect their decisions about abortion (Sjögren 1988).

9. In our survey, 96 percent of geneticists said they would not tell a woman's husband that he is not the biological father of her child. Instead, most (81 percent) would tell the woman alone, so that she could use the information to plan the rest of her reproductive life, and would let her decide whether to tell her husband (Wertz and Fletcher 1989b, 16; Wertz at al. 1990).

10. A policy of *revealing* fetal sex only on request was recently instituted in prenatal diagnostic laboratories in the Birmingham region of England, not because parents were requesting sex selection, but because some parents complained that they wished they had not known the fetus's sex. In 1987–88, when the information was no longer made available as a matter of course, of 3,883 amniotic fluid analyses there were only 95 (2.5 percent) parental requests to know fetal sex (Maj Hulten, East Birmingham Hospital, Birmingham, U. K., personal communication, 1989).

REFERENCES

Asch, Adrienne. 1989. Reproductive technology and disability. In *Reproductive laws for the 1990s*, Sherrill Cohen and Nadine Taub, eds. Clifton, NJ: Humana Press.

Bayles, Michael D. 1984. *Reproductive ethics*. Englewood Cliffs, NJ: Prentice-Hall.

Coutelle, Charles, Carolyn Williams, Alan Handyside, Kate Hardy, Robert Winston, and Robert Williamson. 1989. Genetic analysis of DNA from single human oocytes: A model for preimplantation diagnosis of cystic fibrosis. *British Medical Journal* 669: 22–24.

Fletcher, John C., Kåre Berg, and Knut Erik Tranøy. 1985. Ethical aspects of medical genetics: A proposal for guidelines in genetic counseling, prenatal diagnosis and screening. *Clinical Genetics* 27: 199–205.

Fraser, F. Clarke. 1974. Genetic counseling. *American Journal of Human Genetics* 26: 636–59.

Fraser, F. Clarke, and C. Pressor. 1977. Attitudes of counselors in relation to prenatal sex determination for choice of sex. In *Genetic counseling*, Herbert A. Lubs and Felix de la Cruz, eds. New York: Raven.

Gilligan, Carol. 1982. *In a different voice: Psychological theory and women's development*. Cambridge, MA: Harvard University Press.

Holmes, Helen Bequaert. 1985. Sex preselection: Eugenics for everyone? In *Biomedical Ethics Reviews*, James Humber and Robert Almeder, eds. Clifton, NJ: Humana Press.

Holmes, Helen Bequaert. 1987. Review of *Gendercide: The implications of sex selection*, by Mary Anne Warren. *Bioethics* (1): 100–110.

Holtzman, Neil A. 1989. *Proceed with caution: Predicting genetic risks in the recombinant DNA era*. Baltimore: Johns Hopkins University Press.

Hoskins, Betty B., and Helen Bequaert Holmes. 1984. Technology and prenatal femicide. In *Test-tube women: What future for motherhood*, Rita Arditti, Renate Duelli Klein, and Shelley Minden, eds. London and Boston: Pandora Press.

Hoskins, Betty B., and Helen Bequaert Holmes. 1985. When not to choose: A case study. *Journal of Medical Humanities and Bioethics* 6 (1): 28–37.

India, Ministry of Welfare. 1985. Child in India: A statistical profile. New Delhi.

Joseph, D. T. 1986. Amniocentesis and fetal feticide in Bombay. Bombay.

Mulvihill, John J., Leroy Walters, and Dorothy C. Wertz. 1989. Ethics and medical genetics in the United States of America. In *Ethics and human genetics: A cross-cultural prespective*, Dorothy C. Wertz and John C. Fletcher, eds. Berlin and New York: Springer-Verlag.

Overall, Christine. 1987. *Ethics and human reproduction: A feminist analysis*. Boston: Allen and Unwin.

Pebley, Anne R., and Charles F. Westhoff. 1982. Women's sex preferences in the United States: 1970 to 1975. *Demography* 19 (2): 177–189.

Postgate, John. 1973. Bat's chance in hell. *New Scientist* 5 April: 12–16.

Powledge, Tabitha. 1981. Unnatural selection: On choosing children's sex. In *The custom-made child: Women-centered perspectives*, Helen B. Holmes, Betty B. Hoskins, and Michael Gross, eds. Clifton, NJ: Humana Press.

Rothman, Barbara Katz. 1986. *The tentative pregnancy: Prenatal diagnosis and the future of motherhood*. New York: Viking.

Ryan, Maura A. 1990. The argument for unlimited procreative liberty: A feminist critique. *Hastings Center Report* 20: 6–12.

Sjögren, Berit. 1988. Parental attitudes to prenatal information about the sex of the fetus. *Acta Obstetrica Gynecologia Scandinavia* 67: 43–46.

Steinbacher, Roberta, and Helen B. Holmes. 1987. Sex choice: Survival and sisterhood. In *Man-made women: How new reproductive technologies affect women*, Gena Corea et al., eds. Bloomington: Indiana University Press, pp. 52–63.

Styron, William. 1980. *Sophie's Choice*. New York: Random House.

U.S. Congress Office of Technology Assessment. 1987. *New developments in biotechnology*. Washington, DC: U.S. Government Printing Office.

Verma, Ishwar Chandra, and Balbir Singh. 1989. Ethics and medical genetics in India. In *Ethics and human genetics: A cross-cultural perspective*, Dorothy C. Wertz and John C. Fletcher, eds. Berlin and New York: Springer-Verlag, pp. 250–270.

Warren, Mary Anne. 1985a. The Ethics of Sex Preselection. In *Biomedical Ethics Reviews*, James Humber and Robert Almeder, eds. Clifton, NJ: Humana Press.

Warren, Mary Anne. 1985b. *Gendercide: The implications of sex selection*. Totowa, NJ: Rowman and Allenheld.

Wertz, Dorothy C., and John C. Fletcher. 1988. Attitudes of genetic counselors: A multi-national survey. *American Journal of Human Genetics* 42: 592–600.

Wertz, Dorothy C., and John C. Fletcher. 1989a. Ethical problems in prenatal diagnosis: A cross-cultural survey of medical geneticists in 18 nations. *Prenatal Diagnosis* 9(3): 145–157.

Wertz, Dorothy C., and John C. Fletcher. 1989b. *Ethics and human genetics: A cross-cultural perspective*. Berlin and New York: Springer-Verlag.

Wertz, Dorothy C., and John C. Fletcher. 1989c. Ethics and genetics: An international survey. *Hastings Center Report* 19, Special Supplement (July/August, 1989): 20–24.

Wertz, Dorothy C., John C. Fletcher, and John J. Mulvihill. 1990. Medical geneticists confront ethical dilemmas: Cross-cultural comparisons among 18 nations. *American Journal of Human Genetics* 46: 1200–1213.

Wertz, Richard W., and Dorothy C. Wertz, 1989. *Lying-In: A history of childbirth in America*, expanded edition. New Haven: Yale University Press.

Westhoff, Charles F., and Ronald R. Rindfuss. 1974. Sex preselection in the United States. *Science* 184: 633–636.

CONTRACT PREGNANCY

❖ ❖ ❖

Cutting Motherhood in Two: Some Suspicions Concerning Surrogacy

HILDE LINDEMANN NELSON
and JAMES LINDEMANN NELSON

Surrogate motherhood—at least if carefully structured to protect the interests of the women involved—seems defensible along standard liberal lines which place great stress on free agreements as moral bedrocks. But feminist theories have tended to be suspicious about the importance assigned to this notion by mainstream ethics, and in this paper, we develop implications of those suspicions for surrogacy. We argue that the practice is inconsistent with duties parents owe to children and that it compromises the freedom of surrogates to perform their share of those duties. Standard liberal perspectives tend to be insensitive to such considerations; we propose a view which takes more seriously the moral importance of the causal relationship between parents and children, and which therefore illuminates rather than obscures the stake that women and children have in surrogacy.

I

If unwanted pregnancies are a problem in our culture, so too is the inability to have children. With the widespread use of the Pill and other contraceptive devices, in conjunction with more relaxed social attitudes toward abortion, women have achieved a measure of control over their pregnancies that their great-grandmothers never dreamed of. Is it any wonder, then, that women and men who have experienced the agonizing frustration of remaining childless despite all their best efforts should turn to medical technology for control over their infertility?

Many infertile couples feel a strong desire to bring into being the children they rear; for them, adoption is distressingly inadequate. They may feel that the bond between them is deepened if they have a biological link to the next generation, or they may simply feel shame at the inability to do something as natural as producing a baby. Some people without partners are content to stay single, but want to have their own—not someone else's—children. The urge to reproduce oneself may relate to the desire to survive one's death; it is surely akin to the artist's urge to make something that will outlast its creator's lifetime.

Whatever the reason, it is clear that people will go to considerable lengths to

Hypatia vol. 4, no. 3 (Fall 1989). © by Hilde L. Nelson and James L. Nelson

have children of their own. When the time-honored method fails, the would-be parents may turn to artificial insemination by donor. This remedy will not meet the case, however, if the prospective mother's reproductive equipment isn't functioning properly, or if her general state of health is so poor as to make childbearing an even more risky business than it is ordinarily. In such a situation, the parents may seek a surrogate mother.

By "surrogate mother" we mean a woman who is hired to bear a child whom she turns over at birth to her employer. Typically, she supplies the egg while the man who purchases her services provides the sperm, but the egg need not be hers. Our concern here is not so much with ménage-à-trois arrangements in which the surrogate participates, along with the contracting couple, in the rearing of the child; we focus instead on standard agreements that grant sole custody to the contracting couple—or, just as likely, the contracting father.

Now, on the face of it, "surrogate mother" is an odd designation for the woman hired to gestate the child. The O.E.D. defines "surrogate" as "a person appointed by authority to act in the place of another"; "mother" as "a woman who has given birth to a child." It would seem, then, that the surrogate mother would actually be someone to whom the child is surrendered, and who will then act in place of the mother. The person who does the surrendering, it seems clear, is a *real* mother, not a surrogate anything.

Common usage indicates that we have a richer conception of motherhood than does the O.E.D.; it includes not only the process of gestation and parturition, but also of nurturing. These strands of the concept are generally tightly braided. Sometimes—as in the case of adoption—the strands come apart, and so we distinguish between a biological and a social sense of mothering.

The evaluation of social vs. biological mothering which is implicit in the "surrogate mother" tag may seem a piece of obfuscation, designed to hide some of the reality involved in this practice, or at least to mute a point that deserves the most careful kind of ethical scrutiny. But we think that there is a sense in which what appears to be an ad hoc conceptual move, designed to hide possibly troubling facts, is actually quite revealing. What our current practice with the label indicates is that we have evaluated the significance of those strands in cases where they come apart and regard the social sense of mothering as so significant that it overrides the biological sense when they conflict. That the social sense of mothering can be seen as an elective response to a pregnancy (whether one's own or another's) may explain what seems to be a widespread tendency to conclude that maternal duties as such rest wholly on our decisions; we shall argue that this is not so.

We maintain a view of parental obligation which is based on the *causal* relationships between parents and their offspring, rather than on any intensional ties; it is, we think, not the *decision* to have children but rather the *fact* of having done so, which primarily creates responsibilities. The leading idea of our view is that in bringing a child into the world, the parents have put it at risk of harm; it is extremely needy and highly vulnerable to a vast assortment of physical and psychological damage. Because they have exposed it to that risk, they have at least a prima facie obligation to defend it; further, they may not transfer their parental duties to another caretaker simply as a matter of choice, for it is the child who holds the claim against both mother and father, and it cannot release them.

In our final section we develop this view by defending it against objection and considering its implications for cases other than surrogacy where the strands of motherhood part. Before that, we show how a causal perspective on parental obligation coheres more comfortably with prominent themes in feminist ethics than more permissive accounts.

II

A causal perspective on parental obligation renders surrogate motherhood morally dubious—certainly a position consistent with much feminist analysis of the issue[1]—but it may not be immediately clear that it does so on feminist grounds. The stress, after all, seems more on a putative right of a child to both her parents' care, than on considerations explicitly involving the interests of women. Christine Sistare has written that a "fundamental moral issue in the surrogacy debate is the nature and extent of women's freedom: their freedom to control their bodies, their lives, their reproductive powers, and to determine the social use of those reproductive capacities" (1988, 228). She goes on to claim that "the question which ought primarily to occupy us, therefore, is this: is there sufficient justification for society to deny to adult women the disposition of their reproductive capacities according to their own desires?" (229).

The question Sistare raises is certainly important. But as we see it, her theoretical reliance on liberal presuppositions not only obscures the significance of the connection between parent and child, it also distorts the goal of women's autonomy by offering a crucially one-sided view of the way in which women's freedom is threatened by surrogacy.

Recent work by Christine Overall suggests two ways in which women's control over their lives is impaired by surrogacy. Overall examines models that are frequently used in thinking about surrogacy—the free market model and the prostitution model—and comes to the conclusion that neither is adequate, because both see surrogacy as a job when in fact it is nothing of the kind. In her view, a job implies the selling of a service or other commodity, and it also implies that the worker has control over the work.

The first half of the definition ought to seem suspicious to academics. Embittered joking aside, there is a certain vulgarity in the attempt to commodify learning: a liberal arts institution can't readily be reduced to an "information delivery system." But surrogacy doesn't seem much like college teaching. There is no special expertise involved, nor any interest in the spiritual or intellectual growth of the person paying the fee. If anything, surrogacy is more like the selling of a service. Yet this will not do either, because the surrogate mother has little if any control over the service she is supposedly selling. Pregnancy and birth are not volitional processes; they are simply natural bodily functions she cannot help. Overall quotes Mary O'Brien's application to motherhood of Marx's distinction between the architect and the bee. The mother cannot use her skills and her imaginative vision to create the baby; "like the bee, she cannot help what she is doing" (1987, 127).

It is this lack of autonomy over the enterprise that pushes surrogacy off the far end of the scale of alienated labor and thus distinguishes it, in Overall's mind, from prostitution. We tend to agree with her that "surrogate motherhood is no more a job than being occupied, for a fee, is a job" (128), but then, "being occupied, for a fee," strikes us as such an apt description of prostitution that we wonder if there mightn't be closer parallels between the two than Overall allows. The prostitute, like the bee, is certainly exercising a natural bodily function, and like the bee she has little autonomy with regard to the act. While there can be an art to erotic activity, it is more often practiced by experienced lovers than by a hooker turning twenty tricks a night. The hooker is renting out her body much as another might rent out a room; she has only slightly more control than the room does over what goes on in there.

If prostitutes and surrogate mothers both resemble the bee more than the architect in the nonvolitional nature of the "jobs" themselves, they also lack control over another aspect of the proceedings, namely, the agreements they make with their clients. As the prostitutes have pimps to set the terms of employment, so the surrogate mothers have their clients' lawyers. Overall directs us to the work of Susan Ince, who has found that surrogate contracts are usually written to favor the contracting father. Acting from a postion of relative wealth, he hires a lawyer to assure the preeminence of his interests over not only the surrogate but also his infertile wife, whose consent is not typically required. It is the father to whom the baby must be delivered, and the primary concern of the contract is to "make certain the child has the sperm and name of the buyer" (Overall 1987, 133).

But we don't suppose that any of this is going to impress Sistare—nor should it, given her assumptions. Supposing there were a well-regulated system of surrogate motherhood—one free of coercion, with legally enforced safeguards built in for the surrogate that set conditions of service that were highly to her advantage. Wouldn't such a system allow women new ways to profit from their abilities, while speaking to the deep needs of those who chose to employ them—including women who wish to be mothers, but who cannot themselves give birth? Aren't Overall's concerns about surrogacy's not being a job beside the point? Women's bodies are their property, and if surrogates are *rentiers* rather than workers, fine: our society allows one to execute contracts to rent property, as well as to render service. Wouldn't Sistare be absolutely right in seeing argument against participation in such an arrangement—still more, argument for making it illegal—as condescending and disrespectful to mature adult women?

Embedded in questions of this sort are the classical liberal values of freedom, self-fulfillment, individual dignity, and the equality of opportunity to pursue one's own interests. These interests are to be defined by the individual, because traditional liberal theory is skeptical regarding the justifiability of establishing political institutions that promote any specific conception of human good.

Now, not all feminists look askance at such skepticism, but it is certainly a rich and powerful theme in much of their thinking. Alison Jaggar, for example, has pointed out a serious problem with liberalism's epistemic posture, which she sees as resulting, at least in part, from "normative dualism," her phrase for the view that "what is especially valuable about human beings is their 'mental' capacity for rationality" (1983, 40). In concentrating on the rationality of our social interaction, in the focus on consensual models such as social contract theory, we have overlooked human biology. "No adequate philosophical theory of human need can ignore the facts of biology: our common need for air, water, food, warmth, etc. Far from being irrelevant to political philosophy, these facts must form its starting point" (Jaggar 1983, 42).

Instead of starting with the facts of human biology, liberal theory has started with "abstract individualism"—a model of autonomous, self-interested entities interacting contractually in pursuit of their own goods. These individuals, untouched by any particular language, culture, or socialization, seem woefully inadequate to the facts of biological existence.

Feminists have perhaps all the more readily seen the shortcomings of abstract individualism in that the abstract individual looked so little like a woman or a child. There is something distinctly hairy-chested about Hobbes's state of nature, about the social contract, about revealed preference theory, about the conception of equality that accords to every rational individual equal rights regardless of gender, economic class, race or age. As Virginia Held remarks, "It stretches credulity even further than most philosophers can tolerate to imagine babies as little rational calculators contracting with their mothers for care" (1987, 120).

Sistare does not deny that the kind of individual autonomy on which she centers has been associated with patriarchal structures of thought. She is, however, confident that the association can be dissolved, claiming that "the admittedly real connections of such phenomena and values are historically contingent" (1988, 228). But, as Cheshire Calhoun has recently pointed out, patriarchal systems of thought such as liberal individualism, or that version of it that serves as Calhoun's example—the "justice perspective" in ethics—have causal as well as logical implications: women and children can perhaps be accommodated within such systems in principle, but in fact, they tend to inculcate a "moral ideology" that blinds us to morally important features of situations—especially to those involving women and children.

As Held considers the drawbacks to the contractual "economic man" model of classical liberal theory, she reaches a conclusion that is shared by many feminists:

> At some point contracts must be embedded in social relations that are noncontractual. . . . Although there may be some limited domains in which rational contracts are the appropriate form of social relations, as a foundation for the fundamental ties which ought to bind human beings together, they are clearly inadequate. (1987, 125, 136)

The contractual model, Jaggar argues, is incapable of providing a "substantive conception of the good life and a way of identifying genuine human needs" (1983, 48).

In the context of surrogacy, contractual models are inappropriate because they tend to leave out the interests of infants, who are not contracting parties. They also distort an important feature of human agency: the freedom to do as we ought. This is not, of course, the kind of freedom that we usually associate with "rational contractors" in pursuit of their own good. It is not egoistic or acquisitive; it is not part of the ideology we naturally associate with the occupants of Hobbes's state of nature. But it is morally significant all the same, and surrogacy contracts are incompatible with it. The most meticulously worded contract Sistare could devise cannot protect the surrogate's freedom, not only because of current patterns of patriarchy, and not only because of the nonvolitional nature of the functioning of her body. These issues of control are serious enough, both for the surrogate and for the prostitute, but there is an even more fundamental control issue at stake for the surrogate, and the contract cannot safeguard it because its relinquishing is an essential element of the contract. This is the control over the rearing of the child. In the rest of this paper, we argue why the surrogate mother may not relinquish this control.

III

In her paper "Begetting, Bearing, and Rearing," Onora O'Neill argues that parental obligations come from voluntary undertakings. In the case of biological parents, it is not always plain what kinds of actions or inactions count as voluntarily undertaking the parental role and its responsibilities, but for her purposes this is not crucially important, for O'Neill's central interest is in clearly elected procreation—which, of course, encompasses surrogacy. Bearers and begetters may, as she sees it, either care for the child themselves, or (leaving abortion, infanticide, and malign neglect to one side) arrange for the competent rearing of the child. Whether these alternatives are morally on a par for O'Neill is not clear.

The problem with this view is that causal responsibility—particularly when it does not result from coercion—is closely linked to moral responsibility. In choosing to give birth, parents bring about the presence of a new individual who is both extremely important and extremely needy. As they brought about these needs, parents are primarily responsible for seeing to their satisfaction. Looked at in this way, procreation is more like running someone over in one's car than like signing a contract. Where I create a vulnerability, I have at least a prima facie obligation to stand by the victim.

O'Neill sees a crucial difference between accident victims and children of unconsenting parents: however neglectful or abusive unconsenting parents are, they do not worsen their children's lives (and therefore they haven't harmed them), since, without the unintentional conception, their children wouldn't exist at all. "Worse" is a comparative judgment, and as comparisons between nonexistence and a given life are thoroughly obscure, we cannot say that the child is worse off.

Let's take this apart. In the first place, if I neglect my children, I make them worse off than they would have been had I not done so. But, as it stands, this does not seem to support a claim of special responsibility to satisfy needs; there are, presumably, any number of people who are the worse for my neglect. Yet in the case of my children, I am causally responsible for their needs, and this causal relationship is sufficient to undergird a special moral responsibility to satisfy them.

As an illustration, consider the following case: suppose a woman is infertile, and can conceive only if she takes a certain drug. Suppose, further, that one of the side-effects of the drug is that, some years after conception, the resulting child will contract a hideous disease unless it is provided with an antidote which the manufacturers are capable of supplying. Is there any doubt that they have a duty to make sure that the antidote is available? The drug didn't make the children any worse off than they would have been, but we would find it reprehensible if the manufacturers denied the child the antidote on those grounds.

Of course, unlike the hypothetical corporation, parents are sometimes incapable of supplying their children's needs. Consider the paradigm instance of "cutting motherhood in two": adoption. When a woman (or more often, a teen-aged child) decides she is unable to care for a baby and either chooses not to have an abortion, or because of her beliefs or social constraints, finds that abortion is not an option, she may bear the baby and then give it up. She is doing what she can to see to it that the baby's needs are met, and this is praiseworthy. Sara Ruddick tells the story of a woman of her acquaintance who gave her baby up for adoption, not because she was *unable* to care for it, but because she figured that the child would have a better life elsewhere than the one she could provide.[2] Ruddick points out that this too is a gesture of care, and one which probably ought to be practiced more often. We regard it as more problematic than Ruddick, for reasons we will develop shortly. But whatever the precise motivation, adoption differs from surrogacy at least in that it is a response to an already-existing pregnancy that is somehow troublesome. Something has gone wrong; the situation has an element of the calamitous about it that calls for extraordinary measures. We don't, after all, casually remark to a friend or a neighbor, "Oh, a new baby. How nice! Are you going to keep this one or give it up for adoption?"

Another instance in which the birth-parent may not rear the child is in the aftermath of divorce. In this case the child cannot live with both its parents simultaneously (although, when feasible, joint custody allows the child participation in both parents' lives). Surrogate mothering (especially where the surrogate provides the egg) is very like a divorce in which the mother consents to give up custody of the child. But as with adoption, a salient difference is that in the aftermath of divorce, the child already exists, and the custody arrangement has come about because something has gone wrong between the parents.

A third case in which the procreative function splits off from childrearing is one we are apt to overlook because it is so familiar to us. This is the case in which one parent (almost always the father) says to the other: "All right, we'll have this baby if that's what you want, but my job is far too demanding to permit me to care for it, so you'll have to raise it." Further along the same spectrum is the case of the unwed father who disclaims any responsibility for the child he has sired, or the man whose sperm is used for Artificial Insemination by Donor.

In this last cluster of cases, the morally significant variable seems to be the consent of the other parent. The father is a scoundrel if he leaves the mother holding the baby; we certainly don't think being a parent is so contractual a matter that fathers can unilaterally absent themselves if they change their minds about whether they're "comfortable" with the commitment. On the other hand, if the mother *wants* to take full responsibility for rearing the child, why shouldn't she? Our answer should be apparent by now: it is because of the debt that the father owes *to the child*.

Setting abandonment to one side, the strands of parenthood typically come apart because the parent cannot undertake the burden of adequate care. In surrogacy cases, this is often not true. The parting does not take place because it is in the child's best interests; it is not on its behalf, but on behalf of others, that the placement is made. What the surrogate mother has done is to put herself in a position where it is extremely difficult—perhaps impossible—to ensure continued adequate care over a period of many years for her child. She has compromised her ability to discharge her obligation to the child, when there was no necessity to drive her to this extreme.

It's natural to reply that if a prospective surrogate mother takes care in the selection of her clients, she has answered this objection. But this is at least questionable. Serious disagreements on what constitutes appropriate treatment of children often break out between adults who have had a great deal of opportunity to get to know one another over a period of years. It is not uncommon, for instance, for divorced women who share the custody of children with ex-spouses to find that their conception of proper care progressively and seriously diverges from their former partners' as time goes on—even if they have known their spouses intimately for years, and reared the children with them for long periods. It seems unlikely that a surrogate mother could get to know the prospective parents as intimately as she knows her ex-spouse.

Besides, the point isn't whether someone else would do as good a job; it's that it's *her* job—and his. A parent on the scene is in a position to continually monitor her own efforts with respect to the child's well-being. She cannot do this for anyone else, especially if she removes herself from daily involvement in the child's life. Her relationship to the agency of others is categorically different from her relationship to her own agency. She can at best *predict* that another person will meet the child's needs; she herself is the only person she can bring to *perform* the required services. To engineer a situation in which the biological father can discharge his responsibility daily, but the mother cannot, is to put her under an obligation to the child that she does not intend to meet. Apart from making deceitful promises to Nazis, there would seem to be few cases where we can legitimately act in such bad faith.

The job falls on those who created the vulnerability, and if this is a social decision that could have been made otherwise, it is not so much a decision about parents and children as it is about something more fundamental: the moral link between cause and culpability. If we are right, it follows that sperm donation too is ethically dubious, and that divorced parents may have a duty to do what they can to stay in close contact with their children. On the other hand, it might be quite all right for a surrogate mother to join the household of an infertile couple and participate, along with the couple, in the upbringing of the child she bears for them. But that would be surrogate motherhood of a different kind. In its typical form, surrogacy seems to us to threaten important ideals and duties that bind us together. The assumptions that underlie the practice seem to hold an impoverished view of the full significance of women's freedom, and an inadequate recognition of the child's moral stake in the matter.

NOTES

An earlier version of this paper benefited greatly from presentation at the Conference on Exploring Feminist Ethics, Duluth, Minnesota, October 1988.

1. See, for example, Andrea Dworkin or Gena Corea. There are, of course, thoughtful feminist voices on the other side of the issue. An instance is Juliette Zipper and Selma Sevenhuijsen.

2. In conversation.

REFERENCES

Baier, Annette. 1986. Trust and antitrust. *Ethics* 96: 231–260.

Calhoun, Cheshire. 1988. Justice, care, gender bias. *Journal of Philosophy* 85(9): 451–463.

Corea, Gena. 1985. *The mother machine: Reproductive technologies from artificial insemination to artificial wombs.* New York: Harper and Row.

Dworkin, Andrea. 1983. *Right-wing women.* New York: Perigree Books.

Held, Virginia. 1987. Non-contractual society: A feminist view. *The Canadian Journal of Philosophy* suppl. vol. 13: 111–137.

Ince, Susan. 1984. Inside the surrogate industry. In *Test-tube women: What future for motherhood?* Rita Arditti, Renate Duelli Klein, and Shelley Minden, eds. London: Pandora Press.

Jaggar, Alison M. 1983. *Feminist politics and human nature.* Totowa, NJ: Rowman and Allenheld.

O'Neill, Onora. 1979. Begetting, bearing and rearing. In *Having children: Philosophical and legal reflections.* Onora O'Neill and William Ruddick, eds. New York: Oxford University Press.

Overall, Christine. 1987. *Ethics and human reproduction: A feminist analysis.* Winchester, MA: Allen and Unwin.

Sistare, Christine T. 1988. Reproductive freedom and women's freedom: Surrogacy and autonomy. *The Philosophical Forum* 19(4): 227–240.

Zipper, Juliette, and Selma Sevenhuijsen. 1987. Surrogacy: Feminist notions of motherhood reconsidered. In *Reproductive technologies: Gender, motherhood and medicine.* Michelle Stanworth, ed. Minneapolis: University of Minnesota Press.

Marxism and Surrogacy

KELLY OLIVER ❖ ❖ ❖

In this essay, I argue that the liberal framework—its autonomous individuals with equal rights—allows judges to justify enforcing surrogacy contracts. More importantly, even where judges do not enforce surrogacy contracts, the liberal framework conceals gender and class issues which ensure that the surrogate will lose custody of her child. I suggest that Marx's analysis of estranged labor can reveal the class and gender issues which the liberal framework conceals.

As the legality of contracting "surrogate mothers" is debated in the courts, supporters are becoming more defensive about the morality of this practice. With no legislation and very little judicial precedent, it is difficult to predict the outcome of any particular case involving surrogacy. That is why Noel Keane, a Detroit lawyer and the first person to organize an agency designed to arrange surrogacy contracts, has been urging legislation to ensure that surrogacy contracts can be enforced.[1]

In the *Matter of Baby* M, the New Jersey Supreme Court ruled that surrogacy contracts are not enforceable.[2] The opinion of the court was delivered by Judge Wilentz, who states that:

> We invalidate the surrogacy contract because it conflicts with the law and public policy of this State. While we recognize the depth of the yearning of infertile couples to have their own children, we find payment of money to a "surrogate" mother illegal, perhaps criminal, and potentially degrading to women. (Wilentz 1988)

While this decision seems like a victory for those opposed to "surrogate motherhood," in practice it does very little to change the exploitation of women who serve as "surrogates." I will argue that the framework within which surrogacy issues have been argued in the courts, and in the *Matter of Baby* M in particular, conceals sex and class issues which are central to the practice of surrogacy. In spite of the New Jersey Supreme Court's invalidation of surrogacy contracts, the precedent set by recent cases, including *Matter of Baby* M, ensures that "surrogates" will lose in court.

The logic of the liberal framework allows judges to justify enforcing surrogacy

Hypatia vol. 4, no. 3 (Fall 1989). © by Kelly Oliver

contracts. And, moreover, even in those cases where judges rule that surrogacy contracts are not enforceable and illegal (e.g., the New Jersey Supreme Court Decision), the liberal framework practically guarantees that custody will be awarded to the father. Thus, within the liberal framework, whether or not the surrogacy contract is enforced, the effect is the same: surrogates always lose. Within this framework, the legitimacy, and even morality, of surrogacy is reduced to the arbitration of rights. Using the jargon of rights, the liberal framework conceals social and class interests behind the illusion of formal equality in contract.

I will suggest that a Marxist framework can bring some of these concealed, yet central, issues to the surface. Especially useful for my purpose is Marx's distinction between estranged and alienated labor. While childbirth may be alienated labor, I will suggest that it becomes estranged labor in the context of the surrogacy contract.[3] In conclusion, I will point to some of the limitations of a Marxist analysis and indicate some of the implications of my analysis for a feminist ethics in general.

THE LIBERAL FRAMEWORK

In the courts, surrogacy debates are framed within the democratic liberal postulation of rights and obligations. Trial lawyers pit the rights and obligations of the "surrogate" against the rights and obligations of the "natural father" and his wife, and the rights of the child.[4] Once the rights and obligations of both parties to the surrogacy contract have been arbitrated, custody disputes are always decided based on the "best interests" of the child.

For example, in the *Matter of Baby M*, while Mary Beth Whitehead's lawyers were arguing for her right to the companionship of her child, William Stern's lawyers were arguing for his right to procreate. For example, the New Jersey Supreme Court decided that Stern's right to procreate did not automatically include the right to custody. Furthermore, the court ruled that procreation through the paid surrogacy arrangement was illegal. The court was convinced that the surrogacy arrangement violated state law which prohibits paid adoptions in spite of the fact that Stern's wife was not a party to the initial contract. (Stern, after all, as proponents of surrogacy argue, need not adopt his own child.) In addition, state policy requires that parental rights remain with the natural parents until at least five days after the baby's birth. Thus, the court ruled that Mary Beth Whitehead retained her parental rights. Parental rights and obligations are defined by law. They can be neither claimed nor relinquished without legal sanction. Of course, this distorts the relationship between parents and children. It covers over the biological relations between parents and children in favor of a legal relationship.

Proponents of surrogacy argue that an "infertile couple" has the right to procreate and a woman has the right to use her body as she pleases. As Gena Corea points out in *The Mother Machine*, it is the man's right to procreate which is protected. "The overriding ethic is that the man's issue be reproduced in the world" (Corea 1985, 223). The wife of the father of the child produced as a result of the surrogacy arrangement remains infertile. Thus, it is simply not true that the surrogacy arrangement primarily benefits the infertile couple, or as some proponents argue, the infertile wife. Surrogacy is not, as the pseudo-feminist argument maintains, one woman helping another to have children. In fact, in some cases the infertile wife already has her own children, and/or she is more or less forced into the arrangement by her husband (Corea 1985, 223–224).

In the courts, the right to procreate has been invoked in order to defend limiting parental rights in the case of semen donors. Almost universally, semen donors can be legally required to relinquish their parental rights. Proponents of surrogacy have argued that if it is legal to require semen donors to relinquish parental rights, then it is legal to require womb and egg donors to relinquish parental rights as well. They argue for equal protection under the law. This argument has been used successfully (and unsuccessfully) in many surrogacy trials.[5]

Andrea Dworkin points out a crucial flaw in the analogy between donating sperm and surrogacy. She argues that there is no comparison between an ejaculate of the body and the body itself. She compares collecting semen to collecting tears from the eye and surrogacy to taking the eye itself (Corea 1985, 226). In an argument which almost suggests a Marxian labor theory of value, the New Jersey Supreme Court realized that the time difference between producing semen and producing a child is enough to destroy the analogy (Wilentz 1988, 1254).

In addition to defending surrogacy arrangements for the benefit of the "infertile couple," proponents defend them for the benefit of women who want to serve as "surrogates." Some people have argued that pregnancy is therapeutic for some women (Corea 1985, 239). All admit, however, that very few women, if any, would perform surrogacy services without payment. Many more proponents defend a woman's right to use her body as she wishes, to freely engage in any contracts which she wishes, to make money in any way in which she wishes. In the end, what they argue is that we live in a capitalist society where market demands dictate propriety.

What this argument overlooks is that the market forces women into surrogacy (Corea 1985, 228–229). Economic concerns cause women to do something which they would not otherwise do. Proponents may respond that most people do things which they would not otherwise do in order to make a living. However, most people do not perform their service 24 hours a day, unless they are slaves. And most people sell only their labor, labor performed by the body, perhaps, but distinguishable from it. "Surrogates," on the other hand, perform their service 24 hours a day and sell their body itself. Every act in which the "surrogate" engages may come under the scrutiny of the contracting couple—what she eats, drinks, and how she plays. She is never off-duty.

Proponents argue that women should have the opportunity to engage in these kinds of arrangements if they want. They argue that women are free to choose; they are not forced into surrogacy arrangements. Andrea Dworkin finds this concern with women's freedom suspicious:

> Again, the state has constructed the social, economic, and political situation in which the sale of some sexual or reproductive capacity is necessary to the survival of women; and yet the selling is seen to be an act of individual will—the only kind of assertion of individual will in women that is vigorously defended as a

matter of course by most of those who pontificate on female freedom. The state denies women a host of other possibilities, from education to jobs to equal rights before the law to sexual self-determination in marriage; but it is state intrusion into her selling of sex or a sex-class-specific capacity that provokes a defense of her will, her right, her individual self—defined strictly in terms of the will to sell what is appropriate for females to sell. (1983, 182)

In addition to the general suspicion that women do not enter into surrogacy contracts completely voluntarily, is the more specific suspicion that women cannot give completely informed consent to relinquish parental rights to their babies before they are born. In response to the Sterns' claim that Mary Beth Whitehead freely gave her consent to relinquish her child under the terms of the contract, Judge Wilentz notes the illusion of consent inherent in surrogacy contracts:

Under the contract, the natural mother is irrevocably committed before she knows the strength of her bond with her child. She never makes a totally voluntary, informed decision, for quite clearly any decision prior to the baby's birth is, in the most important sense, uninformed, and any decision after that, compelled by a pre-existing contractual commitment, the threat of a lawsuit, and the inducement of a $10,000 payment, is less than totally voluntary. (1988, 1248)

Thus, many of the supposed benefits to the "surrogate" are illusory. The illusion is created through the presuppositions of the liberal framework operating within a capitalist patriarchal society. Within the liberal framework all people are considered equal with equal rights. They all operate autonomously and have the freedom to exercise their rights as long as they don't interfere with the rights of others. In this framework, the surrogacy contract is seen as an agreement between two or more equal parties. There is an equal exchange, money paid for services rendered.

The lower court's opinion in the "Baby M" case provides a striking example of this attitude. According to Judge Sorkow, this contract is a contract for services between two equal parties who freely enter the agreement. There is no question of possible financial coercion or an uninformed decision: "The male gave his sperm; the female gave her egg in their preplanned effort to create a child—thus a contract" (Sorkow 1987, 74). "Once conception has occurred the parties [sic] rights are fixed, the terms of the contract are firm . . . " (75). "A price for the service each was to perform was struck and a bargain reached" (74).[6]

The liberal framework, then, with its emphasis on equal rights, overlooks important gender-specific and class differences between the parties to the surrogacy contract. In fact, as I have said earlier, *the contract would not exist if the parties were equal.* The woman must give more than her egg in order to gestate a child—an important gender difference; and, as I have argued earlier, without the class difference, women would not enter into surrogacy contracts. Within this framework, the surrogacy contract is always biased in favor of the financially secure male.

What this analysis shows is that the liberal framework which arbitrates surrogacy on the basis of rights allows judges to justify enforcing surrogacy contracts.[7] It protects the "infertile couple's" right to procreate while limiting the surrogate's parental rights. It defends the surrogate's right to enter the contract because she is free to use her own body as she pleases. Yet, it limits her freedom over her body once she enters the contract: "Once conception has occured the parties rights are fixed . . . " Within the liberal framework, the individuals involved are free. There is no consideration of financial coercion: "A price is struck and a bargain reached." In the case of surrogacy, however, the surrogate's freedom is an illusion. And, the arbitration of rights serves to cover over central social and class issues which make surrogacy contracts a possibility.

Although the New Jersey Supreme Court ruled that surrogacy contracts are unenforceable and perhaps criminal, its justifications for that ruling moved them out of the liberal framework. In fact, their opinion points up contradictions in what might be called an "enlightened liberal" framework.[8] Insofar as it is "enlightened," however, it is not really liberal. As soon as the liberal position begins to consider the ways in which an individual is constructed by his or her class and gender, it has moved away from presumptions about human nature that are central to the liberal position. Central to the liberal framework is the presumption that the individual is prior to society and all that individuals are equal and free. This argument need not be developed here since this is Alison Jaggar's critique of what she calls "liberal feminism" in her monumental *Feminist Politics and Human Nature* (1983, 27–48, 174–203).

More importantly, for my argument, even the New Jersey Supreme Court moved back into the liberal framework in its custody decision. Supposedly, the rights of both mother and father were considered equally and custody was based on the "best interests" of the child. However, as I will demonstrate, the way in which the "best interests" of the child are decided in these situations, covers over the socioeconomic situation which gave rise to the initial contract. The contract would not exist if the parties to it were equal. It seems, given the way in which both New Jersey courts defined "best interests," that the surrogacy contract would not exist if the child's "best interests" were not already owned by the father. Thus, whether or not surrogacy contracts are enforced, the effect is the same. The "infertile couple" gets custody of the child.[9]

For example, in the *Matter of Baby M*, after the rights clash was resolved in favor of Whitehead, the court awarded custody of "Baby M" based on the child's "best interests." Even in the 1986 case of *Surrogate Parenting Associates v. Commonwealth of Kentucky*, where the Supreme Court of Kentucky ruled that surrogacy contracts are not in violation of either paid adoption laws or state requirements for relinquishing parental rights, the court ruled that custody disputes would be decided on the basis of the child's "best interests." In other words, although surrogacy contracts are not illegal, they may be avoidable (Leibson 1986, 209). However, even in a case where the "surrogate" refuses to relinquish parental rights and the contract is made void, custody will be decided based on the child's best interests.

The way in which "best interests" are decided in court, however, practically ensures that "surrogates" will lose custody disputes. The very structure of the surrogacy arrangement guarantees that the contracting couple is more likely to gain custody. First, the fact that the "surrogate" enters into a contractual agreement to give up her child makes her an unfit mother. How could a good mother agree to give up her child? The lower court in the case of "Baby M" used this sort of reasoning in order to grant custody to Mr. Stern. The trial court concluded that while the Sterns "wanted" the baby, Mary Beth Whitehead's motivation to have a child was not because she wanted to be a parent. In part, the "best interests" of the child were determined by who "wanted" her before she was conceived (Johnson 1987, 1345–6).

Second, the child's "best interests" are determined, in large part, by the financial security of the disputing parties. Obviously, in the surrogacy arrangement the contracting couple is more likely to be financially secure than the "surrogate." Although they may have other motivations, women who agree to surrogate contracts do so primarily in order to make money (Corea 1985, 228–30). The reason that women enter into surrogate contracts, then, is because they are not financially secure.

In the case of "Baby M," the lower court judge, Judge Sorkow, noted that the Whiteheads' house was too small and that Mary Beth Whitehead's concern for her daughter's education was suspect in light of Mrs. Whitehead's lack of education. In contrast, the Sterns had a new house and could provide the child with "music lessons," "athletics," and a certain college education (Sorkow 1987, 74–75). Although the New Jersey Supreme Court made it clear that their primary task was not to ensure the growth of a new member of the "intelligentsia," they decided custody on the same sort of suspect grounds (Wilentz 1988, 1260).

The two overriding reasons for granting the Sterns custody in the *Matter of Baby* M were first the Whiteheads' finances and second Mary Beth Whitehead's attitude toward her daughter. [10] Whereas Judge Wilentz noted that the Whiteheads' "finances were in serious trouble," the Sterns' "finances are more than adequate, their circle of friends supportive, and their marriage happy" (Wilentz 1988, 1258–9). Whereas Mary Beth Whitehead demonstrated contempt for professional psychological counseling, the Sterns endorsed it. Whereas the court doubted Mary Beth Whitehead's "ability to explain honestly and sensitively to Baby M—at the right time—the nature of her origin," the Sterns, the court decided, "are honest; they can recognize error, deal with it, and learn from it. . . . When the time comes to tell her about her origins, they will probably have found a means of doing so that accords with the best interests of Baby M" (Wilentz 1988, 1258–9).

The Judge also noted Mary Beth Whitehead's "omniscient" attitude toward her daughter. This attitude was evidenced by her claim that "she alone knew what the child's cries meant." Due to her attitude, the court maintained that "Baby M's life with the Whiteheads promised to be too closely controlled by Mrs. Whitehead" whereas the Sterns would encourage the child's "independence" (Wilentz 1988, 1259).

It seems obvious that the financial need which motivates women to serve as "surrogates," combined with the high price of surrogate services through agencies, points to a class issue at the heart of surrogacy arrangements. Of course the contracting couple will be more financially secure than the "surrogate." Otherwise, the contract would not exist in the first place. In addition, the problems which the court identified with Mary Beth Whitehead's attitude are also, at least in part, the result of the surrogacy contract itself.

First her "contempt" for professional psychotherapy may well be a class issue. While academics and upper-middle-class Americans have become accustomed to the "benefits" of psychotherapy, most poor and lower-middle-class Americans simply cannot afford it. Usually it is quite expensive. Even when assistance is available for such therapy, most Americans do not use it. Mary Beth Whitehead is not alone in her "contempt" for professional psychologists. Many people are suspicious of the "benefits" of psychotherapy. In addition, many people believe that only insane people need professional help. Also, the fact that psychotherapy is not prevalant among certain classes probably leads to the attitude toward professional psychology which the court identified as "contempt."

Second, the issue of honesty "when it comes time to tell Baby M about her origins" seems impossible to predict. The court based its evaluation of Mary Beth Whitehead's honesty on her refusal to give up "Baby M" and her "omniscient" attitude toward her. Yet both Mary Beth Whitehead's actions and attitudes were, in large part, caused by the severity of the situation in which her child was taken away from her by the police. It is certainly no wonder that Mary Beth Whitehead felt possessive about her daughter and claimed that only she knew what the child's cries meant. On what grounds did the court prove her wrong in this claim? They did not even consider the possibility that she was right.

Thus, the "omniscient" attitude identified by the courts is another product of the surrogacy arrangement. Mary Beth Whitehead's parental rights were threatened by the surrogacy arrangement and she had to defend those rights. She was forced to demonstrate that there was a natural bond between herself and her baby. She had to argue that she was the natural mother and not merely the surrogate mother of "Baby M." In this position of course she appeared possessive.

Moreover, why wasn't the Sterns' honesty challenged? They had broken the law and Mr. Stern had intentionally signed a contract designed to circumvent the law. In fact, in New Jersey, they may be guilty of a criminal offense (Wilentz 1988, 1227). In addition, the surrogacy arrangement provides a new birth certificate which, upon completion of adoption procedures, identifies the father's wife as the mother of the child (Keane 1987). This arrangement, whereby the birth certificate is actually falsified, does not suggest the honesty necessary to tell the child about her origins "when the time comes."

Finally, the issue of independence and Mary Beth Whitehead's control of "Baby M" may also be a result of the surrogacy arrangement. First, in some sense, it was Mary Beth Whitehead's control of "Baby M" which was threatened by the surrogacy contract. Thus, perhaps she was defensive about her control. Second, perhaps independence is a class issue. The emphasis on the child's independence may be a middle class priority. It is possible that in poor to lower class households, interdependence is more appropriate for financial security.[11]

It is important to note that Mary Beth Whitehead was never judged an unfit mother. In fact, all agreed that she was a good and loving mother to her children (Wilentz 1988, 1239). Thus, it was not her qualifications as a mother, but as a member of the bourgeoisie, that were challenged. Overall, it is virtually inherent to the surrogacy arrangement that the child's "best interests" are served by granting custody to the father. The deciding factor in custody disputes (after fitness as a parent), financial security, is also the motivating factor for surrogacy in the first place.

I should note that a couple of other factors do come to play in the custody decision. First, an obvious result of the class difference between surrogates and contractors is that contractors can afford more expensive and influential custody lawyers. A related issue is who has custody while the surrogacy case is tried. In Mary Beth Whitehead's case, the law sided with the existing contract, granted the Sterns custody, and forceably took the baby away before Mary Beth Whitehead could respond with any legal action herself. Of course, Mary Beth Whitehead did not have her own personal attorney. The Sterns, on the other hand, had access to legal help that could get them what they wanted immediately. In spite of the illegal contract which gave rise to the initial custody decision, the fact that the Sterns had had custody of the child longer than Mary Beth Whitehead became a factor in the final custody decision. Given the class and gender bias evidenced by both New Jersey courts, it seems unlikely that we can assume that pretrial judges will grant temporary custody to surrogates. However, now that surrogacy contracts have been ruled unenforceable, there is more hope for favorable pretrial custody decisions in New Jersey than in other states.

It is interesting to note the New Jersey Supreme Court's statement that their ruling alone would discourage surrogacy contracts. There was no mention of prosecuting the Sterns for breaking the law, even though the court maintained that theirs was a serious crime, punishable by 3–5 years in prison (Wilentz 1988, 1241). In some sense, the Sterns were *rewarded* for breaking the law through custody of "Baby M." The court cited the precedent that the use of illegal adoption does not mean the denial of adoption (Wilentz 1988, 1257). With this precedent and the court's present action, it is difficult to see how their decision will discourage surrogacy arrangements.

In sum, the liberal framework allows judges to justify enforcing surrogacy contracts. And, even when judges do not enforce surrogacy contracts, custody decisions ensure that the surrogate loses in court. Custody decisions are based on socioeconomic issues which are covered over. The class difference that leads to the surrogacy contract in the first place ensures that the contracting couple will get custody of the child. The "best interests" of the child, as they have been set out in courts, are classist. In the *Matter of Baby M*, in particular, custody was decided on the basis of financial security, access to education, music lessons, and psychotherapy.

THE MARXIST FRAMEWORK

Using a Marxist framework in order to analyze surrogacy arrangements can provide insights hidden by the liberal framework. A Marxist framework can diagnose class issues and even, at least indirectly, gender issues. Within the Marxist framework, the parties to this contract are not autonomous equals. Rather, each party enters the contract from a particular context and in a particular relationship to the "means of production." The contract itself, set up within capitalist patriarchy, hides these relationships.

Important to my analysis of surrogacy is Marx's distinction between alienated and estranged labor.[12] The example of surrogacy very clearly points up this distinction. Marx makes a distinction between *entfremdung*, estranged or foreign, and *verausserung*, alienated or outer. Whereas, according to Marx, *verausserung* is a natural (and healthy) human relation to the world (including the human relationship to itself), *entfremdung* is a distorted (and unhealthy) relation to the world. Although this Marxist framework may not be useful in every context, it can diagnose surrogacy arrangements in a more insightful way than the liberal framework. In fact, surrogacy provides a quintessential example of what Marx means by estranged labor.

In Marx's scenario, human beings are unique in that they can act not only for the good of themselves and their species, but also for the good of all species. Human beings are in the fractured position of being both individual beings and social beings at once. Marx calls this unique position "species-being" (1975, 327–30, 347, 350–1, 369, 386–91; 1975a, 176, 220, 226). In order to realize that we are in this position, according to Marx, we must first be able to separate ourselves from the outside world. This alienated relationship is what enables the human being to see itself, ultimately, as a social being, as species-being. However, when this relationship is inverted and the separation of self exists for the sake of covering up species-being, then the relationship is one of estrangement (Marx 1975b, 266–7; 1975, 326–7).

Surrogacy arrangements, as they are defended in the courts and elsewhere, are estranged relationships in this sense. Proponents of surrogacy, as I have argued, maintain that each party to the surrogacy contract is an autonomous agent with the right to exercise his/her freedom. This covers up the social context in which these individuals operate and are constructed. It covers up the fact that this is a social transaction which results from particular economic and social structures which, I have argued above, perpetuate sexism and classism. The Marxist framework, however, insists that we look at these social factors which construct the so called "autonomous individuals."

Specifically, Marx talks about the difference between *estranged* labor and *alienated* labor (1975, 342, 361, 384). According to Marx, it is natural and necessary that humans take that which they produce to be outside themselves. From their capacity to produce and *verausserung*, humans can, according to Marx, see that they are in a unique relationship to the world. Alienation, then, can reveal the species-being of humans. In this relationship to their labor, humans eat, sleep, procreate—stay alive—in order to maintain themselves so that they can actualize their uniquely human capacity to be social, manifest in labor. According to Marx, it is not necessary that human beings are estranged from that which they produce. Not all labor is estranged labor.[13]

I would like to note two important differences between other forms of labor in general and surrogacy. First, as I have already mentioned, surrogates do not merely sell their labor for 8 hours a day. Rather, surrogates, in a sense, sell *at least* 10 months out of their lives which will affect their bodies for the rest of their lives. Surrogacy is a 24-hour-a-day job which involves every aspect of the surrogate's life. Second, whereas much of Marx's analysis of estranged labor applies only metaphorically to other forms of labor, it applies literally to surrogacy. In fact, in some ways, because of the relationship between the body and labor in surrogacy, the surrogate is *doubly estranged.*

In *Economic and Philosophical Manuscripts*, Marx suggests that there are four characteristics of estranged labor. First, the worker is estranged from nature and her products. Second, the worker is estranged from herself and the process of production. Third, the worker is estranged from the social aspect of her work and her life. And, fourth, the worker is estranged from other people (1975, 326–332).

1. Marx suggests that the worker is estranged from her product. Since the worker's very subsistence is dependent on the product, she is, in some sense, a slave to her product. In the case of the paid surrogate, if she doesn't produce, she doesn't get paid. Marx argues that the product does not appear to the worker as the result of her "dialogue with nature" (1975, 328). Rather, it seems hostile to her. Marx suggests that human beings can engage in a dialogue with inorganic nature. We need to in order to live. Nature, says Marx, is our "inorganic body." In estranged labor, we are estranged from our inorganic body. It becomes a set of commodities which we must produce on demand.

In the case of surrogacy, the estrangement is even more pernicious. The surrogate is not merely estranged from the "product," the child, or nature, her "inorganic body." In the case of surrogacy, the product is not part of the "inorganic body" of nature. Rather, the "product," the child, is itself an organic body created out of another organic body. The surrogate, then, is doubly estranged. She is estranged from her organic body and the body of the child insofar as they appear within the economy of inorganic nature. And, she is estranged from inorganic nature insofar as it appears as a set of commodities to be exchanged. In addition, and most obviously, the surrogate is estranged from the "product." The surrogacy contract creates the resulting baby as a commercial product which exists for the sake of the exchange.

2. The second characteristic of estranged labor is that the worker is estranged from herself and the process of production. In general, within the surrogacy arrangement, the "surrogate" is treated as a machine whose services can be exchanged for money. As Marx maintains, in the exchange of human labor for money within capitalism, the human being is treated as a machine. Capitalism, argues Marx, turns the worker into a fragment of a person, an appendage of a machine (1977, 799). This is clearly the case in surrogacy arrangements. The "surrogate" is seen, and sees herself, as a fragment of a woman, a womb and/or egg. Her body itself is seen as a machine which can be rented out. Unlike other workers, she is not an appendage of a machine. She is the machine. Her body becomes the machinery of production over which the contractor has ultimate control. In spite of the liberal framework's insistence to the contrary, she does not have rights equal to those of her contractor.

The child appears as a commodity which can be bought and sold. The "surrogate" assumes a passive role in this transaction. Her active function as the mother of the child is covered over. Rather, she is seen as the passive incubator whose purpose and obligation is to produce and relinquish a flawless product no matter what physical and/or psychological pain she may suffer. Once she has signed the contract, she is no longer free to do as she pleases. She cannot have an abortion unless the doctor agrees that she is in great danger without one (Corea 1985, 241–2). She can be forced to have a cesarean against her will (Corea 1985, 243).[14] The surrogate, then, is estranged from her own body and her own pregnancy.

As Gena Corea points out, "surrogates' " estranged representations of themselves are striking in their testimonies (1985, 213–245). Many of them maintain that the babies merely resided in their bodies and were not their babies. The "infertile couple" was merely using her womb. The "infertile couple" has control over her womb and ultimately her life. The surrogate is not even free when she eats, sleeps, or makes love.

Unlike other workers whom Marx describes, the surrogate cannot even feel free when she is satisfying her bodily desires. Marx complains that workers only feel free when they are engaging in animal pleasures—eating, drinking, sleeping, having sex. This, he says, covers over their potential as human beings, the potential which separates them from the animals. According to Marx, workers do not feel free when they are working, producing, doing what animals cannot do (1975, 327).

Once again, the surrogate is doubly estranged. She is not only estranged from her potential as a human being (insofar as she does not feel free when she is working), but also from her animal pleasures (insofar as she does not feel free because these are also controlled by the contract). Marx complains that in estranged labor, the worker feels human when she is engaging in animal pleasures and feels like an animal when engaging in human production (1975, 327). This, he says, is the distortion of estranged labor. The surrogate, however, always feels like an animal. Even her human production is only animal reproduction.

3. The third characteristic of estranged labor is that the worker is estranged from her existence as a social being. In the estranged relationship, the human being labors (is social) in order to eat, sleep and procreate—stay alive. Labor (being social) is necessary in order to stay alive. Here the relationship is reversed: labor, the unique human capacity to interact with the world, is turned into a means with which to maintain the "animal function."[15] Marx argues that whereas alienation reveals the "species-being" of humans, estrangement conceals "species-being":

> For in the first place labour, *life activity, productive life* itself appears to man only as a *means* for the satisfaction of a need, the need to preserve physical existence. But productive life is species-life. It is life-producing life. The whole character of a species, its species-character, resides in the nature of its life activity, and free conscious activity constitutes the species-character of man. Life itself appears only as a *means of life*. (Marx 1975, 328)

Estranged labor conceals the social character of all human experience. The social, or the unique human experience of being both social and individual, becomes merely a means to life. Labor, according to Marx, should point to the social character of all human experience. Human consciousness is social. It is this consciousness which liberates humans from purely animal functions. Which is not to say that "animal functions" are not human or that humans are not animals. Rather, it points to a difference between the way other animals perform their "animal functions" and the way in which humans perform their animal functions. This difference is based on the human capacity for social exchange.

In the case of surrogacy, the social constitution of the "animal functions" is covered up.[16] The surrogacy contract covers up the social constitution of reproductive practices. This is obvious in the arguments of proponents who invoke the 14th amendment in their claim to a right to privacy. The right to privacy implies that each individual (the woman who rents out her womb, and the man who buys her services) has rights which originate in her/his autonomous position with respect to her/his own body.[17] This shuts out the possibility that those rights and even perceptions of those bodies are social and already implicated in the oppressive structures of patriarchal capitalism.

In the surrogacy situation, in a literal sense, "life itself appears only as a means to life." The "surrogate" maintains her own life, watches what she eats, what she does, so that she can produce the child in exchange for the money that she needs in order to sustain her own life. Moreover, what she produces is life itself, the life of a child. Thus, the creation of life and the sustenance of life becomes a *means* by which to live, or "make a living."

The surrogacy arrangement, as an estranged relationship, merely appears to give the surrogacy more control over her "animal functions." In this estranged form, it conceals the way in which it transforms the animal functions into social exchange. Insofar as the individuals are considered apart from their social context, the surrogacy arrangement distorts the exchange. A woman's freedom to exchange her reproductive services for money may appear to be a liberation from purely animal functions. It may seem as though she has turned an animal function into purely human function—animals do not make this kind of social exchange. However, insofar as the social construction of the exchange is covered up, a situation which appears to empower the "surrogate" in reality disempowers her.[18]

As Marx points out, "the Roman slave was held by chains; the wage-labourer is bound to his owner by invisible threads. The appearance of independence is maintained by a constant change in the person of the individual employer, and by the legal fiction of a contract" (1977, 719). The "surrogate," as I have already argued, is not only forced into the contract due to financial insecurity, but also, in some cases, subject to constant contractual restrictions on her diet and activity. She is, in this sense, a slave. Her "freedom" is an illusion created by estranged labor.

It is not the case that the "surrogate" freely exchanges her services in an equal trade for money as the liberal framework suggests—"a price struck and a bargain reached." Rather, as the Marxian framework reveals, this exchange distorts the reality of the exchange. Marx's critique, of course, is that within capitalism, human exchange is estranged. In a contradictory movement, capitalism both distorts the human as social being and human as individual being. Or, as I have previously said, it covers over species-being.

On the one hand, the estranged exchange turns the social activity of work and exchange into a means for individual existence. The worker engages in social exchange in order to afford food, shelter, etc.—in order to maintain her individual existence. On the other hand, the estranged exchange reduces every individual into an equal which can be exchanged within the labor force. Through money, human beings and their products can be translated into equally exchangeable commodities; they are not truly individuals. Thus, the estranged exchange not only turns the social activity of work into a means for individual subsistence, but also, turns each individual into an equal, or nonindividual. This is the illusion of estranged exchange. It covers over the socioeconomic factors which make the individual susceptible to the contract in the first place.

Now we can see why the surrogacy situation is so drastically misrepresented within the liberal (estranged) framework. The surrogacy arrangement appears to be an exchange of equals—service for money. It is this premise which leads proponents to the ridiculous arguments that the mother and father have equal roles in procreation because an egg equals sperm—or, that sperm donors should have the same rights as womb donors. Through the mediation of money, wombs, eggs, sperm, gestational services, etc. can be equalized and substituted for each other. For example, if one sperm sample is worth $10, and one gestational service is worth $10,000, then 1,000 sperm samples are equal to one gestational service. As Carol Gilligan says, it becomes a simple math problem with humans (1982).

Like other workers, individual women can be substituted for each other. If one "surrogate" doesn't work out, the contractors can simply hire another one. However, in what I take to be the most obvious estrangement in the surrogate arrangement, one birth mother can be substituted for another. The attempt to conceal the real relationship in the surrogate situation becomes obvious through the practice advertised by Noel Keane whereby the birth certificate is falsified after the adoption proceedings are completed (Keane 1987). The father's wife is misrepresented as, exchanged for, the child's natural mother.

The liberal framework, with its autonomous individuals, covers over what Marx calls "species-being." The emphasis on the free choice of the individual covers over the social context of the surrogacy arrangement, while the emphasis on the equal rights of all individuals involved actually covers over their individuality. Within the liberal framework, individuals are equal and therefore interchangeable without regard to important social differences, e.g., class and gender.

4. The fourth characteristic of estranged labor, according to Marx, is that the worker is estranged from other people. She takes her estranged relation to nature, herself, and her species-being, to be the natural relation for everyone. She sees everyone in this estranged relation. In the case of surrogacy, all children are seen as commodities and all women the producers of children. Of course, this is not to say that the practice of surrogacy has caused these attitudes. However, surrogacy certainly perpetuates them. Another possible result of the surrogacy arrangement is that children will see themselves as commodites.[19] They will see themselves as the result of a commercial exchange. Human beings will appear as the result of commercial contracts—the result of services rendered.

Marx's analysis of estranged labor has helped to reveal that the "surrogate" mother is the real mother of the child. She is not, as she appears, a machine producing a commodity for exchange. The relationship between the mother and child is not the relationship between a producer and a commodity. This is a distortion. In this distorted relationship, the "surrogate" is not renting her womb, but selling herself and her child. She is not free either when she enters the contract or after. Her pregnancy is not her own. She is not an autonomous participant in the contract equal to other participants. Rather, she is caught up in her socioeconomic situation which leads to the surrogacy arrangement.

Now we can see how issues of class and gender were covered up in the *Matter of Baby M*. The custody decision in particular can be reread as the result of an estranged representation of the surrogacy situation. Both the "surrogate" and the father of the child were (mis)represented as equals with equal rights to the child. Within the liberal framework, as I have argued, the class difference inherent in the surrogate contract ensured from the start that they were not equal and did not have equal rights to the child.

In the New Jersey Supreme Court's statement, the surrogacy contract was (mis)represented as not affecting the custody decision. Although the New Jersey Supreme Court ruled that the contract was illegal and would not enter into their custody decision, as I have argued, the class difference which motivated the contract in the first place was also responsible for the factors which became significant in deciding custody. The financially secure male's best interests were (mis)represented as the "child's best interests." Thus, even in this case, where the court ruled that the contract was illegal, the representation of the surrogacy arrangement is estranged and the social construction of the arrangement and the relationships which facilitate the arrangement are covered over. My use of Marx's analysis of estranged labor reveals that the factors which ensure that the surrogate loses custody of her child are built into the contract itself.

AFTERWORD

Some feminists have argued that Marx's analysis of production should be applied to reproduction.[20] However, at the same time that Marx's notion of estranged labor reveals relationships which the liberal framework conceals, the notion that reproduction can be treated like production may perpetuate the very structure which it proposes to undermine. The analogy between reproduction and production can turn children into products and mothers into the machinery of production. In the case of surrogacy, viewing the mother as the means of production is partially responsible for the exploitation of "surrogates." Talking about the surrogate's body as the means of production implies that the child is a product. Moreover, it may cover over the fact that the surrogate does not just control or not control the means of production: her body. She *is* her body. Thus, although feminists who argue for the analogy between production and reproduction intend to put women in control of the means of reproduction, the effect may be to turn women into the machinery of the production of children. A discourse intended to liberate may actually oppress.

This is true of medical technology as well. Reproductive technology which appears to liberate women may actually oppress women (Donchin 1986). This is especially true when medical institutions import the discourse of economics. For example, when doctors and scientists talk about guaranteeing a better product as a result of cesarean sections, women become machinery and children become products (Corea 1985, 17). Or, in the case of surrogacy, women become womb renters, supposedly, in order to "alleviate infertility" in the "infertile couple."

The treatment of women, or the current ethics of reproduction, which results from this view of women as machines, reproduction as production, and children as products, promotes the exploitation of women. In diagnosing surrogacy, I have used a particular reading of Marx which is concerned not with the production of commodities, but rather with the production of self-representations and representations of people in general. Although this diagnosis is useful in order to reveal the estranged representation of the surrogacy arrangement, it cannot pinpoint one cause of this estrangement. The institution of surrogacy, like any other, is a complex of many factors which interact in ways that are not always predictable or even comprehensible.

What this analysis suggests for a feminist ethics in general is that we must use old frameworks in new ways in order to create ways in which to reveal women's exploitation. We must also create new frameworks which can reveal oppression which is concealed by traditional frameworks. At the same time, we must continue to re-examine our own frameworks in order to be flexible enough to revise them if it becomes obvious that they oppress rather than liberate.

Unlike traditional ethics, feminist ethics cannot be a rigid system. Rather it must change with the changing situation of women within patriarchal societies. An ethic which is appropriate for one context may not be appropriate for another. An example might be a crude Marxist analysis of the workers' relations to the means of production in capitalism, which may work in the context of some workers' struggles, but becomes oppressive when applied to women's relations to reproduction. In some sense, a feminist ethics must be a guerilla ethics that strategically works to undermine patriarchal values wherever they oppress women. It must be an ethics that changes with the site of oppression.

NOTES

1. Most of the potential enforcement problems involve one of three situations, variations of which have appeared in court in recent legal history. First, the "surrogate" does not abide by her prenatal agreement not to use alcohol, tobacco, or drugs while pregnant (Keane 1981, 107). Second, the "surrogate" may refuse to give up the child after it is born (A v. C 1978 Fam. 170; Matter of Baby M 537 A 2d. 1227 N.J. 1988). Third, the father can refuse custody of the child after it is born (Malahoff v. Stiver 1983).

2. The Matter of Baby M, as it is called by the New Jersey Supreme Court, is the appeal of Mary Beth Whitehead in order to challenge the Superior Court's decision that her surrogacy contract with William Stern was valid and custody of "Baby M" should go to the contracting father, William Stern. The original contract between Mary Beth Whitehead and William Stern was signed in February 1985. In March 1986, "Baby M" was born. Whitehead refused to relinquish the baby to Stern. Early in 1987, William Stern sued Mary

Beth Whitehead for custody of "Baby M" and sought the enforcement of the surrogacy contract. Both were awarded to him. The Supreme Court reached a decision on Whitehead's appeal on February 3, 1988. They held that the surrogacy contract was invalid, but awarded custody of "Baby M" to William Stern.

3. Some feminists have suggested that this enslavement and estrangement are inherent to motherhood in general (Allen 1984; Beauvoir 1953). If this is so, then there is nothing unique about the surrogacy arrangement. However, in her article "Possessive Power," Janet Farrell Smith points to the difference between estranged and alienated motherhood—what she calls the difference between "alienated" and "alienable" (Smith 1986). Smith argues that while the experience of motherhood and the mother/child relationship is necessarily alienable, it is not necessarily alienated. She argues that alienated motherhood is the product of patriarchal constructions of motherhood. I agree with Smith that estrangement is not inherent to motherhood itself, even if it is inherent to motherhood within a capitalist patriarchal society. I will suggest, however, that surrogacy is the quintessence of capitalist patriarchy's estranged construction of motherhood.

4. In most cases the courts assume, and some commercial agencies insist, that the contracting agent is a heterosexual married man. Often the contracting agent is referred to as the "infertile couple." And the desire for a child is referred to as the "infertile couple's desire to have *their own* children" (Wilentz 1988, 1234), even though the father's wife is not biologically related to the child. The surrogate's services are said to "alleviate infertility" (Eaton 1986, 717), even though the father's wife remains infertile.

5. E.g., this argument was used successfully in: *Surrogate Parenting Associates v. Commonwealth of Kentucky*, 1986; *Stern v. Whitehead*, New Jersey Superior Court 1987; *Syrkowski v. Appleyard*, Michigan Supreme Court 1985. It was unsuccessful in *The Matter of Baby M*, New Jersey Supreme Court 1988.

6. As Sandra Johnson points out, "services are something you *do*; pregnant is something you *are*. Pregnancy changes a woman's entire body—she is not merely renting her womb— and has significant impact on her psyche as well" (1987, 1345).

7. For example, this was the logic used by the Kentucky Supreme Court and the New Jersey Superior Court (Leibson 1986; Sorkow 1987).

8. In her/his helpful comments, one of the *Hypatia* reviewers called both the New Jersey Supreme Court opinion and the opinion of others who hold this position, e.g., George Annas (1986, 1987, 1988), an "enlightened liberal" position.

9. If the surrogacy contract is not enforced and the surrogate's parental rights are not relinquished, then the father's wife may not be able to officially adopt the child. However, in New Jersey, at least, as the Supreme Court points out, illegal adoption does not mean denial of adoption. In addition, the court need not grant the surrogate visitation rights if it is not in the "best interests" of the child. See my arguments below. In addition, I would like to note that even the "enlightened liberal" position of many philosophers, specifically George Annas, endorses the custody process of the status quo, thereby covering over the socioeconomic issues which give rise to the surrogacy contract in the first place (Annas 1986, 1987, 1988).

10. I should mention that Mary Beth Whitehead's husband during the Superior Court trial had a drinking problem. By the time of the Supreme Court trial, Mary Beth Whitehead had divorced Mr. Whitehead and remarried. However, her remarriage was not a factor in the custody decision.

11. Some feminists (e.g., Carol Gilligan 1982) have argued that the emphasis on independence is also a gender issue. They argue that while males are socialized to be independent, females are socialized to be interdependent. This is possibly true for poor families as well: whereas middle to upper classes are socialized to be independent, poor to lower classes are socialized to be interdependent and take care of each other. It may be that only as a group can they survive financially.

12. It is crucial to note that this distinction is not as available to English readers of Marx. The English translations, while some are more faithful than others, all tend to translate

entfremdung and *verausserung* both as "alienation." In German, *entfremdung* means foriegn while *verausserung* means outer. I learned this important distinction from Gayatri Spivak in her lectures on Marx at the University of Pittsburgh, Fall 1987. In fact, this article was inspired by her emphasis on that distinction. For this, and so much more that I learned from her, I am grateful.

13. For Marx, exchanges that took place under a precapitalist barter system, exchanges which were the result of labor, were not estranged. Most labor, taken out of the capitalist economy of exchange, can be merely alienated (in the good sense) and not estranged. It is questionable whether or not this is true, however, for surrogacy. One difference between other forms of labor and surrogacy, might be that surrogacy is necessarily estranged labor. Within Marx's analysis, other forms of labor, even within capitalism, have a use-value apart from their exchange value which can be produced without estrangement. For example, a friend can cook a meal for you without becoming estranged from her labor. On the other hand, if she works as a cook in the cafeteria, when she cooks meals there, she is estranged from her labor. However, at least according to Marx's analysis, if a friend has a baby for you, even if you don't pay her, isn't she still, in some sense, estranged from her labor? Although I am perplexed by this question and not conviced that the answer is yes, I'm also unwilling to admit that the answer is no.

14. Unfortunately, forced cesareans are not unique to surrogacy arrangements. Court orders can be obtained within an hour or two in order to force women, against their will, to undergo a cesarean (Ladd 1988).

15. While this remark clearly suggests a denigration of the "animal functions" which, within feminist discourse, seems male-biased, Marx does maintain that "eating, drinking, procreating, etc., are also genuine human functions. However, when they are abstracted from other aspects of human activity and turned into final and exclusive ends, they are animal" (1975, 327).

16. This is true in Marx's writings as well. Marx does not develop the social nature of "animal functions" in humans.

17. Privacy is a complex issue that I cannot go into here. For a discussion of its complexities, one of the *Hypatia* reviewers led me to Schoeman (1984).

18. This is Marx's insight into the situation of the worker. The worker thinks that she is empowered through her ability to sell her labor to the capitalist in exchange for money. However, as Marx points out, the worker, in an important sense, sells herself into slavery. Since it is the capitalist who accumulates wealth, it is the worker who must continue to work. And, as Marx points out, the worker does not really work for a wage. The worker extends credit to the capitalist. That is, the worker works and is not paid until later. She is not paid, in fact, until she has already made the capitalist enough money to pay her. In essence, she pays herself and then pays the capitalist (1977, 278, 712).

19. Mary Gibson, among others, talks about the harmful effects of surrogacy on children (1988).

20. E.g., Evelyn Reed, Margaret Benston, and Catherine MacKinnon; a modified version is presented by Heidi Hartmann and Gayle Rubin.

REFERENCES

Allen, Jeffner. 1984. Motherhood: The annihilation of women. In *Mothering: Essays in feminist theory.* Joyce Trebilcot, ed. Totowa, NJ: Rowman & Allenheld.

Annas, George. 1988. Death without dignity for commercial surrogacy: The case of Baby M. *Hastings Center Report* 18(2): 21–24.

Annas, George. 1987. Baby M: Babies (and justice) for sale. *Hastings Center Report* 17(3): 13–15.

Annas, George. 1986. The baby broker boom. *Hastings Center Report* 16(3): 30–31.

Beauvoir, Simone de. 1953. *The second sex.* H. M. Parshley, trans.. NY: Knopf.

Corea, Gena. 1985. *The mother machine.* NY: Harper & Row.

Dworkin, Andrea. 1983. *Right-wing women.* NY: Perigee Books.

Eaton, Thomas. 1986. Comparative responses to surrogate motherhood. *Nebraska Law Review* 65: 686–725.

Gibson, Mary. 1988. The legal and moral status of surrogate motherhood. Paper presented at the American Philosophical Association Eastern Division Meeting, Washington D.C., December.

Gilligan, Carol. 1982. *In a different voice.* Cambridge: Harvard University Press.

Jaggar, Alison. 1983. *Feminist politics and human nature.* Totowa, NJ: Rowman & Allanheld.

Johnson, Sandra. 1987. The Baby "M" decision: Specific performance of a contract for specially manufactured goods. *Southern Illinois University Law Journal* 11: 1339–1348.

Keane, Noel (with Dennis Breo). 1981. *The surrogate mother.* NY: Everest House.

Keane, Noel. 1987. Paper presented at the seminar on Surrogate Motherhood. Berry College. Rome, Georgia. April.

Ladd, Rosalind. 1989. Woman in labor: Some issues about informed consent. *Hypatia* 4(3): 37–45. Also in this volume.

Leibson, J. 1986. *Surrogate Parenting Associates Inc. v. Commonwealth of Kentucky.* Supreme Court of Kentucky. Ky., 704, South West Reporter, 2nd Series, 209.

Marx, Karl. 1977. *Capital* Vol. I. Ben Fowkes, trans. NY: Random House.

Marx, Karl. 1975. Economic and philosophical manuscripts. In *Early Writings.* Quintin Hoare, ed. R. Livingstone and G. Benton, trans. NY: Random House.

Marx, Karl. 1975a. Critique of Hegel's doctrine of the state. In *Early Writings.* Quintin Hoare, ed. R. Livingstone and G. Benton, trans. NY: Random House.

Marx, Karl. 1975b. Excerpts from James Mill's *Elements of political economy.* In *Early writings.* Quintin Hoare, ed. R. Livingstone and G. Benton, trans. NY: Random House.

Schoeman, Ferdinand, ed. 1984. *Philosophical dimensions of privacy.* Cambridge: Cambridge University Press.

Smith, Janet Farrell. 1986. Possessive power. *Hypatia* 1(2): 103–120.

Sorkow, Harvey R. 1987. *Stern v. Whitehead.* New Jersey Superior Court. 217, N.J., Super., 313, 525, A.2d 1128.

Wilentz, C. J. 1988. *The matter of Baby "M".* New Jersey Supreme Court. N.J., 537, Atlantic Reporter, 2nd Series, 1234.

Selling Babies and Selling Bodies

SARA ANN KETCHUM ❖ ❖ ❖

I will argue that the free market in babies or in women's bodies created by an institution of paid surrogate motherhood is contrary to Kantian principles of personhood and to the feminist principle that men do not have—and cannot gain through contract, marriage, or payment of money—a right to the sexual or reproductive use of women's bodies.

The "Baby M" case turned into something approaching a national soap opera, played out in newspapers and magazines. The drama surrounding the case tends to obscure the fact that the case raises some very abstract philosophical and moral issues. It forces us to examine questions about the nature and meaning of parenthood, of the limits of reproductive autonomy, of how the facts of pregnancy should affect our analysis of sexual equality,[1] and of what counts as selling people and of what forms (if any) of selling people we should honor in law and what forms we should restrict. It is this last set of questions whose relevance I will be discussing here. One objection to what is usually called "surrogate motherhood" and which I will call "contracted motherhood" (CM) or "baby contracts"[2] is that it commercializes reproduction and turns human beings (the mother and/or the baby) into objects of sale. If this is a compelling objection, there is a good argument for prohibiting (and/or not enforcing contracts for) commercial CM. Such a prohibition would be similar to laws on black market adoptions and would have two parts, at least: 1) a prohibition of commercial companies who make the arrangements and/or 2) a prohibition on the transfer of money to the birth mother for the transfer of custody (beyond expenses incurred) (Warnock 1985, 46–7). I will also argue that CM law should follow adoption law in making clear that pre-birth agreements to relinquish parental rights are not binding and will not be enforced by the courts (the birth mother should not be forced to give up her child for adoption).[3]

CM AND AID: THE REAL DIFFERENCE PROBLEM

CM is usually presented as a new reproductive technology and, moreover, as the female equivalent of AID (artificial insemination by donor) and, therefore, as an extension of the right to privacy or the right to make medical decisions about one's own life. There are two problems with this description: 1) CM uses the same technology as AID—the biological arrangements are exactly the same—but intends

Hypatia vol. 4, no. 3 (Fall 1989). © by Sara Ann Ketchum

an opposite assignment of custody. 2) No technology is necessary for CM as is evidenced by the biblical story of Abraham and Sarah who used a "handmaid" as a birth mother. Since artificial insemination is virtually uncontroversial[4] it seems clear that what makes CM controversial is not the technology, but the social arrangements—that is, the custody assignment. CM has been defended on the ground that such arrangements enable fertile men who are married to infertile women to reproduce and, thus, are parallel to AID which enables fertile women whose husbands are infertile to have children. It is difficult not to regard these arguments as somewhat disingenuous. The role of the sperm donor and the role of the egg donor/mother are distinguished by pregnancy, and pregnancy is, if anything is, a "real difference" which would justify us in treating women and men differently. To treat donating sperm as equivalent to biological motherhood would be as unfair as treating the unwed father who has not contributed to his children's welfare the same as the father who has devoted his time to taking care of them. At most, donating sperm is comparable to donating ova; however, even that comparison fails because donating ova is a medically risky procedure, whereas donating sperm is not.

Therefore, the essential morally controversial features of CM have to do with its nature as a social and economic institution and its assignment of family relationships rather than with any technological features. Moreover, the institution of CM requires of contracting birth mothers much more time commitment, medical risk, and social disruption than AID does of sperm donors. It also requires substantial male control over women's bodies and time, while AID neither requires nor provides any female control over men's bodies. Christine Overall (1987, 181–185) notes that when a woman seeks AID, she not only does not usually have a choice of donor, but she also may be required to get her husband's consent if she is married. The position of the man seeking CM is the opposite; he chooses a birth mother and his wife does not have to consent to the procedure (although the mother's husband does).[5] The contract entered into by Mary Beth Whitehead and William Stern contains a number of provisions regulating her behavior, including: extensive medical examinations, an agreement about when she may or may not abort, an agreement to follow doctors' orders, and agreements not to take even prescription drugs without the doctor's permission. Some of these social and contractual provisions are eliminable. But the fact that CM requires a contract and AID does not reflects the differences between pregnancy and ejaculation. If the sperm donor wants a healthy child (a good product), he needs to control the woman's behavior. In contrast, any damage the sperm-donor's behavior will have on the child will be present in the sperm and could, in principle, be tested for before the woman enters the AID procedure. There is no serious moral problem with discarding defective sperm; discarding defective children is a quite different matter.

COMMODIFICATION

There are three general categories of moral concern with commercializing either adoption (baby selling) or reproductive activities. The three kinds of argument are not always separated and they are not entirely separable:

1) There is the Kantian argument, based on a version of the Second Formulation of the Categorical Imperative. On this argument, selling people is objectionable because it is treating them as means rather than as ends, as objects rather than as persons. People who can be bought and sold are being treated as being of less moral significance than are those who buy and sell. Allowing babies to be bought and sold adds an extra legal wedge between the status of children and that of adults, and allowing women's bodies to be bought and sold (or "rented" if you prefer) adds to the inequality between men and women. Moreover, making babies and women's bodies available for sale raises specters of the rich "harvesting" the babies of the poor. 2) Consequentialist objections are fueled by concern for what may happen to the children and women who are bought and sold, to their families, and to the society as a whole if we allow an area of this magnitude and traditional intimacy to become commercialized. 3) Connected to both 1 and 2 are concerns about protecting the birth mother and the mother-child relationship from the potential coerciveness of commercial transactions. These arguments apply slightly differently depending on whether we analyze the contracts as baby contracts (selling babies) or as mother contracts (as a sale of women's bodies), although many of the arguments will be very similar for both.

Selling Babies: The most straightforward argument for prohibiting baby-selling is that it is selling a human being and that any selling of a human being should be prohibited because it devalues human life and human individuals. This argument gains moral force from its analogy with slavery. Defenders of baby contracts argue that baby selling is unlike selling slaves in that it is a transfer of parental rights rather than of ownership of the child—the adoptive parents cannot turn around and sell the baby to another couple for a profit (Landes and Posner 1978, 344). What the defenders of CM fail to do is provide an account of the wrongness of slavery such that baby-selling (or baby contracts) do not fall under the argument. Landes and Posner, in particular, would, I think, have difficulty establishing an argument against slavery because they are relying on utilitarian arguments. Since one of the classic difficulties with utilitarianism is that it cannot yield an argument that slavery is wrong in principle, it is hardly surprising that utilitarians will find it difficult to discover within that theory an argument against selling babies. Moreover, their economic argument is not even utilitarian because it only counts people's interests to the extent that they can pay for their satisfaction.

Those who, unlike Landes and Posner, defend CM while supporting laws against baby-selling, distinguish CM from paid adoptions in that in CM the person to whom custody is being transferred is the biological (genetic) father. This suggests a parallel to custody disputes, which are not obviously any more appropriately ruled by money than is adoption. We could argue against the commercialization of either on the grounds that child-regarding concerns should decide child custody and that using market criteria or contract considerations would violate that principle by substituting another, unrelated, and possibly conflicting, one. In particular, both market and contract are about relations between the adults involved rather than about the children or about the relationship between the child and the adult.

Another disanalogy cited between preadoption contracts and CM is that in preadoption contracts the baby is already there (that is, the preadoption contract is offered to a woman who is already pregnant, and, presumably, planning to have the child), while the mother contract is a contract to create a child who does not yet exist, even as an embryo. If our concern is the commodification of children, this strikes me as an odd point for the *defenders* of CM to emphasize. Producing a child to order for money is a paradigm case of commodifying children. The fact that the child is not being put up for sale to the highest bidder, but is only for sale to the genetic father, may reduce some of the harmful effects of an open market in babies but does not quiet concerns about personhood.

Arguments for allowing CM are remarkably similar to the arguments for legalizing black-market adoptions in the way they both define the problem. CM, like a market for babies, is seen as increasing the satisfaction and freedom of infertile individuals or couples by increasing the quantity of the desired product (there will be more babies available for adoption) and the quality of the product (not only more white healthy babies, but white healthy babies who are genetically related to one of the purchasers). These arguments tend to be based on the interests of infertile couples and obscure the relevance of the interests of the birth mothers (who will be giving the children up for adoption) and their families, the children who are produced by the demands of the market, and (the most invisible and most troubling group) needy children who are without homes because they are not "high-quality" products and because we are not, as a society, investing the time and money needed to place the hard to adopt children. If we bring these hidden interests to the fore, they raise a host of issues about consequences—both utilitarian issues and issues about the distribution of harms and benefits.

Perhaps the strongest deontological argument against baby-selling is an objection to the characterization of the mother-child relationship (and, more generally, of the adult-child relationship) that it presupposes. Not only does the baby become an object of commerce, but the custody relationship of the parent becomes a property relationship. If we see parental custody rights as correlates of parental responsibility or as a right to maintain a relationship, it will be less tempting to think of them as something one can sell. We have good reasons for allowing birth-mothers to relinquish their children because otherwise we would be forcing children into the care of people who either do not want them or feel themselves unable to care for them. However, the fact that custody may be waived in this way does not entail that it may be sold or transferred. If children are not property, they cannot be gifts either. If a mother's right is a right to maintain a relationship (see Ketchum 1987), it is implausible to treat it as transferrable; having the option of terminating a relationship with A does not entail having the option of deciding who A will relate to next—the right to a divorce does not entail the right to transfer one's connection to one's spouse to someone else. Indeed, normally, the termination of a relationship with A ends any right I have to make moral claims on A's relationships. Although in giving up responsibilities I may have a responsibility to see to it that someone will shoulder them when I go, I do not have a right to choose that person.

Selling Women's Bodies: Suppose we do regard mother contracts as contracts for the sale or rental of reproductive capacities. Is there good reason for including reproductive capacities among those things or activities that ought not to be bought and sold? We might distinguish between selling reproductive capacities and selling work on a number of grounds. A conservative might argue against commercializing reproduction on the grounds that it disturbs family relationships,[6] or on the grounds that there are some categories of human activities that should not be for sale. A Kantian might argue that there are some activities that are close to our personhood[7] and that a commercial traffic in these activities constitutes treating the person as less than an end (or less than a person).

One interpretation of the laws prohibiting baby selling is that they are an attempt to reduce or eliminate coercion in the adoption process, and are thus, based on a concern for the birth mother rather than (or as well as) the child. All commercial transactions are at least potentially coercive in that the parties to them are likely to come from unequal bargaining positions and in that, whatever we have a market in, there will be some people who will be in a position such that they have to sell it in order to survive. Such concerns are important to arguments against an open market in human organs or in the sexual use of people's bodies as well as arguments against baby contracts of either kind.

As Margaret Radin suggests (1987, 1915–1921), the weakness of arguments of this sort—that relationships or contracts are exploitative on the grounds that people are forced into them by poverty—is that the real problem is not in the possibility of commercial transactions, but in the situation that makes these arrangements attractive by comparison. We do not end the feminization of poverty by forbidding prostitution or CM. Indeed, if we are successful in eliminating these practices, we may be reducing the income of some women (by removing ways of making money) and, if we are unsuccessful, we are removing these people from state protection by making their activities illegal. Labor legislation which is comparably motivated by concern for unequal bargaining position (such as, for example, minimum wage and maximum hours laws, and health and safety regulations) regulates rather than prevents that activity and is thus less vulnerable to this charge. Radin's criticism shows that the argument from the coerciveness of poverty is insufficient as a support for laws rejecting commercial transactions in personal services. This does not show that the concern is irrelevant. The argument from coercion is still an appropriate response to simple voluntarist arguments—those that assume that these activities are purely and freely chosen by all those who participate in them. Given the coerciveness of the situation, we cannot assume that the presumed or formal voluntariness of the contract makes it nonexploitative.

If the relationship of CM is, by its nature, disrespectful of personhood, it can be exploitative despite short-term financial benefits to some women. The disrespect for women as persons that is fundamental to the relationship lies in the concept of the woman's body (and of the child and mother-child relationship) implicit in the contract. I have argued elsewhere (1984) that claiming a welfare right to another person's body is to treat that person as an object:

> An identity or intimate relation between persons and their bodies may or may not be essential to our metaphysical understanding of a person, but it is essential to a minimal moral conceptual scheme. Without a concession to persons' legitimate interests and concerns for their physical selves, most of our standard and

paradigm moral rules would not make sense; murder might become the mere destruction of the body; assault, a mere interference with the body . . . and so on. We cannot make sense out of the concept of assault unless an assault on S's body is ipso facto an assault on S. By the same token, treating another person's body as part of my domain—as among the things that I have a rightful claim to—is, if anything is, a denial that there is a person there. (1984, 34–35)

This argument is, in turn, built on the analysis of the wrongness of rape developed by Marilyn Frye and Carolyn Shafer in "Rape and Respect" (1977):

The use of a person in the advancement of interests contrary to its own is a limiting case of disrespect. It reveals the perception of the person simply as an object which can serve some purpose, a tool or a bit of material, and one which furthermore is dispensable or replaceable and thus of little value even as an object with a function. (341)

We can extend this argument to the sale of persons. To make a person or a person's body an object of commerce is to treat the person as part of another person's domain, particularly if the sale of A to B gives B rights to A or to A's body. What is objectionable is a claim—whether based on welfare or on contract—to a right to another person such that that person is part of my domain. The assertion of such a right is morally objectionable even without the use of force. For example, a man who claims to have a *right* to sexual intercourse with his wife, on the grounds of the marriage relationship, betrays a conception of her body, and thus her person, as being properly within his domain, and thus a conception of her as an object rather than a person.

Susan Brownmiller in *Against Our Will* (1975) suggests that prostitution is connected to rape in that prostitution makes women's bodies into consumer goods that might—if not justifiably, at least understandably—be forcibly taken by those men who see themselves as unjustly deprived.

When young men learn that females may be bought for a price, and that acts of sex command set prices, then how should they not also conclude that that which may be bought may also be taken without the civility of a monetary exchange? . . . legalized prostitution institutionalizes the concept that it is a man's monetary right, if not his divine right, to gain access to the female body, and that sex is a female service that should not be denied the civilized male. (391, 392)

The same can be said for legalized sale of women's reproductive services. The more hegemonic this commodification of women's bodies is, the more the woman's lack of consent to sex or to having children can present itself as unfair to the man because it is arbitrary.

A market in women's bodies—whether sexual prostitution or reproductive prostitution—reveals a social ontology in which women are among the things in the world that can be appropriately commodified—bought and sold and, by extension, stolen. The purported freedom that such institutions would give women to enter

into the market by selling their bodies is paradoxical. Sexual or reproductive prostitutes enter the market not so much as *agents* or subjects, but as commodities or
objects. This is evidenced by the fact that the pimps and their counterparts, the
arrangers of baby contracts, make the bulk of the profits. Moreover, once there is
a market for women's bodies, all women's bodies will have a price, and the woman
who does not sell her body becomes a hoarder of something that is useful to other
people and is financially valuable. The market is a hegemonic institution; it determines the meanings of actions of people who choose not to participate as well
as of those who choose to participate.

Contract: The immediate objection to treating the Baby M case as a contract
dispute is that the practical problem facing the court is a child custody problem
and to treat it as a contract case is to deal with it on grounds other than the best
interests of the child. That the best interests of the child count need not entail
that contract does not count, although it helps explain one of the reasons we should
be suspicious of this particular contract. There is still the question of whether the
best interests of the child will trump contract considerations (making the contract
nonbinding) or merely enter into a balancing argument in which contract is one
of the issues to be balanced. However, allowing contract to count at all raises some
of the same Kantian objections as the commodification problem. As a legal issue,
the contract problem is more acute because the state action (enforcing the contract)
is more explicit.

Any binding mother contract will put the state in the position of enforcing
the rights of a man to a women's body or to his genetic offspring. But this is to
treat the child or the mother's body as objects of the sperm donor's rights, which,
I argued above, is inconsistent with treating them as persons. This will be clearest
if the courts enforce specific performance[8] and require the mother to go through
with the pregnancy (or to abort) if she chooses not to or requires the transfer of
custody to the contracting sperm-donor on grounds other than the best interests
of the child. In those cases, I find it hard to avoid the description that what is
being awarded is a person and what is being affirmed is a right to a person. I think
the Kantian argument still applies if the court refuses specific performance but
awards damages. Damages compensate for the loss of something to which one has
a right. A judge who awards damages to the contracting sperm donor for having
been deprived of use of the contracting woman's reproductive capacities or for being
deprived of custody of the child gives legal weight to the idea that the contracting
sperm donor had a legally enforceable *right* to them (or, to put it more bluntly, to
those commodities or goods).

The free contract argument assumes that Mary Beth Whitehead's claims to her
daughter are rights (rather than, for example, obligations or a more complex relationship), and, moreover, that they are alienable, as are property rights. If the
baby is not something she has an alienable right to, then custody of the baby is
not something she can transfer by contract. In cases where the state is taking
children away from their biological parents and in custody disputes, we do want
to appeal to some rights of the parents. However, I think it would be unfortunate
to regard these rights as rights to the child, because that would be to treat the
child as the object of the parents' rights and violate the principles that persons

and persons' bodies cannot be the objects of other people's rights. The parents' rights in these cases should be to consideration, to nonarbitrariness and to respect for the relationship between the parent and the child.

CONCLUDING REMARKS

The Kantian, person-respecting arguments I have been offering do not provide an account of all of the moral issues surrounding CM. However, I think that they can serve as a counter-balance to arguments (also Kantian) for CM as an expression of personal autonomy.[9] They might also add some weight to the empirical arguments against CM that are accumulating. There is increasing concern that women cannot predict in advance whether or not they and their family[10] will form an attachment to the child they will bear nor can they promise not to develop such feelings (as some on the contracts ask them to do). There is also increasing concern for the birth-family and for the children produced by the arrangement (particularly where there is a custody dispute). A utilitarian might respond that the problems are outweighed by the joys of the adopting/sperm donor families, but, if so, we must ask: are we simply shifting the misery from wealthy (or wealthier) infertile couples to poorer fertile families and to the "imperfect" children waiting for adoption?

These considerations provide good reason for prohibiting commercialization of CM. In order to do that we could adopt new laws prohibiting the transfer of money in such arrangements or simply extend existing adoption laws, making the contracts non-binding as are pre-birth adoption contracts (Cohen 1984, 280–284) and limiting the money that can be transferred. There are some conceptual problems remaining about what would count as prohibiting commodification. I find the English approach very attractive. This approach has the following elements: 1) it strictly prohibits third parties from arranging mother contracts; 2) if people arrange them privately, they are allowed; 3) the contracts are not binding. If the birthmother decides to keep the baby, her decision is final[11] (*and* the father may be required to pay child-support; that may be too much for Americans); 4) although, in theory, CM is covered by limitations on money for adoption, courts have approved payments for contracted motherhood, and there is never a criminal penalty on the parents for money payments.[12]

NOTES

An earlier version of this paper was presented at the Eastern Division Meetings of the American Philosophical Association in 1987. Work on this paper was supported by an ACLS/ Ford Foundation grant and was performed while I was a Fellow in Law and Philosophy at Harvard Law School. I want to thank the following people for enlightening and lively discussions on the issue and helpful comments on an earlier draft of the paper: Elizabeth Bartholet (and the students in her seminar on Adoption and New Reproductive Technologies in the Spring of 1987), Frank Michelman, Martha Minow, Lewis Sargentich, and Cass Sunstein.

1. In "Is There a Right to Procreate?" (1987a), I argue that there is an asymmetry between the right not to reproduce (as in the right to access to abortion and contraception) and the right to reproduce in that a decision to reproduce (unlike a decision not to reproduce) involves two other persons—the person who is to be produced and the person who is the other biological parent. Thus, the claim of a privacy right to reproduce is a claim to a right to make decisions about other people's lives, and those people's rights and interests must be weighed in the balance. Furthermore, I will argue (and this paper is part of that argument) that issues of reproductive privacy cannot be entirely separated from issues of sexual equality.

2. Terms such as "surrogate mother" and "renting a womb" are distortions—the surrogate mother *is* the mother, and she is giving up her child for adoption just as is the birth mother who gives up her child for adoption by an unrelated person. This language allows the defenders of paternal rights to argue for the importance of biological (genetic) connection when it comes to the *father's* rights, but bury the greater physical connection between the mother and the child in talk that suggests that mothers are mere receptacles (shades of Aristotle's biology) or that the mother has a more artificial relationship to the child than does the father or the potential adoptive mother. But, at the time of birth, the natural relationship is between the mother and child. (I discuss this issue further in "New Reproductive Technologies and the Definition of Parenthood: A Feminist Perspective" [1987]). A relationship created by contract is the paradigm of artificiality, of a socially created relationship, and the most plausible candidate for a natural social relationship is the mother-child bond. I will be using "contracted motherhood" and "baby contracts" (a term offered by Elizabeth Bartholet) rather than "surrogate motherhood" and "surrogacy." I will use "baby contracts" as the more general term, covering paid adoption contracts as well as so-called surrogate mother arrangements. I have not yet found a term that is either neutral between or inclusive of the motherhood aspects and the baby-regarding aspects.

3. She may still lose a custody fight, since the male of the adopting couple is the genetic father of the child, but in that case, she would still be the legal mother of the child and have a right to maintain a relationship.

4. I do not mean to suggest that there are no moral problems with AID. See Krimmel (1983) for an approach that presents arguments against both.

5. Indeed, there is a technical reason for her not to sign the contract. The wife of the sperm donor in CM intends to adopt the resulting child. If she is a party to the contract, it would be more difficult to avoid the conclusion that the arrangement exchanges money for adoption and is thus contrary to baby-selling laws.

6. Robert C. Black (1981) argues, in response to an argument of this sort, that: "In any realistic view of the situation, the only true 'family' whose future is at stake is the one the child is predestined to enter—that of the childless married couple—not the *nominal, intentionally temporary 'family'* represented by the surrogate mother" (382, emphasis added). Surely, this is a disingenuous response. Mary Beth Whitehead's family is just as much a family as the Sterns' (and it is larger); even if we are to ignore her, we must consider the interests of her children (what effect does it have on them that their half-sister is being sold to another family?) and her husband and the integrity of the family unit. Some surrogates report problems their children have with the arrangement in "Baby M: Surrogate Mothers Vent Feelings," by Iver Peterson (1987).

7. This is the position that Margaret Radin (1987) develops and relies on in "Market-Inalienability." "Market-inalienability ultimately rests on our best conception of human flourishing . . . " (1937). Radin's article provides a very thorough discussion of and argument for prohibiting commodification of personal services.

8. M. Louise Graham (1982) argues that traditional contract doctrine and precedent would prohibit requiring specific performance against the birth mother:

> The rule that a contract for distinctly personal, nondelegable services will not be enforced
> by specific performance is nearly universal. The reasons given for the refusal to enforce are

the difficulty of gauging the quality of any performance rendered, prejudice against a species of involuntary servitude, and a reluctance to force a continued relationship between antagonistic parties. (301)

9. See, for example, Joan Hollinger (1985, 865–932) for a well developed analysis of new reproductive technology issues as pure (or almost pure) autonomy issues.

10. One former surrogate reports that her daughter (11 at the time of the birth and now 17) is still having problems: "Nobody told me that a child could bond with a baby while you're still pregnant. I didn't realize then that all the times she listened to his heartbeat and felt his legs kick that she was becoming attached to him." Another quotes her son as having asked, "You're not going to give them me, are you?" (Peterson 1987, B1).

11. This presupposes a presumption in favor of the birth-mother as custodial or deciding parent. I have argued for that position on the grounds that, at the time of birth, the gestational mother has a concrete relationship to the child that the genetic father (and the genetic mother, if she is not the gestational mother) does not have (Ketchum 1987). Without that presumption and without a presumption of sale or contract, each case would be subject to long custody disputes.

12. This, I think, helps us get around Radin's double-bind problem (1987, 1915–1921).

REFERENCES

Black, Robert. 1981. Legal problems of surrogate motherhood. *New England Law Review* 16 (3): 380–392.

Brownmiller, Susan. 1975. *Against our will: Men, women, and rape.* New York: Simon and Schuster.

Cohen, Barbara. 1984. Surrogate mothers: Whose baby is it? *American Journal of Law and Medicine* 10: 243–285.

Frye, Marilyn, and Carolyn Shafer. 1977. Rape and respect. In *Feminism and philosophy.* Mary Vetterling-Braggin, Frederick A. Elliston, and Jane English, eds. Totowa, N.J.: Littlefield, Adams and Co.

Graham, M. Louise. 1982. Surrogate gestation and the protection of choice. *Santa Clara Law Review* 22: 291–323.

Hollinger, Joan Heifetz. 1985. From coitus to commerce: Legal and social consequences of noncoital reproduction. *Michigan Journal of Law Reform* 18: 865–932.

Ketchum, Sara Ann. 1987. New reproductive technologies and the definition of parenthood: A feminist perspective. Presented at Feminism and Legal Theory: Women and Intimacy, a conference sponsored by the Institute for Legal Studies at the University of Wisconsin-Madison.

Ketchum, Sara Ann. 1987a. Is there a right to procreate? Presented at the Pacific Division Meetings of the American Philosophical Association.

Ketchum, Sara Ann. 1984. The moral status of the bodies of persons. *Social Theory and Practice* 10: 25–38.

Krimmel, Herbert. 1983. The case against surrogate parenting. *Hastings Center Report* 13 (5): 35–39.

Landes, Elizabeth A., and Richard M. Posner. 1978. The economics of the baby shortage. *Journal of Legal Studies* 7: 323–348.

Overall, Christine. 1987. *Ethics and human reproduction.* Boston: Allen & Unwin.

Peterson, Iver. 1987. Baby M: Surrogate mothers vent feelings. *New York Times*, March 2, 1987: B1 and B4.

Radin, Margaret. 1987. Market-Inalienability. *Harvard Law Review* 100: 1849–1937.

Warnock, Mary. 1985. *A question of life: The Warnock report on human fertilization and embryology*. Oxford: Basil Blackwell.

Commodification or Compensation: A Reply to Ketchum

H. M. MALM ❖ ❖ ❖

I defend the permissibility of paid surrogacy arrangements against the arguments Sara Ketchum advances in "Selling Babies and Selling Bodies." I argue that the arrangements cannot be prohibited out of hand on the grounds that they treat persons as objects of sale, because it is possible to view the payments made in these arrangements as compensation for the woman's services. I also argue that the arguments based on exploitation and parental custodial rights fail to provide adequate grounds for prohibiting the arrangements.

The practice of surrogate motherhood raises at least three sorts of moral questions.[1] First, there are questions about the nature of surrogate motherhood itself. Is there something inherently wrong, for example, with intentionally becoming pregnant when one does not intend to raise the child? Second, there are questions about the status of the arrangements when they involve a transfer of money. Is it morally wrong for one person to offer, and another person to accept, payment for being a surrogate mother? What is being purchased? Third, there are questions about the legal status of the arrangements. Should they be regarded as binding contracts?

Sara Ketchum (this volume) addresses questions of the second sort in "Selling Babies and Selling Bodies." She argues for a ban on paid surrogacy arrangements by arguing that persons are not the sort of thing that may be bought, sold, or rented. In one sense Ketchum's arguments are successful. She has shown us, or perhaps reminded us of *why* it is wrong to treat persons as objects of sale. In another sense they are unsuccessful. For while she intends her arguments to provide grounds for prohibiting paid surrogacy arrangements, she has not argued that these arrangements *do in fact* treat persons as objects of sale. That is, while she has defended premise 1 in the following argument, she has not defended premise 2.

1. It is morally wrong to treat persons, including babies, as objects of sale.
2. Paid surrogate motherhood arrangements treat persons as objects of sale.
3. Therefore, paid surrogacy arrangements are morally objectionable.

Hypatia vol. 4, no. 3 (Fall 1989). © by H. M. Malm

The failure to defend premise 2 is not simply a failure to defend the obvious. Though it is possible that the payments made in paid surrogacy arrangements are payments for the baby, or for the use of the woman's body, it is also possible that they are not. They may be payments for the woman's services—compensation, that is, for the efforts and risks of bearing a child, e.g., not drinking coffee or alcohol for nine months, not engaging in enjoyable but potentially dangerous activities, for the risks involved in giving birth, and for the effort it may take to return her body to the condition it was in prior to pregnancy.

In this essay I develop the distinction between compensating a woman for her services, and paying a woman for the use of her body, and then evaluate some of Ketchum's arguments in its light. I argue that since this distinction allows us to reject premise 2, we cannot prohibit paid surrogacy arrangements on the grounds that they treat persons as objects of sale. I then discuss some of Ketchum's arguments that can be offered against the compensation-view of the payments. I argue that they too provide inadequate grounds for prohibiting the arrangements.[2]

I

Ketchum's acceptance of premise 2 can be seen in the structure of her essay and in some of its particular passages. After introducing the topic of paid surrogacy arrangements, she distinguishes three sorts of arguments that may be raised against the commodification of persons.

> 1) There is the Kantian argument . . . [that] selling people is objectionable because it is treating them as means rather than ends, as objects rather than persons. . . . 2) Consequentialist objections are fueled by concern for what may happen to the *children and women who are bought and sold.* . . . 3) Connected to both 1 and 2 are concerns about protecting the birth mother and the mother-child relationship from the potential coerciveness of commercial transactions. These arguments apply slightly differently *depending on whether we analyze the contracts as baby contracts (selling babies) or as mother contracts (as a sale of women's bodies),* although many of the arguments will be very similar for both. (emphasis added; Ketchum, above, 286)

She then offers a number of particular arguments explaining why it is wrong to treat persons as objects of sale, and concludes by claiming "these considerations provide good reason for prohibiting commercialization of [surrogate motherhood]" (Ketchum, above, 291). But absent from Ketchum's discussion is an argument that *connects* paid surrogacy arrangements *with* the commodification of persons. Without this argument, even the most forceful arguments about the wrongness of selling people cannot do the work she wants them to do.

The question before us may be stated as follows: Are we committed to viewing the payments made in paid surrogacy arrangements as payments for either the baby itself or for the use of the woman's body? To see that we are not, it will be helpful if we first grant, as Ketchum does, that the payments made are not necessarily for the baby itself, and then examine what Ketchum finds wrong with paying a woman for the use of her body:

> The disrespect for women as persons that is fundamental to the [surrogacy] relationship lies in the concept of the woman's body . . . implicit in the contract. I have argued elsewhere . . . that claiming a welfare right to another person's body is to treat that person as an object. . . . [T]reating another person's body as a part of my domain—as among the things that I have a rightful claim to— is, if anything is, a denial that there is a person there. . . . We can extend this argument to the sale of persons. To make a person or a person's body an object of commerce is to treat the person as part of another person's domain, particularly if the sale of A to B gives B rights to A or to A's body. . . . (Ketchum, above, 288–289)

Ketchum seems to be assuming that if I pay you to bear a child for me, then I acquire a right to your body, treat you as an object of my domain, and (or) deny that you are a person. But this assumption is flawed. It fails to take into account the difference between (a) my paying you for *me* to use your body in a way that benefits me, and (b) my paying you for *you* to use your body in a way that benefits me. The difference between these two is important because it determines whether my payments to you give me a right to your body, and thus whether they treat your body as an object of commerce and you as less than a person. To illustrate it, suppose that you own a lawnmower. (I do not mean to suggest that women's bodies are on a par with machines.) If I need to have my lawn mowed then I may (a) pay you for *me* to use your lawnmower to mow my lawn, in which case I *rent* your lawnmower from you, or (b) pay you for *you* to use your lawnmower to mow my lawn, in which case I pay you for your *services*. In the former case I acquire a right to your lawnmower—the right to use it for a limited period of time. In the latter case I do not. Any right I have here is at most a right to insist that you do with your lawnmower what you said you would. But that is not a right to your lawnmower.

When we apply this distinction to the issue of surrogate motherhood we see that there is no need to view the payments to the woman as payments for the use (i.e., rental) of her body—the customer does not acquire a space over which he (or she)[3] then has control. He may not paint it blue, keep a coin in it, or do whatever else he wishes provided that he does not cause permanent damage. Instead, the woman is being paid for *her* to use her body in a way that benefits him— she is being compensated for her services.[4] But this does not treat her body as an object of commerce, or her as less than a person, any more than does my paying a surgeon to perform an operation, a cabby to drive a car, or a model to pose for a statue. My payments to the surgeon do not give me a right to her arm, make her an object of my domain, nor deny that she is a person. Indeed, recognizing that persons can enter into agreements to use their own bodies in ways that benefit others *reaffirms* their status as persons—as agents—rather than denies it. Given this, we cannot prohibit paid surrogacy arrangements on the grounds that they involve the buying and selling or renting of babies and women's bodies.

II

Though Ketchum does not address the compensation-view of the payments, some of her arguments against paid surrogacy arrangements may seem to stand even given that view:

> Perhaps the strongest deontological argument against baby-selling is an objection to the characterization of the mother-child relationship . . . that it presupposes. Not only does the baby become an object of commerce, but the custody relationship of the parent becomes a property relationship. If we see parental custody rights as correlates of parental responsibility or as a right to maintain a relationship, it will be less tempting to think of them as something one can sell. We have good reasons for allowing birth-mothers to relinquish their children because otherwise we would be forcing children into the care of people who either do not want them or feel themselves unable to care for them. However, the fact that custody may be waived in this way does not entail that it may be sold or transferred. If children are not property, they cannot be gifts either. (Ketchum, above, 287)

As this passage suggests, one may object to paid surrogacy arrangements on the grounds that (a) since they require that custody of the child be *transferred* (by sale or gift) from one person to another, then (b) they require that we view the parent-child relationship as a property relationship. And that is morally objectionable.

Let us grant that the parent-child relationship is not a property relationship, as well as adopt Ketchum's suggestion that parental custodial rights be viewed as rights to maintain a relationship. The problem with the above argument is that there is nothing in the nature of surrogate motherhood arrangements that requires that custody be transferred rather than waived. In order for one parent to gain sole custody of a child, he or she need not acquire the other parent's parental custodial right, such that he or she would then have two parental custodial rights—two rights to maintain a relationship—when before he or she had only one. Instead, one parent may obtain sole custody of a child merely by the other parent's *waiving* his or her custodial right. The one would then have sole custody because he or she is then the only one *with* custody. But his or her right to maintain a relationship has not, somehow, doubled in size. (This is supported by the fact that a judge is not required to find a parent with sole custody *twice* as unfit as a parent who shares custody, before she would be justified in removing a child from that parent's care. Indeed, we may think it should be just the reverse.)

Another way to object to paid surrogacy arrangements, given the compensation-view of the payments, is to argue that there is an important moral difference between compensating a woman for the efforts and risks of bearing a child, and compensating a woman for the efforts and risks of, say, mowing a lawn, posing for a drawing, or performing an operation. But making this argument requires that we can explain what that difference is, and the differences suggested by Ketchum seem to me to be inadequate. She writes:

We might distinguish between selling reproductive capacities and selling work on a number of grounds. A conservative might argue against commercializing reproduction on the grounds that it disturbs family relationships, or on the grounds that there are some categories of human activities that should not be for sale. A Kantian might argue that there are some activities that are close to our personhood and that a commercial traffic in these activities constitutes treating the person as less than an end (or less than a person). (Ketchum, above, 288)

Ketchum's first suggestion, that paid surrogacy arrangements disturb family relationships (while typical forms of work do not?), won't draw an appropriate line because many forms of work run that risk. Laura Purdy (1989) points out that women risk their lives and health by building bridges, working on farms, and even working for the postal service. Yet few of us would regard the disruption of the family that would be occasioned by the woman's death or serious illness as legitimate grounds for prohibiting women (or mothers) from these jobs. Further, divorce, remarriage, and adoption all risk disruption of the family, yet we would not want to deny a woman these options simply because she is a mother.

The second suggestion, that "some categories of human activities should not be for sale," is also inadequate. In order to make use of it, we would have to know what these categories are or at least how to distinguish them from others. But Ketchum does not tell us. Her comment that "some activities are close to our personhood . . . " is likewise of little help. (It is not clear whether this is offered as a third suggestion or as way to clarify the second.) If, on the one hand, it refers to those activities that distinguish persons from other beings, then reproduction is certainly not one of them. On the other hand, if it refers to those activities that we *identify* with—those by which we conceive of ourselves—then it is a mistake to think that all women (or all women in their child-bearing years) conceive of themselves as essentially child-bearers. What we do with some parts of our lives need not define who we are; a woman who is paid to bear a child for another need not conceive of herself as essentially a child-bearer any more than a woman who is paid to teach a college course need conceive of herself as essentially a teacher.

Perhaps there are ways to mark an important moral difference between compensating a woman for the efforts and risks of bearing a child, and compensating her the efforts and risks of typical (and unobjectionable) ways that she uses her body to benefit others. But Ketchum has not told us what they are. And without that information we cannot use the difference in a case against surrogate motherhood.

The last objection I will address focuses on coercion and exploitation. Ketchum writes:

All commercial transactions are at least potentially coercive in that the parties to them are likely to come from unequal bargaining positions and in that, whatever we have a market in, there will be some people who will be in a position such that they have to sell it in order to survive. Such concerns are important to arguments . . . against [baby selling and surrogate contracts]. (Ketchum, above, 288)

It is true that offers to enter into paid surrogacy arrangements are *potentially* coercive. It is also true that by permitting these offers we increase the risk that poor women will be exploited. The question, however, is whether these risks provide adequate grounds for prohibiting paid surrogacy arrangements. The following four points should help to show that they do not.[5]

First, as John Robertson (1983, 28) discusses, offers to be paid to bear a child for another are not "unjustly" coercive. They do not leave the recipient worse off than before the offer was made. (For contrast, consider the gunman's "Your money or your life" offer which does leave the recipient worse off.) Second, there is evidence that the opportunity to be paid for one's services in bearing a child has not been widely exploitive of poor women. Statistics indicate that the "average surrogate mother is white, attended two years of college, married young, and has all the children she and her husband want."[6] These are not the characteristics of the group we envision when we express concerns about protecting the poor from exploitation.

Third, though it is possible that the opportunity to be paid for one's services in bearing a child *will become* widely exploitive of poor women (as the arrangements increase in popularity), the same may be true of any opportunity to be paid for one's services. Yet we would not serve the interests of poor women in general if, in the efforts to protect them from exploitation, we prohibited them the means of escaping poverty. (Ketchum recognizes this point and cites Radin (1987, 1915) in its defense.)

Finally, the concern about exploitation and coercion seems to presuppose that the act of bearing a child for another is so detestable, so degrading, that few women would enter into the arrangements were they not forced to do so out of economic necessity. But the statistics mentioned above suggest that this is not the case. Further, some women enjoy being pregnant and may view their act as altruistic.[7] They are doing for another what that other cannot do for him or herself, and thereby allowing that other to know the joys (and pains) of raising an offspring. And if our aim is to protect those women who *do* view bearing a child for another as degrading, but nonetheless feel forced to do so out of economic necessity, then we can protect those women by putting restrictions on who can *enter into* paid surrogacy arrangements—we do not need to prohibit the arrangements entirely. One may object that such restrictions would be *unfair* because they would prohibit poor women from doing something that other women were allowed to do. But that seems to presuppose that the restrictions would be denying poor women a good, rather than protecting them from a harm, which, if true, would suggest that our initial concerns about coercion and exploitation were misguided.

NOTES

1. Though I will continue to use the lay term "surrogate motherhood," it is a misleading name for the practice it identifies. In typical cases (i.e., those not involving embryo transfer)

the woman bearing the child is both the genetic mother of the child and the birth mother. The only "mother" role she does not (intend to) fulfill is the social one. Were this enough to render her a surrogate mother then we should have to refer to women who relinquish their children for adoption, and to men who donate sperm to sperm banks, as "surrogate mothers" and "surrogate fathers." The term seems to be rooted in the oppressive notion that a woman's proper role in life is to be a child-bearer for a mate. Were that the case, then the woman being paid to bear a child could be viewed as a surrogate for another woman.

2. Some of the arguments I discuss are also discussed (and some in more detail) in my "Paid surrogacy: Arguments and responses" (1989). Also, it is worth noting that my arguments defend only the permissibility of the arrangements. Their legal enforcement is a separate issue.

3. Though I use the masculine pronoun when referring to a customer of surrogate motherhood arrangements, the customer need not be male. A woman with ova but no uterus may wish to have one of her ova fertilized, in vitro, with sperm from a sperm bank and then pay another woman to carry the conceptus to term. The possibility that a woman may be a customer of surrogate mother arrangements counsels against our objecting to these arrangements on the grounds that they treat women as "fungible baby-makers for men whose seed must be carried on" (Radin 1987, 1935). (Radin makes this objection within the context of our current gender ideologies.)

4. Laura Purdy (1989) raises the possibility that "lurking behind objections to surrogacy is some feeling that it is wrong to earn money by letting your body work, without active effort on your part. But this would rule out sperm selling as well as using women's beauty to sell products and services." Notice that on the compensation-view of the payments the woman is not being paid for something her body does. She is being compensated for the efforts she must make, and the risks she incurs, in the nine month process of bearing a child.

5. Purdy (1989) offers some different, and in many ways more detailed, responses to the argument from exploitation.

6. The statistics are from "Surrogate motherhood: A practice that's still undergoing birth pangs," Los Angeles Times, March 22, 1987. Radin (1987) cites them as well.

7. Radin rejects this point on the grounds that "even if surrogate mothering is subjectively experienced as altruism, the surrogate's self-conception as nurturer, caretaker, and service-giver might be viewed as a kind of gender-role oppression" (Radin 1987, 1930). I respond to this claim in "Paid surrogacy: Arguments and responses."

REFERENCES

Ketchum, Sara. 1984. The moral status of the bodies of persons. Social Theory and Practice 10: 25–38.

Ketchum, Sara. 1989. Selling babies and selling bodies: Surrogate motherhood and the problem of commodification. Hypatia, 4(3): 116–127. Also in this volume.

Malm, H. M. 1989. Paid surrogacy: Arguments and responses. Public Affairs Quarterly 3 (2): 57–66.

Purdy, Laura. 1989. Surrogate mothering: Exploitation or empowerment? Bioethics 3 (1): 18–34.

Radin, Margaret. 1987. Market inalienability. Harvard Law Review 100 (8): 1849–1937.

Robertson, John. 1983. Surrogate mothers: Not so novel after all. Hastings Center Report 13 (5): 28–34.

Notes on Contributors

Nora Kizer Bell is currently Professor and Chair of the Department of Philosophy at the University of South Carolina. She holds adjunct professorships in the USC Schools of Medicine and Public Health and is resident ethicist at School of Medicine teaching hospitals. A member of the Board of the National Leadership Coalition on AIDS and a commissioner on the South Carolina Commission on Aging, her current research deals primarily with AIDS and aging issues.

Jeannine Ross Boyer has practiced in the Veterans Administration Medical System, as a public health nurse, and as a nurse clinician in a sexually transmitted diseases clinic; she has also often lectured on ethical aspects of nursing. She is currently employed as a consultant on medical issues by Holmen and Oistad, Attorneys at Law, in St. Cloud, MN.

Joan C. Callahan is Associate Professor of Philosophy at the University of Kentucky. She has published a number of papers on ethics and social philosophy, is editor of *Ethical Issues in Professional Life* (Oxford University Press, 1988), and is coauthor with James W. Knight of *Preventing Birth: Contemporary Methods and Related Moral Controversies* (University of Utah Press, 1989).

John C. Fletcher is Professor of Biomedical Ethics and Religious Studies at the University of Virginia. He is also Director of the Center for Biomedical Ethics in UVA's Health Sciences Center. An Episcopal minister by background, he received his Ph.D. in Christian Ethics from Union Theological Seminary in 1969. Dr. Fletcher served as Chief of the Bioethics Program in the Warren G. Magnuson Clinical Center of the National Institutes of Health from 1977–87.

Sara T. Fry is Associate Professor at the University of Maryland at Baltimore. She has authored articles in biomedical ethics and nursing ethics. She is coauthor of *Case Studies in Nursing Ethics* and is currently working on a book on the protection of privacy in health care. She teaches courses in the philosophy of science, epistemology, and health care ethics.

Helen Bequaert Holmes has a Ph.D. in genetics and is currently an independent scholar and editor. She was a coeditor of *Birth Control and Controlling Birth: Women-Centered Perspectives* and *The Custom-Made Child? Women-Centered Perspectives*. Her research is on feminist technology assessment and ethical analysis in reproductive medicine.

Sara Ann Ketchum has a Ph.D. in philosophy from the University of Michigan and has taught philosophy at several colleges, including SUNY/College at Oswego, Dartmouth, and Rollins College in Winter Park, Florida. Her research and publications have focused on feminist theory, medical ethics, and moral and political issues related to sexual and racial equality. A member of the class of 1991 at Harvard Law School, she plans to start work at the U.S. Department of Justice (Tax Division) in fall 1991.

James W. Knight is a Professor of Animal Science (Reproductive Physiology) at Virginia Tech. He has authored or coauthored over one hundred scientific articles on various aspects of reproductive physiology/endocrinology and is coauthor with Joan C. Callahan of *Preventing Birth: Contemporary Methods and Related Moral Controversies* (University of Utah Press, 1989).

ROSALIND EKMAN LADD is Professor of Philosophy at Wheaton College (Massachusetts) and lecturer in pediatrics in the Brown University Program in Medicine, and has served on ethics committees at two local hospitals. She has published a number of articles in medical ethics and is coauthor, with E. N. Forman, of *Ethical Dilemmas in Pediatrics: A Case Study Approach* (Springer Verlag, 1991).

JUDITH LORBER is Professor of Sociology at Brooklyn College and the Graduate School, City University of New York. She is the author of *Women Physicians: Careers, Status and Power* (Tavistock/Methuen, 1984), and numerous journal articles on women and health care. Her current research is on the organization of in vitro fertilization clinics and couples' experiences with the new reproductive technologies. She was founding editor of *Gender & Society*, official publication of Sociologists for Women in Society.

H. M. MALM is an Assistant Professor of Philosophy at Loyola University of Chicago. During recent years, while employed by the University of Nebraska, she taught courses in the Philosophy Department and the Medical School, and cotaught courses in the Law School. Her research focuses on an individual's rights and duties within society, with emphasis on the right of autonomy and the duty to prevent harm.

DON MARQUIS received his Ph.D. from Indiana University and is Professor of Philosophy at the University of Kansas, Lawrence, Kansas. His primary research area is medical ethics. Most of his recent publications have been concerned with the ethics of experimentation in medicine.

JULIEN S. MURPHY is an Associate Professor of Philosophy and member of the Women's Studies faculty at the University of Southern Maine. She has published numerous articles in continental philosophy and feminist philosophy of medicine.

HILDE LINDEMANN NELSON is Associate Editor of the *Hastings Center Report*. She has taught rhetoric and critical thinking in the Department of American Thought and Language at Michigan State University and at the College of St. Benedict's, a school for women in Minnesota. She has recently published an extensive critical notice of Nel Noddings's *Women and Evil* in *Bioethics Books*, and is currently at work on a book with James Lindemann Nelson on medicine and the ethics of the family.

JAMES LINDEMANN NELSON is currently writing on maternal-fetal relationships, as well as completing a project on animal research ethics jointly funded by the NSF and NIH. He has been a consultant to Veterans Administration Medical Centers in Minnesota, and an Associate Professor in the Center for Ethics and Humanities in the Life Sciences at Michigan State University. Currently, he is Associate for Ethical Studies at the Hastings Center and (in Sara Ruddick's sense) mother to six children.

KELLY OLIVER is Assistant Professor of Philosophy at The University of Texas at Austin. She has published articles on Nietzsche, Foucault, and various aspects of feminist theory. Her book, *Unraveling the Double-bind: Julia Kristeva's Theory of the Subject*, is forthcoming in 1992.

LAURA M. PURDY is Associate Professor of Philosophy at Wells College; she has also held the Irwin Chair at Hamilton College and has taught at Cornell University. Her research is mainly in applied ethics and feminism, and her book *In Their Best Interest? The Case against Equal Rights for Children* is forthcoming from Cornell University Press.

SUE V. ROSSER is a Director of Women's Studies at the University of South Carolina at Columbia and Professor of Family and Preventive Medicine in the Medical School. She has edited collections and written extensively on the theoretical and applied problems of women and science, including the books *Teaching about Science and Health from a Feminist Perspective: A Practical Guide*; *Feminism within the Science and Health Care Professions: Overcoming Resistance*; and *Female Friendly Science*.

SUSAN SHERWIN is Professor of Philosophy at Dalhousie University, Halifax, Nova Scotia. After too many years in administrative work, she is now trying to devote herself to her principal academic interests in feminist ethics and health care ethics; she has published several articles in these areas and her book on feminist medical ethics, *Patient No Longer*, has been published by *Temple University Press*.

BETTY A. SICHEL is Professor of Philosophy of Education at Long Island University, C. W. Post Campus, Brookville, New York. She has published in such journals as *Philosophy and Phenomenological Research*, *Educational Theory*, and *Journal of Moral Education*. Her recent book, published by Temple University Press, is entitled *Moral Education: Ideals, Community, and Character*.

MARY ANNE WARREN currently teaches in the Philosophy Department at San Francisco State University. She has published many articles in applied ethics and feminist philosophy and two books: *The Nature of Woman: An Encyclopedia and Guide to the Literature* (Edgepress, 1980) and *Gendercide: The Implications of Sex Selection* (Littlefield Adams, 1985).

VIRGINIA L. WARREN is an Associate Professor of Philosophy at Chapman College. She serves on a hospital ethics committee, and has taught seminars for health care professionals at local hospitals. She wrote the guidelines for nonsexist language for the American Philosophical Association, and has published articles on ethics, Kierkegaard, and masochism. Her current research topics include autonomy, world hunger, and elitism in higher education.

SUSAN WENDELL is Associate Professor of Philosophy and Women's Studies at Simon Fraser University. She and David Copp edited *Pornography and Censorship* (Prometheus Books, 1983). She has published articles on discrimination, equality of opportunity, pornography, and liberal feminism. She has chronic fatigue immune dysfunction syndrome.

DOROTHY C. WERTZ is a medical sociologist with an interdisciplinary background in social ethics, social anthropology, and the study of religion and society. She is Senior Scientist at the Shriver Center for Mental Retardation and Research Professor in the Health Services Section at the Boston University School of Public Health. Her publications include *Lying-In: A History of Childbirth in America* (1977; enlarged ed. Yale University Press, 1989); and articles on interpersonal communication and interpretation of risk in genetic counseling.

Index